THIRD EDITION

PRINCIPLES OF GROUP FITNESS INSTRUCTION

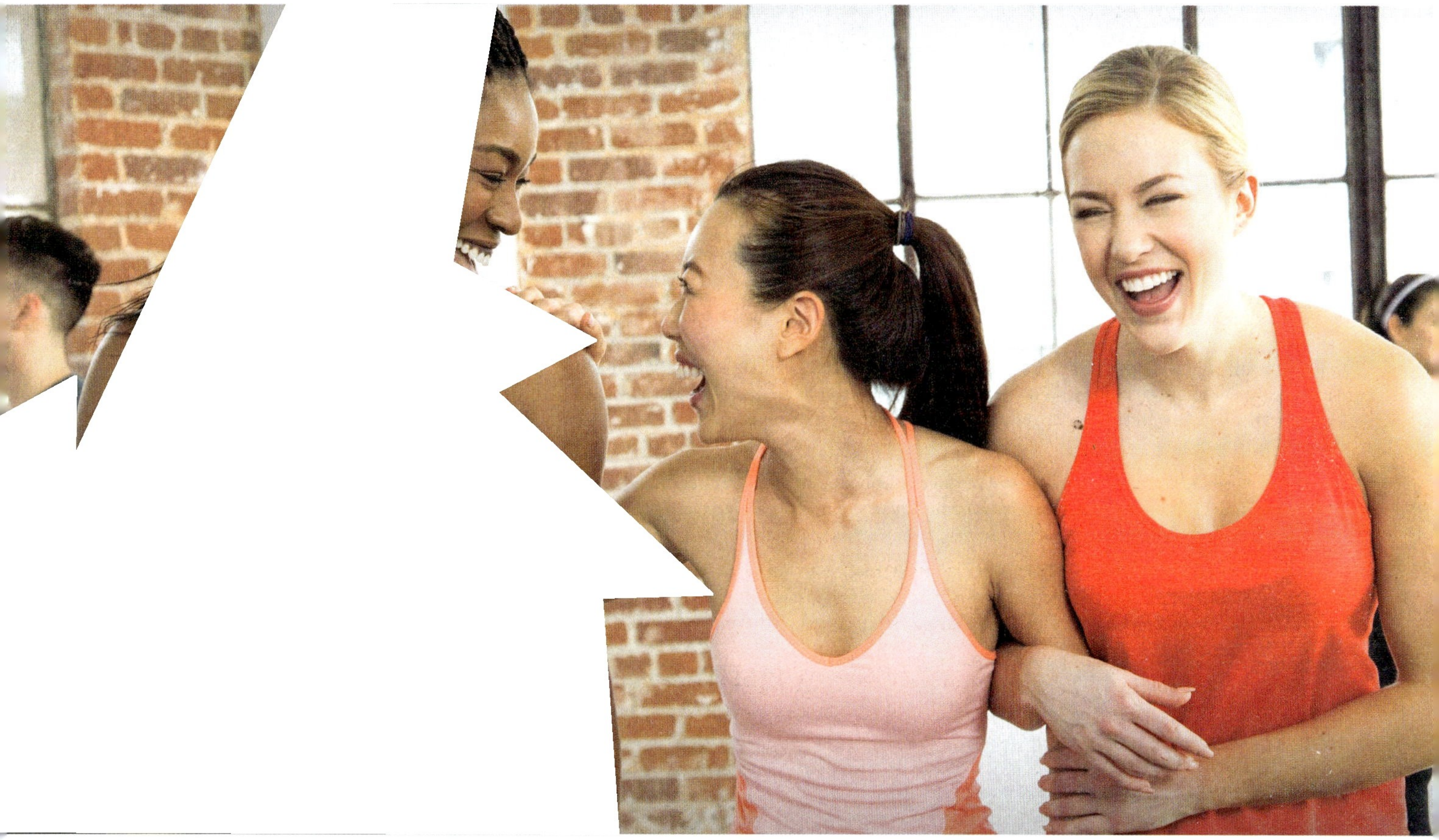

Editor

Richard Fahmy, MS

Content Development and Production Manager

Athletics and Fitness Association of America

Gilbert, Arizona

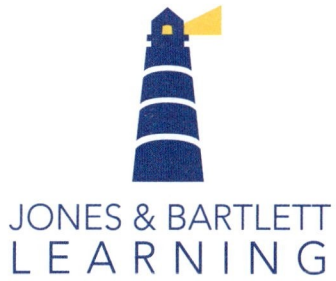

JONES & BARTLETT LEARNING

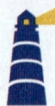

World Headquarters
Jones & Bartlett Learning
25 Mall Road
Burlington, MA 01803
978-443-5000
info@jblearning.com
www.jblearning.com

National Academy of Sports Medicine
355 E. Germann Road
Suite 201
Gilbert, AZ 85297
800-460-6276

Jones & Bartlett Learning books and products are available through most bookstores and online booksellers. To contact Jones & Bartlett Learning directly, call 800-832-0034, fax 978-443-8000, or visit our website, www.jblearning.com.

Substantial discounts on bulk quantities of Jones & Bartlett Learning publications are available to corporations, professional associations, and other qualified organizations. For details and specific discount information, contact the special sales department at Jones & Bartlett Learning via the above contact information or send an email to specialsales@jblearning.com.

Production Credits

Vice President, Product Management: Marisa R. Urbano
Vice President, Content Strategy and Implementation: Christine Emerton
Director, Product Management: Matthew Kane
Product Manager: Whitney Fekete
Director, Content Management: Donna Gridley
Manager, Content Strategy: Orsolya Gall
Content Strategist: Summer Ibrahim
Director, Project Management and Content Services: Karen Scott
Manager, Project Management: Jackie Reynen
Project Manager: Jennifer Risden
Program Manager: Alex Schab
Senior Digital Project Specialist: Angela Dooley

Director, Marketing: Andrea DeFronzo
Director, Marketing: Brian Rooney
Content Services Manager: Colleen Lamy
Procurement Manager: Wendy Kilborn
Composition: S4Carlisle Publishing Services
Text and Cover Design: NASM
Senior Media Development Editor: Troy Liston
Rights & Permissions Manager: John Rusk
Rights Specialist: Robin Silverman
Cover Images: Courtesy of Athletics and Fitness Association of America
Printing and Binding: Lakeside Book Company

Library of Congress Cataloging-in-Publication Data

Names: Fahmy, Rich, editor.
Title: Principles of group fitness instruction / Editor: Richard Fahmy, MS Content Development and Production Manager, Athletics and Fitness Association of America, Gilbert, Arizona.
Description: Third edition. | Burlington, MA : Jones & Bartlett Learning, [2025] | Includes bibliographical references and index.
Identifiers: LCCN 2023013870 | ISBN 9781284281750 (hardcover)
Subjects: LCSH: Physical fitness--Handbooks, manuals, etc. | Personal trainers--Handbooks, manuals, etc.
Classification: LCC GV481 .P777 2025 | DDC 613.7--dc23/eng/20230331
LC record available at https://lccn.loc.gov/2023013870

6048

Printed in the United States of America
27 26 25 24 23   10 9 8 7 6 5 4 3 2 1

Deciding to become an AFAA Group Fitness Instructor means that you are committed to creating life-changing group fitness experiences. Congratulations, and welcome. This is a profession that values individuals like you—community-builders, life-long learners, and party-starters—people who have discovered the power of moving together and want to share it with others.

The AFAA group fitness credential you are embarking on recognizes that what Group Fitness Instructors *do* is lead movement, but what we *provide* is so much more. Your classes will be a catalyst for transformation. You will empower people to enjoy physical activity, maybe for the very first time. You will create spaces where people discover self-confidence and belonging. You will be the best part of someone's day—the thing that helps them through major life challenges.

As you work through this credential, keep that vision in mind. The information and self-reflections will help you make that vision real. Embrace the opportunity to approach each aspect of leading group fitness with education and intention. Every choice you make can contribute to the life-changing impact you will have: how you welcome people to class, the music you play, the words you use, the care you bring to making each workout safe and effective, and the relationships you build where you teach.

I've been a certified Group Fitness Instructor for more than 20 years, and it has been more rewarding than I ever imagined. The time you put in now will lead to professional moments you will savor: the satisfaction when a participant thanks you for making exercise fun, the pride when you coach a group beyond what they knew they were capable of, the feeling when the epic playlist you put together drives people to give it their all, and the joy of seeing newcomers become enthusiastic regulars who bring friends and family to class. You'll have moments after class, packing up your gear, when you can't help but grin—because you just shared the best part of yourself with a room full of people who are glad you showed up for them.

Thank you for helping to create the future of group fitness. We need you for the unique gifts and perspectives you bring. I hope that this process celebrates every *why* that drives you and gives you the *how* to do it with confidence.

Best,

Kelly McGonigal, PhD
AFAA Certified Group Fitness Instructor
Research Psychologist
Author, *The Joy of Movement*

AFAA's *Principles of Group Fitness Instruction* prepares instructors for their final exam and teaches skills necessary to effectively lead complete group fitness experiences. Our content is founded in the notion that the best way to connect with participants is through thoughtful and engaging movement rooted in evidence and best practice. This text meets learners where they are to elevate their knowledge and skills in fitness and participant engagement and helps them facilitate exciting and effective group fitness classes.

New Content

Based on feedback from past learners and fitness professionals, this new textbook includes revised and refreshed content and has been updated throughout from the previous edition:

- **Updated layout and table of contents.** This revised textbook organizes content into the four distinct domains of group fitness principles and topics focused on presenting information in a logical, helpful way for the aspiring Group Fitness Instructor.
- **New illustrations and photos.** This textbook includes updated imagery to bring principles and concepts to life.
- **Updated chapter content**. All the topics in this textbook have been updated to include new information and updated research provided and reviewed by the most well-respected health, wellness, and fitness professionals in the industry.
- **Glossary of terms**. We have updated our glossary to include a larger number of terms and definitions.

Program Learning Objectives

As you progress through your Group Fitness Instructor program, you will work toward achieving competency in the following areas:

- Demonstrate comprehension of fundamental concepts related to exercise science as they apply to the group fitness setting.
- Design a well-structured and engaging fitness class or workout for a diverse group of participants that is both safe and effective.
- Demonstrate key instruction, cueing, presentation, and participant-engagement techniques necessary for effective group classes.
- Demonstrate key traits of professionalism as a Group Fitness Instructor.
- Demonstrate the key skills and knowledge required to be a Group Fitness Instructor.

MANAGING EDITOR

Rich Fahmy
MS, NASM-CPT, CES, PES, CWC

LEAD REVIEWERS

Emily Booth
BM, AFAA-GFI, NASM-CPT

Ayla Donlin
EdD, MS, ACSM-CPT, ACE-CHC, FNS

Dana Monson
BS

Nicole Pinto
MA, ACSM-CEP, NSCA-CES, TSAC-F

AUTHORS

Emily Booth
BM, AFAA-GFI, NASM-CPT

Candice Campbell
MS, CSCS, ACSM-CPT, NASM-CES

Jill Drummond
NASM-CPT, ACE-CPT

Cassandra Hirschberg-Brown
BS, NASM-CPT, AFAA-GFI

Kristen Sokel
BA, NASM-CPT, AFAA-GFI

PRODUCT TEAM

Jeri Dow
Senior Instructional Designer

Rich Fahmy
Content Development and Production Manager

Ashley Fuller
Senior Content Developer

Steve Myers
Product Manager

Melissa Schimmel
Project Manager

SPECIAL THANKS

Thank you to all the teams across AFAA, Nurture Digital, and Reflection Software who had a hand in this content. You were instrumental in bringing this experience to life.

Please take a few moments to look through this User's Guide, which will introduce you to features that will enhance your learning experience:

Learning Objectives open each chapter and present learning goals to help you focus and retain the crucial information discussed.

Sidebars, set in the margins, highlight the definitions of key terms that are presented in the chapter. The key terms are bolded throughout the chapter for easy reference.

Helpful Hint boxes help you retain information by providing an easy way to learn it or memory tips.

Instructor Tip boxes provide practical application of the concepts with clients from the perspective of a Group Fitness Instructor.

Critical boxes provide key information that learners need to know before moving on to the next section or warnings about the content being discussed.

Check It Out boxes provide you with fun or interesting information in relation to the discussed content.

Practice This boxes give you activities to practice on your own.

Getting Technical boxes dive more deeply into the content being discussed.

SECTION 1

PROFESSIONALISM

CHAPTER 1

WELCOME TO GROUP FITNESS

LEARNING OBJECTIVES

The intent of this chapter is to explore your *what* and *why* as you learn about common characteristics of Group Fitness Instructors and gain a deeper understanding of the roles you will serve as expert, leader, motivator, performer, and employee. This chapter provides foundational benefits of group fitness classes across all formats and introduces you to the instructor mindset of inclusivity, a concept explored throughout this course.

After reading this content, students should be able to demonstrate the following objectives:

- **Identify** the hallmarks of a successful AFAA Group Fitness Instructor.

- **Identify** the importance of trust in establishing and nurturing the Group Fitness Instructor's various professional relationships.

- **Describe** the group fitness participant's explicit and implicit needs and motivations.

- **Identify** the importance of inclusivity in creating a welcoming and engaging experience.

Lesson 1: Group Fitness Instructors

Introduction

Who is a Group Fitness Instructor? Depending on an individual's personal experiences, background, and age, the answer to that question (and the image it brings to mind) might include everything from a hyped-up rockstar to a stopwatch-wielding drill sergeant. As group fitness has evolved from its dance-based origins in the late 1960s, so have the individuals and modalities associated with it.

Today, group fitness can mean very different things to different people. Some enjoy dancing to Latin beats, whereas others prefer pedaling a bike to pulsing bass in a cycle studio. Some are drawn to the mindful experience of yoga practice, whereas others want to "leave it all on the

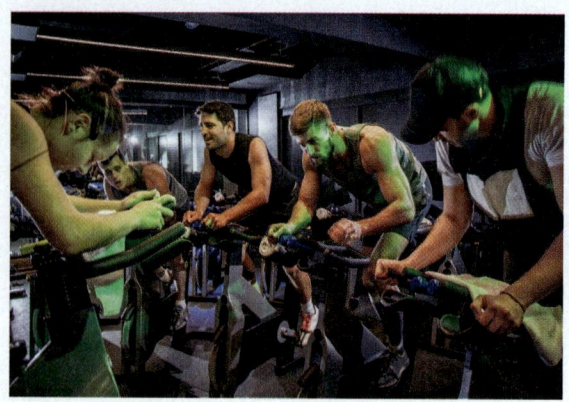
© Bojan Milinkov/Shutterstock

floor" in a boot camp class. Many enjoy participating in all manner of group classes, with favorites that shift from year to year. This is great news for both participants and instructors. With so many ways to exercise together (whether live or virtual or in a large commercial facility, a small private studio, or a public park), there are more opportunities than ever for aspiring Group Fitness Instructors to touch lives doing what they love.

However, beneath the exciting diversity of formats, goals, delivery styles, and environments under the group fitness umbrella, successful instructors possess a common foundation of knowledge, characteristics, and behaviors. Regardless of format or personal style, a Group Fitness Instructor is a leader, coach, motivator, educator, and performer—all at the same time.

What Brought You Here and Why?

There is great variety in the types of classes instructors may opt to teach, and there is also a variety of reasons instructors may have for teaching. Many instructors move from the front row to the front of the class because they enjoy the group fitness experience so much that they are compelled to share it with others. Some choose to become instructors to earn extra income and get paid to do something they value: exercise. Others may perceive that they have something unique to offer that is missing from the classes they have experienced. All of these are common motivations for choosing to become an instructor. Career motivations feed into a sense of meaningful work. As research on this topic grows, a consensus has emerged that when work has a sense of significance, it contributes to a broader purpose; allows for self-realization; and results in greater motivation, commitment, and personal well-being (Martela & Pessi, 2018). Although there is certainly no right or wrong reason for teaching, knowing what brought you here, and why, is an important consideration as you begin this journey. Not only will it motivate you to persevere when you feel challenged by concepts in this course, but it will also help you craft a vision and plan for the kind of instructor you want to become.

Consider a recipe for a favorite dish. Some individuals may prefer a little more spice and others a little more salt, but the fundamental recipe still contains the same basic ingredients. The goal of the Athletics and Fitness Association of America (AFAA) is to provide Group Fitness Instructors with the fundamental knowledge and tools, the recipe, to create and deliver engaging, effective, inclusive, and professional group fitness experiences. By beginning this coursework, you have taken the first step.

⚙ PRACTICE THIS

Visualize your ideal Group Fitness Instructor. (You likely have an actual individual that immediately comes to mind.)

- What are the defining traits and behaviors of the ideal Group Fitness Instructor? List them out.
- Which do you think are most important and why?
- Which do you think you already possess?
- Which do you think might be your greatest areas of opportunity?

THE ROLE OF CREDENTIALING IN YOUR JOURNEY

As an aspiring instructor, you may be thinking, "Why exactly do I need to have a credential?" After all, you love group fitness, attend lots of classes, and could probably do one of your favorite instructor's routines by heart. Perhaps you have already been asked to step in and teach a class or two and it went well. The participants had a good time, and you loved the feeling of being at the front of the room. Why then, should you devote your valuable time and financial resources to earning a credential? Because you want to be a professional.

By definition, a *professional* is someone "characterized by or conforming to the technical or ethical standards of a profession" who participates "for gain or livelihood in an activity or field of endeavor often engaged in by amateurs . . . that requires special education, training, or skill" (Merriam-Webster, n.d.). In discussing the role of credentials for Group Fitness Instructors, these are important points to explore.

To clarify, simply enjoying, participating in, or even being good at an activity is not the same as having the ability to effectively teach it to others. For example, some individuals are naturally talented singers. They have an innate ability to sing on key, project their voice, and clearly articulate every lyric. However, just because they can sing well does not mean they have the knowledge, skill, or ability to coach someone who struggles to stay on pitch, breathe from their diaphragm, or memorize the words to a song. To learn those skills, an individual would need to hire a professional vocal coach.

In the same way, many professional Group Fitness Instructors make teaching classes look easy. They move perfectly to the music, perform every exercise with ease, and communicate every cue to keep the class in unison. However, under the surface, this requires a significant amount of knowledge and skill. They may have the natural ability to move with grace and strength on their own, but the key difference lies in their ability to help *others* do it, too, especially when the stakes of *not* doing it well have the potential to cause harm.

Earning and maintaining a professional credential or certification allows someone to make the jump from enthusiastic participant to paid professional, providing both the technical knowledge to deliver safe, effective classes and the ethical standards to do so as a responsible member of the greater fitness industry. With this education, you can confidently create and deliver classes that adhere to the foundational

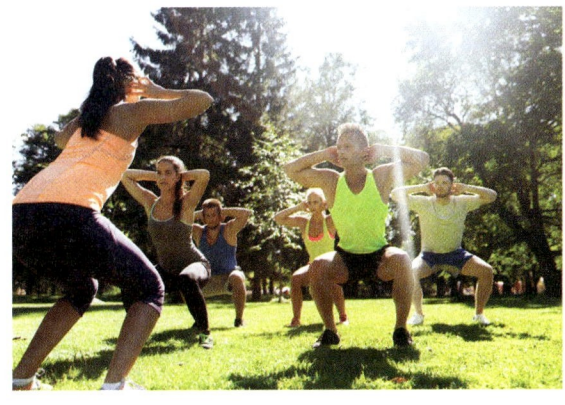

© Ground Picture/Shutterstock

⚙ PRACTICE THIS

In his book *Start with Why*, leadership consultant Simon Sinek (2009) outlines the importance of determining your *why* before you proceed to *what* and *how*. As a Group Fitness Instructor, knowing and remembering why you started this journey is an incredibly valuable tool that will keep you focused throughout your instructor journey. Not only will it help you become the instructor you strive to be, but it will also help you attract the kinds of employers, mentors, and participants who will support you in it.

Take a few moments to jot down the specific reasons that led you to become an instructor. Then, evaluate how those reasons might help shape your approach to teaching and your personal instructor brand.

principles of exercise science with a credibility that instructors without a credential or certification lack. You can effectively balance the principles of human movement, how the body works, and what types of exercises elicit the best results while still producing a creative and fun experience for your participants. And when participants have fun, avoid injury, and reap the benefits of a well-designed class, they will come back for more, which leads to the next benefit of certification and credentialing.

Being credentialed is good for business; both for you, the instructor, and for the facility in which you teach. A credential significantly increases your employment opportunities by signaling to hiring managers that you are committed to education and growth and adhering to industry standards. In most reputable facilities, it is not just desired, but required for employment. Hiring credentialed instructors not only helps ensure a standard of quality but also affects a facility's liability in the event of an incident. In the competitive fitness landscape, having a reputable credential can set you apart from the masses by instilling confidence in both prospective employers and potential participants.

Along with knowledge of how and what to teach, earning a credential offers credibility and expands professional aptitude. The knowledge gained through the acquisition (and maintenance) of a group fitness certification or credential not only will provide you with the foundation to create safe, effective classes for participants, but it can also help you set and achieve new goals of your own. The leadership, communication, and relationship-building skills learned can be applied in business and personal interactions beyond the group fitness environment. Moreover, as a credentialed Group Fitness Instructor, you will be connected to the greater fitness community and all the emerging research, opportunities, relationships, and experiences associated with it.

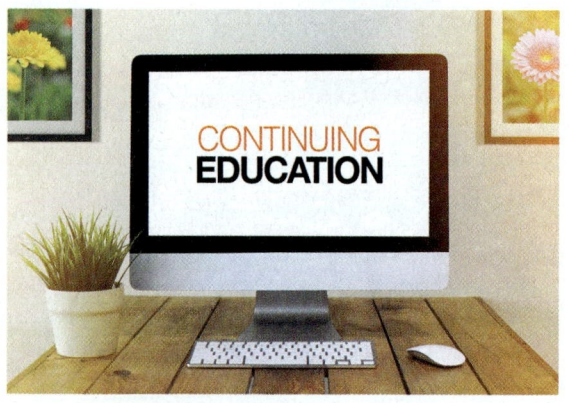

© Adha Ghazali/Shutterstock

REQUIREMENTS BEYOND CERTIFICATION

Although becoming a credentialed Group Fitness Instructor is a vital first step in your journey, it is only the beginning. Beyond the knowledge you gain through the initial process, you have access to an ever-growing body of new research, technology applications, and exciting format evolutions that will provide new insight and opportunities throughout your career. These include keeping your credential(s) current with continuing education, improving your skills in one or more areas of specialization, and adhering to the safety standards and protocols established by your employer.

Staying current with the latest research and industry trends is an essential requirement beyond certification or credentialing, and it applies to all fitness professionals. You would be uneasy receiving treatment from a healthcare professional unfamiliar with updated safety protocols and treatment options. Likewise, your participants deserve a qualified Group Fitness Instructor who keeps their education on best practices current. This requires that you achieve a minimum number of **CONTINUING EDUCATION UNITS (CEUs)** over a 2-year renewal period. Depending on your interests, availability, and budget, many diverse continuing education topics are available for you to choose from as well as a variety of mediums to access them.

For example, you may decide that you want to learn more about working with the expanding active aging population, teaching outdoor classes, or improving your virtual teaching skills. You may decide that you want to earn a specialty certification such as yoga, kickboxing, or indoor cycling that requires additional knowledge and skill. Perhaps you want to learn about emerging trends or a new type of equipment to enhance the classes you already teach. Whatever your interests, you can almost certainly find an approved workshop, training, or conference to learn about it. Some of the most popular options include in-person and online conferences or workshops where you take a full day to immerse yourself in one or more topics. Other popular options include being quizzed on articles from approved industry publications or enrolling in specialty certification courses. Regardless, whether you choose to do it in person or online or whether you choose one specific focus or multiple, it is not only easy to meet your continuing education requirements, but also immensely beneficial to keep you informed and inspired.

Related to the topic of continuing education is the distinction between **PRIMARY CERTIFICATION/CREDENTIAL** and **SPECIALTY CERTIFICATION**. Similar to other professions where advanced credentials are required to perform specific jobs (e.g., general medicine versus neurosurgery), if you want to teach a format such as Pilates, indoor cycling, kickboxing, yoga, aqua, a **BRAND-SPECIFIC FORMAT**, or any other discipline that requires a specific set of knowledge and skills, then you, too, will need to pursue a specialty certification. Fortunately, the acquisition and maintenance of a new specialty certification will almost always fulfill the continuing education requirements needed to keep your primary certification or credential current, making it a rewarding experience (**Figure 1.1**).

A final but important requirement beyond certification (unless you are independently teaching out of your home or another personal venue) is adhering to the policies and procedures outlined by the organization or facility at which you teach. This will often include maintaining

PRIMARY CERTIFICATION/ CREDENTIAL

A foundational group fitness certification that addresses the essential knowledge, skills, and abilities that every group fitness instructor should possess to operate within their scope of practice.

SPECIALTY CERTIFICATION

Formats created and managed by businesses, education providers, corporate club chains, private studios, and even individual instructors in specific fitness disciplines or with specific equipment.

BRAND-SPECIFIC FORMAT

A specialized group fitness training to prepare instructors to teach formats that require knowledge and skill beyond the scope of a primary certification, such as indoor cycling.

Multi-Day Conferences
Acquire CEUs learning from a variety of educators on diverse topics; in person or virtual.

Educational Articles
Professional industry-specific publications offer the opportunity to read articles, take a quiz, and receive CEUs.

In-Person Workshops
Half or full-day immersion training about a specific topic, type of equipment, or a specialty format.

CEU TYPES/ RESOURCES

Online Courses
Many industry leaders offer continuing education courses that can be completed at your own pace online.

Specialty Certifications
Earn a significant number of CEUs while simultaneously obtaining a specific required certification.

FIGURE 1.1 Common Continuing Education Types/Resources

a valid CPR/AED certification (which you also need to maintain your AFAA Group Fitness Instructor status) as well as any other codes of conduct, class delivery guidelines, and employee policies. By performing the actions required of all credentialed Group Fitness Instructors in a consistent and timely manner, you will not only establish yourself as a reliable, well-informed, and respected member of the fitness industry, but you will also expand your own knowledge and opportunities.

Characteristics of a Group Fitness Instructor

Although every instructor has unique qualities that influence their personal teaching style, there are several fundamental characteristics that successful Group Fitness Instructors possess (**Infographic 1.1**). At the most basic level, an instructor is someone who teaches something. In the case of group fitness, that means teaching movement. However, teaching movement is only the beginning. As anyone who has been subjected to an uninteresting or uninspiring teacher can attest, learning is difficult in the absence of motivation or interest in the subject. Engaging in regular exercise can be challenging for a significant number of individuals, so a Group Fitness Instructor must capture and maintain the attention of the group long enough for them to reap its benefits (Kravitz, 2012). To do that, in addition to creating an effective workout, instructors must also be able to communicate clearly to a variety of fitness levels and personalities; use music to motivate, energize, and coordinate movement; and foster a caring community that inspires consistent participation.

LEADER/EXPERT

The primary role of a Group Fitness Instructor is to lead a group (large or small) through movement with the goal of improving or maintaining fitness. However, leading a group and being a leader are not quite the same. Consider the difference between a manager who simply assigns tasks with little regard for their employees' personal skill sets, life circumstances, or career aspirations and one who inspires employees to grow by challenging them with new projects, performing thoughtful reviews, and recognizing individual achievements. Although both managers perform the same fundamental job, the latter is likely to inspire greater loyalty and, ultimately, better results for both the individuals they manage and the organization for which they work. In the same way, an effective leader in the group fitness environment does more than simply demonstrate exercises while shouting out general instructions and hoping the class follows along. In group fitness, great leaders are not only confident role models capable of delivering an effective workout, but they are also inspiring, compassionate, and committed to serving the individuals in their charge. They put participants' needs ahead of their own and are purposeful in their actions. In addition, they seek to become experts who understand not only how to perform movements themselves, but also why, when, and how to teach them in a way that leads to participant success (Kravitz, 2012).

PROFILE OF A GROUP FITNESS INSTRUCTOR

Group Fitness Instructors fill many roles.

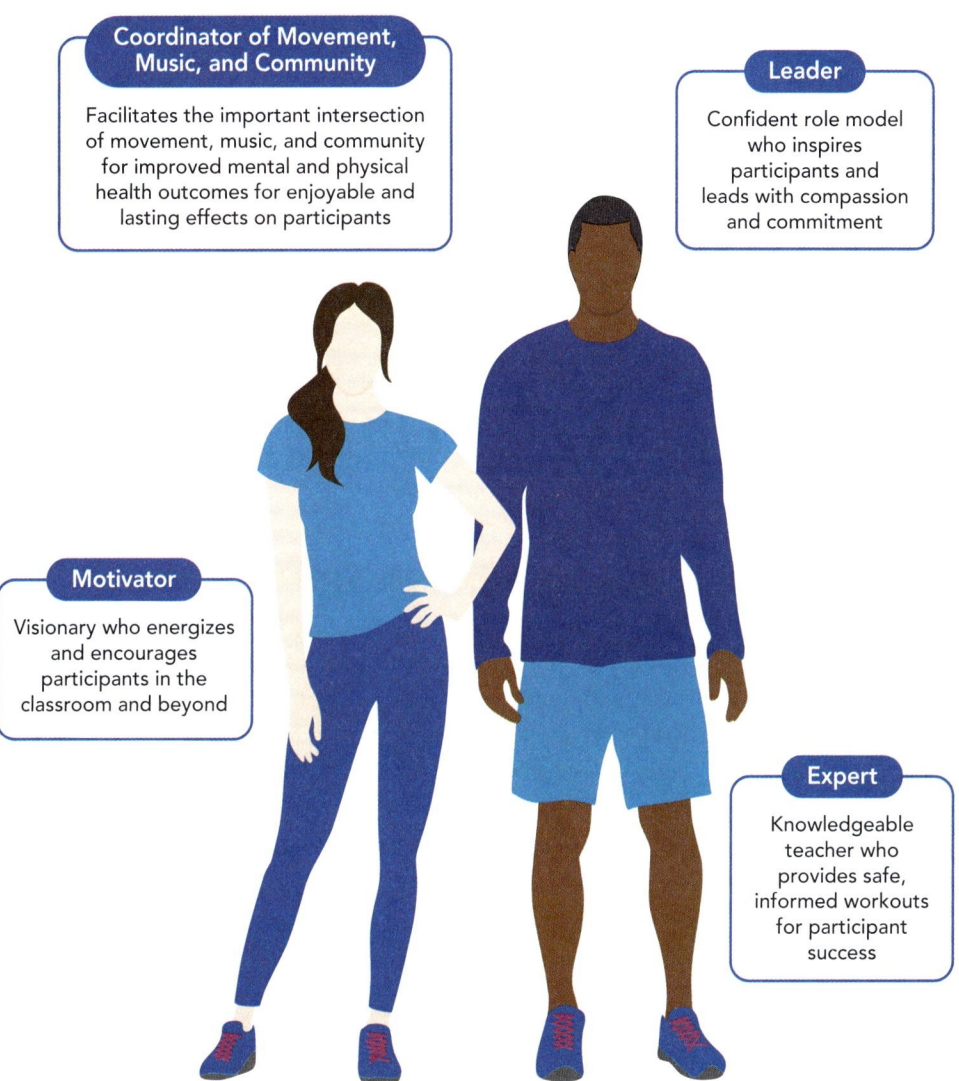

Coordinator of Movement, Music, and Community

Facilitates the important intersection of movement, music, and community for improved mental and physical health outcomes for enjoyable and lasting effects on participants

Leader

Confident role model who inspires participants and leads with compassion and commitment

Motivator

Visionary who energizes and encourages participants in the classroom and beyond

Expert

Knowledgeable teacher who provides safe, informed workouts for participant success

INFOGRAPHIC 1.1 Profile of a Group Fitness Instructor

✓ CHECK IT OUT

Although it may be attractive to approach teaching group fitness as a means to be paid to work out, great instructors should be prepared to sacrifice their personal workouts in service of their participants. For example, if an instructor is focused on performing at maximal effort in an interval or exercise, it is very difficult for them to simultaneously coach and monitor participants. If you are breathless, it is difficult to cue; if you are doing the most challenging progression, you cannot demonstrate more accessible options. A better strategy is to perform personal workouts on your own (or in another instructor's class) so that you can devote your attention to the safety and success of participants when you are teaching.

MOTIVATOR

In addition to being a leader and expert, one of the most important characteristics that Group Fitness Instructors demonstrate is their ability to motivate participants both in the class environment and beyond. Although the importance of movement for overall health and well-being is well-known, it is often challenging for many individuals to self-motivate, especially when they first begin an exercise program. Instructors can be instrumental in that process by sharing a vision, providing encouragement, and helping participants learn to motivate themselves, which can lead to better long-term outcomes (Teixeira et al., 2012).

INSTRUCTOR TIP

Providing real-life applications and imagery can be a very effective strategy to motivate participants. For example, "I know that loaded barbell may look heavy, but with one plate on each side, it is 20 pounds. How many of you have a child you carry around that weighs 20 pounds? Or a heavy suitcase, or grocery bags? How great will it feel to unload your car in one trip or to carry your suitcase up the stairs instead of waiting in line for the escalator at the airport? If you train to do it here, you'll be able to do it there!"

COORDINATOR OF MOVEMENT, MUSIC, AND COMMUNITY

Three of the most important features that make group fitness unique and attractive are the combined elements of movement, music, and community (**Figure 1.2**). Each of these can lead to improved physical and mental health outcomes independently, but together they can form an even more powerful tool. The health benefits of regular exercise are well-documented for both physical and mental well-being (Warburton et al., 2006). Music has been shown to not only improve exercise endurance but to also increase motivation and enjoyment while doing it (Karageorghis, 2017). Research studying the value of social connections and community continues to emerge, demonstrating its vital role in health and happiness (Eastwick, 2021). As a Group Fitness Instructor, you have the opportunity to coordinate all of this into a single experience, fostering an environment that can have profound immediate as well as lasting effects on participants' well-being (Centers for Disease Control and Prevention [CDC], 2019). To do this effectively, instructors must not only understand the benefits of each but also maximize them by coordinating movement with intentionally selected music and thoughtful, community-building behaviors.

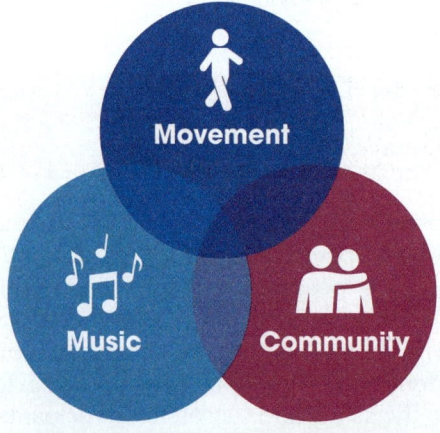

FIGURE 1.2 Instructor as Coordinator

Lesson 2: Benefits of Group Fitness

Benefits of Group Fitness

The popularity of group fitness as an exercise category is undeniable. For any dedicated group fitness participant, the accountability, commitment, community, and desire to be guided in movement alongside like-minded others yields benefits that cannot be replicated alone. From being more motivated to show up, to working harder while exercising, to feeling more relaxed afterward, exercising with others can contribute to improvements in consistency, performance, and enjoyment (Irwin et al., 2012).

Accountability

One of the most powerful benefits of group fitness classes is the many forms of accountability they create. Attending a regularly scheduled class provides the structure and consistency necessary to form lasting habits, making exercise a dedicated priority rather than one more thing to squeeze in before work or at the end of a long day. In addition, it also provides accountability during the workout. It is much harder to stop and walk during a run with a partner, and it is much harder to quit during class when you are surrounded by others who are also uncomfortable but refusing to give in (Feltz et al., 2011). Finally, when the experience is led by a **PARTICIPANT-CENTERED** instructor who knows your name and notices your absence, you may be less likely to miss for fear of disappointing them.

Commitment

As with accountability, group fitness can also improve participants' commitment to exercise, making it a valuable part of everyday life rather than a dreaded task that must be performed. Studies have shown that **INTRINSIC MOTIVATION**, the kind of motivation that comes from the sense that you are accomplishing something personally satisfying (like doing 10 push-ups on your toes) rather than from an external reward (like a new set of exercise clothes) is more likely to result in long-term changes (Teixeira et al., 2012). When participants experience the reward of growing stronger and accomplishing new skills, it strengthens their commitment and supports a pattern of consistency that is essential to creating healthy habits that last.

Sense of Community

The sense of community experienced in group fitness classes provides another unique and powerful benefit. Strong social connections have been shown to improve brain health, reduce risk for chronic disease, lower stress, bolster mood, increase longevity, and enhance performance (Eastwick, 2021). Considering that these are also many of the known benefits of exercise (CDC, 2019), it is not hard to understand why exercising in a group is so effective for overall health and well-being.

PARTICIPANT-CENTERED

Creating, modifying, and teaching workouts for the needs and goals of your participants.

INTRINSIC MOTIVATION

The driving force behind actions taken for inherent enjoyment, interest, and the pleasure of doing them and the satisfaction one receives from them.

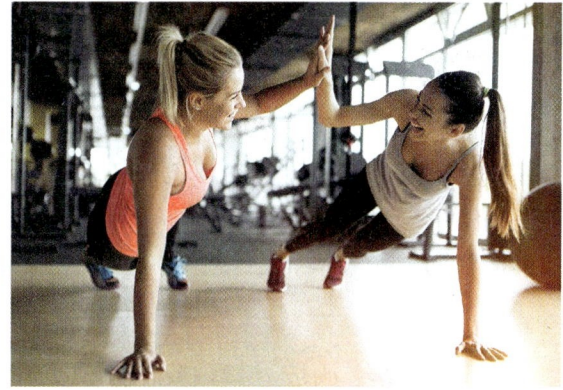

© NDAB Creativity/Shutterstock

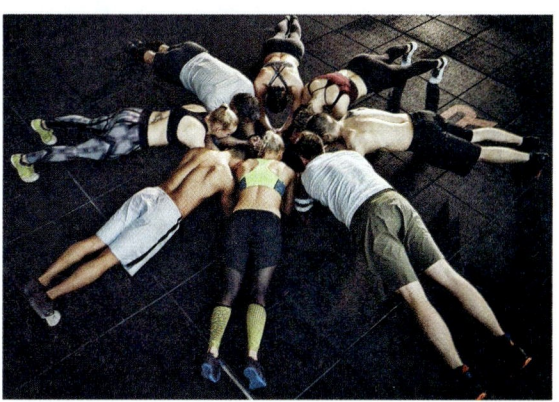

© Ground Picture/Shutterstock

Volitional Movement Versus Prescribed Movement

Physical activity is an effective intervention for the prevention and treatment of obesity, diabetes, and other diseases, yet many people still find it difficult to exercise. Even when it is recommended or prescribed by a healthcare provider, exercise can feel like a chore, or worse, a punishment. However, when exercise aligns with individual preferences, lifestyle, and attitudes, it can result in better adherence and outcomes (Aboagye, 2017).

Through the variety of approaches, environments, and modalities that exist within group fitness, it is possible to engage more people with more activities they enjoy and value. As a Group Fitness Instructor, you play a pivotal role in helping participants shift their attitude toward movement from a reluctant "have to" (i.e., prescribed) to an enthusiastic "want to" (i.e., volitional). By offering participants options and encouraging them to make good personal choices, group fitness can empower individuals to develop a more positive relationship with exercise and, therefore, regular participation.

Health Benefits of Fitness

For individuals, families, and the community at large, the health benefits of being physically fit are profound and far-reaching. Although lifestyle-related health conditions can place a strain on individuals, families, the economy, and the healthcare system, many of these negative consequences can be reduced or avoided with regular exercise (CDC, 2019; World Health Organization, 2009). The health benefits of fitness are listed in **Figure 1.3**.

Group Fitness Instructors can play an important role in helping more people reap these benefits by providing safe, effective classes that educate participants about the many ways that physical fitness can improve their health and quality of life.

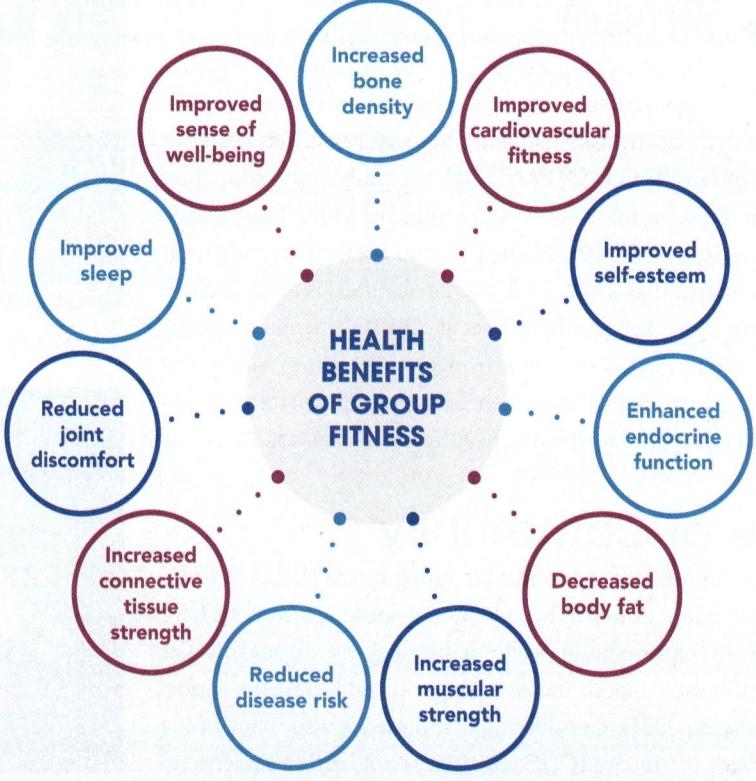

FIGURE 1.3 Health Benefits of Fitness

Lesson 3: Trust and Participants

The Role of Trust

As the activities encompassed under group fitness continue to expand and evolve, so do the depth and volume of the essential knowledge, skills, and abilities required to deliver it. As any passionate group fitness participant will attest, exercising together in a group (large or small) is often more motivating and fun than doing it alone, especially when there is an energetic, inspiring instructor to lead it. An instructor removes the guesswork for participants, providing structure and purpose for the exercises they perform. They trust that their instructor is not only knowledgeable but also has their best interest at heart. Group Fitness Instructors have a responsibility to ensure that they deserve the trust their participants place in them. At AFAA, we value that trust and recognize its role in an integrated web that includes our commitment to our instructors, the employers they work for, the participants in their classes, and the community at large.

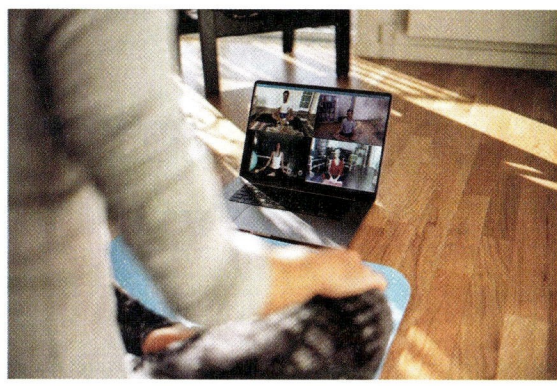

© Jacob Lund/Shutterstock

Trust in AFAA

At AFAA, we believe that group fitness fulfills a demonstrated need for fitness, community, and health. In service of that belief, we are committed to maintaining a standard of quality that our professionals can take pride in. Starting in 1983 with the creation of AFAA's Basic Exercise Standards and Guidelines and following up with our first textbook shortly thereafter, we have continued to evolve and elevate our educational standard for fitness professionals worldwide.

As a proven leader in fitness education, we believe in evidence-based movement practices supported by science. Considering the abundance of confusing, and often misleading, information circulating in the health and fitness space, we recognize that it can be difficult to discern fact from fiction. To that end, AFAA is continually evaluating research and trends and refining and adapting our products to ensure that they meet the needs of our professionals. By collaborating with industry experts and leaders to deliver content instructors can rely on, it is our goal to consistently provide our professionals with information and resources they can trust to design their classes, continue their education, and grow their careers.

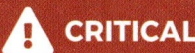 **CRITICAL**

The proliferation of social media has turned many unqualified *influencers* into *fitness experts*. As a responsible, trustworthy instructor, use a critical eye when sifting through the overwhelming number of fads and trends promoted online. A good rule is that if it sounds too good to be true, it probably is. Before adopting a technique or advocating for a new or "game-changing" methodology, be sure to consult a multitude of credible resources to ensure that you are not contributing to the spread of misleading and confusing information about health and fitness.

We believe our professionals have something unique and valuable to offer participants, and we want to ensure that they are supported in their efforts to do so. Participants rely on their instructors to deliver safe, effective, engaging, and inclusive classes. In turn, instructors rely on their education and training to deliver on that expectation. We value the investment you have made in AFAA to obtain your education as well as the value you add to the AFAA brand as a Group Fitness Instructor. Because your success is our success, we strive to invest in new ways to help our professionals (and the participants they serve) achieve their goals.

From Employer to Employee

Unless you opt to teach independently (e.g., out of your home or as the owner of a studio), another trusting relationship exists between you and your employer. Whether you are working for a commercial facility, a boutique, a corporate wellness environment, or a community recreation center, you will be joining a team with an organizational structure determined by someone other than you. With that in mind, it is important to learn and adhere to their policies, procedures, and expectations. Although you may not always like or agree with every policy or decision, if you accept a position, it is your responsibility to conduct your classes according to the standards set forth by your supervisor or company. For example, if the policy is to arrive 15 minutes prior to the class start to set up and greet participants, then arriving 5 minutes before class is a breach of that trust. If you are responsible for finding a substitute instructor in your absence, then you must ensure that your class is covered before going out of town. If there are specific brand guidelines required for certain class formats, then you must adhere to them. By acting with integrity and according to expectations, you will earn the trust and respect of your employer as well as the participants in your classes.

From Instructor to Participant

Trust between you and the participants in your class(es) is important and personal. Fortunately, it is also the relationship over which you have the most control. By becoming an instructor, you have accepted a significant responsibility that involves the health and well-being of others. With that in mind, you must do your best to keep every participant you encounter as safe and supported as possible.

To do that, it is vital that you always work within your **SCOPE OF PRACTICE** and strive to maximize benefits while minimizing risks. Because you are the leader at the front of the class, participants will inherently trust you to make good decisions about the movements and methods you select. It is your responsibility to honor that trust. Participants often do not know whether a movement feels difficult simply because it is challenging or because it is harmful, so you must be clear in how you communicate proper performance to ensure that they understand the difference. Before introducing a popular new movement or exercise from social media, check with a credible resource to make sure it aligns with safe and effective principles. Before repeating a statistic or "fact" from a trendy blog, check multiple sources to confirm that it is accurate. Participants will believe what you say and mimic what you do, so choose your words thoughtfully and strive to be a role model in all interactions before, during, and outside of class. When you treat participants with respect, know what you know (as well as what you do not know), and act within your scope of practice, you will not only earn the trust of your participants, but you will also deserve it.

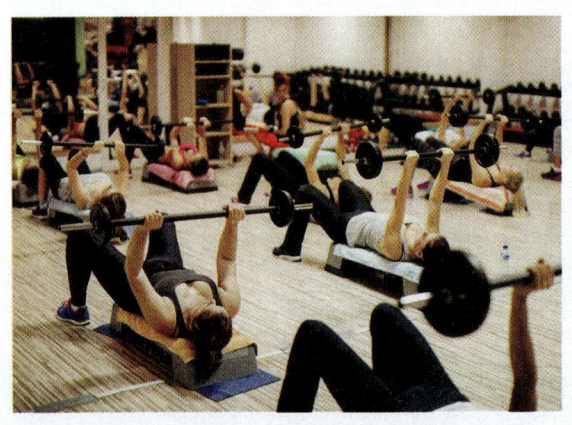

© Shevtsovy/Shutterstock

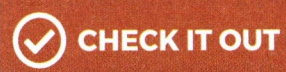

CHECK IT OUT

As a Group Fitness Instructor, it is important to know where your responsibilities begin and end. Like all health professionals, Group Fitness Instructors focus on one area of practice and work within set guidelines that are standardized and legally defined by national and state agencies. This is called the scope of practice and refers to what an instructor can legally and ethically do in their role, including the knowledge, skills, processes, and limitations for which they should be held accountable.

The tasks and responsibilities of an AFAA instructor include the following:

- Preparing and delivering fun, safe, evidence-based workouts for participants
- Dynamically reacting to group or individual needs by providing modifications for fitness level
- Providing energy, enthusiasm, and optimism to create positive associations with exercise
- Maintaining CPR/AED certification
- Answering participant questions but avoiding one-on-one recommendations
- Referring personal health questions out to appropriate providers

These guidelines exist to protect you and your participants and should always be followed.

From Instructor to Instructor

In your career as an instructor, another of your most valuable relationships will be with fellow instructors (**Figure 1.4**). Whether they are your managers, your mentors, or your colleagues, nurturing trusting relationships with them will lead to greater satisfaction and success for you. In the best circumstances, they can be great allies and supporters; at their worst, they can be contentious competitors who make your job more difficult. Although you cannot be responsible for the outcome of every situation or for the behavior of others, you can control your own behavior.

Simple ways to earn trust and fellowship include taking and promoting others' classes, subbing for an instructor in need, teaching in accordance with established guidelines, and being willing to give and receive constructive feedback. For example, by stepping up to help another instructor when they need a substitute, they are more likely to do the same for you.

TRUST AMONG INSTRUCTORS

T ··· Take others' classes

R ··· Reliably adhere to guidelines

U ··· Understand the value of feedback

S ··· Sub whenever you are able

T ··· Team teach

FIGURE 1.4 Instructor-to-Instructor Trust

By taking other instructors' classes, you not only have an opportunity to learn something new but also to demonstrate support for your colleagues. That spirit of support will often be reciprocated in kind, resulting in a culture of teamwork and mutual benefit. When you teach in a manner that aligns with the organization's standards instead of going rogue, you promote consistency and trust in the program that benefits everyone involved, including you. And when you graciously accept feedback, you are more likely to be trusted when you deliver it.

As a community within a community, the instructor-to-instructor relationship has the potential to be one of the most inspiring and enriching of your career, but it must be built on a foundation of mutual trust and respect.

✓ CHECK IT OUT

Team teaching, or teaching with another instructor, can be one of the most effective (and fun) methods to gain experience, improve skills, and build relationships. When team teaching, be sure to plan ahead with the other instructor regarding who will teach each section and ensure that the entire experience is cohesive from start to finish (that includes everything from exercise selection to music coordination). Approach it as a respectful partnership rather than a competition and use it as an opportunity to create a special, one-of-a-kind experience for you, your teaching partner, and the participants.

Participants

Without participants, there is no group fitness. Sometimes, as a Group Fitness Instructor, it is easy to be distracted by individual desires (such as social media recognition, personal fitness goals, or career aspirations); however, never lose sight of the fact that if you choose to lead others, your responsibility to them must come first. To do that, recognize that every individual in your classes also brings with them a unique set of values, experiences, limitations, and personal goals that may be very different from your own. Although it is impossible to know the distinct needs and motivations of every participant encountered, it is important to be aware of how your choices can affect them and to develop effective strategies to support their success. Group fitness exists because of the participants. Instructors must get to know participants, learn their needs, and provide experiences that meet those needs to the best of their ability.

Who Are the Participants?

Teaching a group fitness class might be likened to teaching in a school where the students range from preschool age to postgraduate level, with new and different students showing up daily. Putting it in this context might be an extreme analogy, but it highlights the potential diversity in demographics, fitness level, and experience that a Group Fitness Instructor may encounter in a single class and throughout their career. Starting from this perspective highlights the importance of being flexible, creative, and inclusive when planning and delivering group fitness classes.

Although it may seem obvious, complex human beings are not all motivated by the same desires (**Figure 1.5**). Some participants come to class because they are die-hard fitness enthusiasts who want to look and perform their best. They are motivated to work hard, learn the most

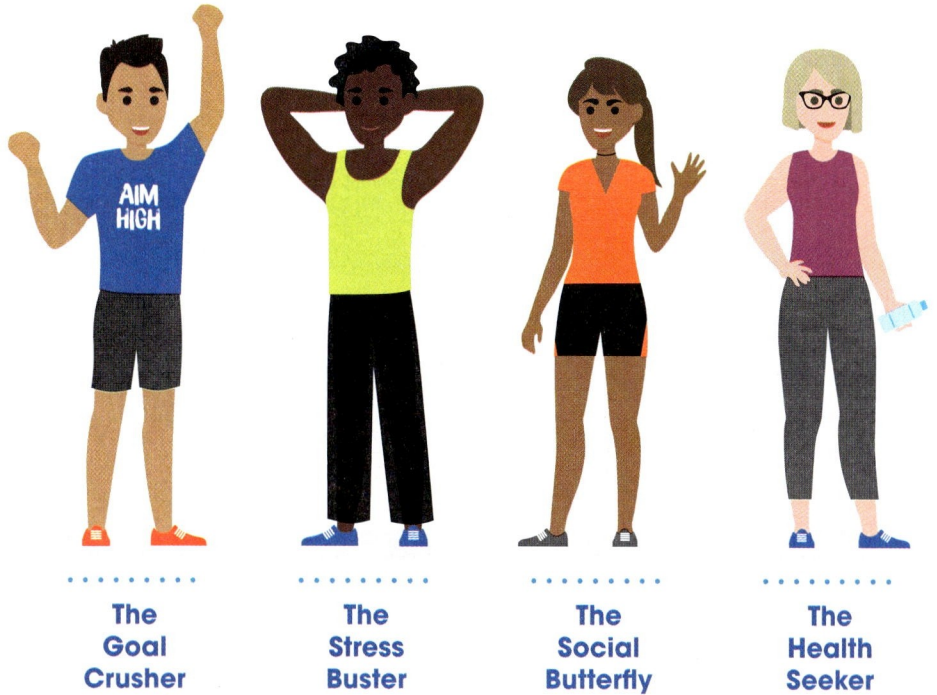

The Goal Crusher

The Stress Buster

The Social Butterfly

The Health Seeker

FIGURE 1.5 Participant Types

effective techniques, and take on the most challenging exercises. Conversely, others are more interested in relieving stress and having fun than in maximizing their performance. Some choose to come because they struggle with motivation on their own but recognize that exercise is essential for their health. Many are primarily drawn to group fitness for the social connections and opportunity to engage with like-minded individuals. Although desired outcomes vary greatly from person to person, fundamentally, each participant wants to feel accomplished in one way or another. For instructors, this is important to remember. Instead of imposing personal goals and values on the participants in your classes, acknowledge, celebrate, and support the diversity that exists among their goals and values. This can be accomplished by not only being aware of these differences but also adopting a more inclusive communication and presentation style to accommodate them.

The Instructor's Relationship with Participants

The relationship between the instructor and the class participants is necessarily bi-directional. In other words, it works both ways. As established, without participants, instructors do not have anyone to teach. And without an instructor, participants have no one to lead them. Instructors can have a tremendously positive effect on the lives of the individuals they teach. It is not uncommon for instructors to receive heartfelt messages of thanks from grateful participants acknowledging the life-changing effects that the instructor has had on them. As an instructor, few things are more rewarding than the confirmation that all your hard work has resulted in such positive outcomes. Participants look to instructors for guidance and leadership. In turn, instructors look to participants to affirm the choice they have made to pursue a career in fitness. When instructors put

thank you

I hope this card isn't too weird, but I wanted to thank you for being the BEST at what you do. I have been rehabbing a serious hip injury since August of last year and cycling was a saving grace. I don't know that I would have truly avoided all the gym activities I was supposed to if I didn't have your rocking/hard/sweaty classes to get me through. My hip is nearly 100% now and I just want to tell you how much you helped me these past 6 months.

Very sincerely – Amy XO

participants first, they will often find that it results in more regular attendance, and with more attendance, instructors are more likely to be rewarded with more and better opportunities to grow their careers.

To become more effective in your approach to communication with others, it is helpful to begin by understanding yourself. The continued practice of self-reflection is an essential component of your growth as an instructor, and by identifying your own personal preferences, goals, and biases you can learn to avoid the pitfall of only communicating with participants whose values match yours. Think about the following reflections and journal on them for future review:

- What is the primary reason you exercise (e.g., to look/perform better, to improve your health, to have fun, to master a new skill)?
- When you are attracted to a particular class format or instructor, what is it, specifically, about the experience and/or the person that you find most compelling?
- Do you choose an instructor because they epitomize an aspirational physique, because they make you laugh, or because you always learn something?
- Do you enjoy classes that are so challenging you struggle to keep up, or do you prefer to turn off your brain and just enjoy the music?
- Are you interested in learning the finer details of the muscles you are working and why, or do you assume that so long as the muscles feel like they are burning it must be good?
- Do you notice when other participants are struggling, or are you so focused on your own workout that you scarcely remember there are others around?
- Do you like to high-five your neighbor and participate in team drills, or are you uncomfortable when encouraged to do so?
- Does it bother you when an instructor starts class late because they were chatting, or are you the person they were chatting with?
- If the instructor ends class a little late, do you leave at the scheduled end time or are you happy to get in a few extra minutes?

No matter how you answered the questions, remember that it is not about what is right or wrong: *they are only personal preferences*. What is important to remember is that however you answered, there are plenty of others who are the complete opposite, and they will also be in your classes. By recognizing your own goals, values, and priorities, you have taken the first step to understanding the importance of acknowledging the many types of participants you will encounter, and, through that awareness, you can develop strategies to communicate better with all of them.

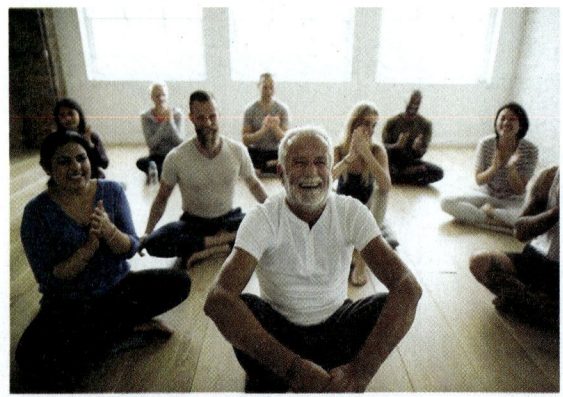

© Rawpixel.com/Shutterstock

Inclusivity

As a mindset, inclusivity is fundamental to the success of both instructors and participants and will be threaded throughout the entirety of this course. Your job as an instructor is to make participants feel welcome and included regardless of their motivations, needs, expectations, perceived limitations, background, experiences, or identity (Pilkington, 2020). A skilled, conscientious instructor can simultaneously honor differences while fostering inclusion. Everything from your choice of language to movement selection can influence the sense of inclusion (or lack thereof) in the classes you teach. By practicing awareness and being intentional in your planning and communication strategy, you can create an environment that allows every individual to feel seen, valued, celebrated, and supported in their fitness goals.

USING INCLUSIVE LANGUAGE

One of the most basic ways to foster an environment of inclusivity is to bring awareness to your body language and word choice. Remember that powerful first impressions can be made before you speak a single word. Smile, make comfortable eye contact, and carry yourself with an open, welcoming posture. When you welcome the participants to class, instead of using words like "ladies and gentlemen" or "boys and girls," consider using words such as "team" or "friends." When cueing movement, avoid the practice of leveling movements in a way that puts participants in categories such as beginner or advanced. Instead, frame movement choices (such as progressions and regressions) as variations that may be appealing to them today. For example, rather than saying, "Next up, lunges! Beginners don't use any weights; advanced folks, pick up your heavy dumbbells and let's see what you've got!" a more inclusive way to frame it might be, "Next up, lunges! You can do them with or without weights, depending on how your body feels today. Either way, let's focus on great form and alignment."

With the great diversity of goals and experience inherent to group fitness, not all participants will come with the same knowledge of terms or context relevant to certain movements, intensity levels, or images (e.g., "In today's class, we are going to climb the hill to Jamestown") that you do. Whenever possible, use simple, consistent, and literal terms so that everyone, not just the regulars, understands the expectations. This also includes when you are communicating a specific movement or method of measuring intensity. Perhaps you have a signature move called the *Sara Special*. If you say, "Okay, get ready for the Sara Special in 3, 2, 1," every participant who does not know what the Sara Special is will be standing there wondering what to do. If you use heart rate zones but not everyone has a heart rate monitor (or knows what their Zone 3 is), it is vital to explain it in terms all participants can understand. In this way, everyone has a chance to feel successful and included rather than confused and left out.

MODIFICATIONS

Providing modifications for movement and intensity targets is one of the best strategies to create an inclusive environment. By offering multiple options for altering an exercise (such as a progression or regression), each member of your class can find something that works for them. To effectively deliver modifications, it is important to make every option valid. Celebrate differences and commend participants for making good personal choices. Instead of saying "If you can't" before showing a regression, try saying "Here's another great option to accomplish the same goal." Instructors rarely know the reasons a participant may choose one movement over another; therefore, to be inclusive, provide them with examples and ideas that empower them to make the right decision for themselves without making them feel excluded in the process.

 INSTRUCTOR TIP

Instead of using the terms *progression* and *regression*, try "We can choose from option A, B, C on this next sequence," "We have a couple different choices for this exercise," or "Choose the version that provides the right mix of challenge and form for you."

SUMMARY

As a Group Fitness Instructor, you have an incredible opportunity to touch countless lives. Through the delivery of effective, science-based workouts you can help improve the health, fitness, and performance of your participants. With an engaging, optimistic, and energizing presence, you can create fun, socially connected experiences that lead individuals to have positive associations with exercise. By using inclusive language and offering thoughtful modifications, you can foster an environment in which all feel welcome. And, by acting with integrity and honoring your scope of practice, you can establish yourself as a respected professional, worthy of trust in the eyes of your participants, your peers, and the greater fitness industry.

REFERENCES

Aboagye, E. (2017, June). Valuing individuals' preferences and health choices of physical exercise. *Pain and Therapy*, 6(1), 85–91. https://doi.org/10.1007/s40122-017-0067-4

Centers for Disease Control and Prevention. (2019). *Lack of physical activity*. https://www.cdc.gov/chronicdisease /resources/publications/factsheets/physical-activity.htm

Eastwick, R. (2021). *The benefits of social connections in fitness: Learn how physical activity and social connection benefit the brain and improve quality of life*. IDEA Health & Fitness Association. https://www.ideafit.com/mind -body-recovery/the-benefits-of-social-connections-in-fitness/

Feltz, D. L., Kerr, N. L., & Irwin, B. C. (2011). Buddy up: The Köhler effect applied to health games. *Journal of Sport & Exercise Psychology*, 33(4), 506–526. https://doi.org/10.1123/jsep.33.4.506

Irwin, B. C., Scorniaenchi, J., Kerr, N. L., Eisenmann, J. C., & Feltz, D. L. (2012). Aerobic exercise is promoted when individual performance affects the group: A test of the Kohler motivation gain effect. *Annals of Behavioral Medicine*, 44(2), 151–159. https://doi.org/10.1007/s12160-012-9367-4

Karageorghis, C. I. (2017). *Applying music in exercise and sport*. Human Kinetics.

Kravitz, L. (2012). *Qualities of top teachers: Engage and encourage your clients and students. Make them hungry for more!* IDEA Health & Fitness Association. https://www.ideafit.com/personal-training/qualities-of-top-teachers/

Martela, F., & Pessi, A. B. (2018). Significant work is about self-realization and broader purpose: Defining the key dimensions of meaningful work. *Frontiers in Psychology*, 9, 363. https://doi.org/10.3389/fpsyg.2018.00363

Merriam-Webster. (n.d.). Professional. In *Merriam-Webster.com*. https://www.merriam-webster.com/dictionary /professional

Pilkington, K. (2020). *Diversity, equity, and inclusion in fitness: What's your strategy? Set your fitness business up for wider reach an inspiration*. IDEA Health & Fitness Association. www.ideafit.com/business/diversity-equity-and -inclusion-whats-your-strategy/

Sinek, S. (2009). *Start with why: How great leaders inspire everyone to take action*. Penguin Group.

Teixeira, P., Carraça, E. V., Markland, D., Silva, M. N., & Ryan, R. M. (2012). Exercise, physical activity, and self-determination theory: A systematic review. *International Journal of Behavioral Nutrition and Physical Activity, 9*, 78. https://doi.org/10.1186/1479-5868-9-78

Warburton, D. E. R., Nicol, C. W., & Bredin, S. S. D. (2006, March). Health benefits of physical activity: The evidence. *Canadian Medical Association Journal, 174*(6), 801–809. https://doi.org/10.1503/cmaj.051351

World Health Organization. (2009). *WHO guide to identifying the economic consequences of disease and injury*. https://www.who.int/publications/i/item/9789241598293

CHAPTER 2

PROFESSIONAL EXPECTATIONS OF A GROUP FITNESS INSTRUCTOR

LEARNING OBJECTIVES

The intent of this chapter is to provide professional expectations in the various roles you will serve as a Group Fitness Instructor across various class types and delivery mediums. This chapter will discuss commonalities found in all group fitness classes, regardless of the format; provide expectations from a participant's perspective; and help identify any oversights you might have as an instructor.

After reading this content, students should be able to demonstrate the following objectives:

- **Identify** the three primary class types in group fitness.
- **Describe** the various delivery mediums for group fitness.
- **Identify** group fitness formats and their characteristics.
- **Describe** the five components of a group fitness workout.
- **Describe** the importance of music to group fitness.
- **Define** bias and its influences on the group fitness class experience.

Lesson 1: Your Role as a Group Fitness Instructor

Introduction

When watching an instructor teach a group fitness class, it can sometimes be amazing to see how the instructor can anticipate what their participants need before they need it. An experienced instructor can smoothly orchestrate the class and participants' moves from the time they walk into the room until they walk out. Your role as an instructor will be to create that experience for your group fitness community. This chapter explores your role as a Group Fitness Instructor and will help you clarify expectations for your career.

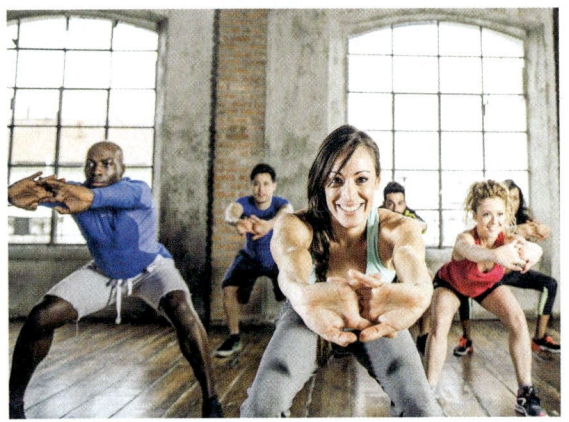

© Oeinchpunch/Shutterstock

Your Role as a Group Fitness Instructor

Becoming a Group Fitness Instructor can be an exciting journey, especially when you have a love for fitness or are passionate about a specific format. This journey starts with understanding your role and expectations as a Group Fitness Instructor as you start your career. These expectations begin with you and extend to your employer and participants. This will make up your group fitness community. As you develop your skills, you will be able to anticipate, meet, and exceed the expectations of your community.

Expectations for Your Career

A Group Fitness Instructor's role is to create and deliver purpose-driven workouts while coaching, assessing, and modifying movement for participants in a group setting. Simply put, you are delivering a fitness experience. Delivering these workouts is the final product. Education, research, preparation, and skill development are where you will do most of the work for your classes.

Initial and continuing education are the foundation upon which classes are built. Understanding the basics of exercise science, the human movement system, and integrated fitness will allow you to do the following:

- Create safe and effective workouts
- Coach form and technique
- Deliver a class that is authentic to the designated format

Use of valid evidence and practices will enable you to deliver classes that are current, effective, and relevant. As fitness trends and classes continue to evolve, being able to research and adapt will extend the life of your career. Updated music trends are equally important to keep the experience fresh and exciting for your participants. This research will create an expanding library of knowledge for you to pull from as you develop your classes.

Regardless of the format or class type, developing material to deliver to your class is the largest part of your role as a Group Fitness Instructor. This includes the following:

- Preparing the class layout
- Building combinations
- Learning and creating choreography
- Sequencing exercises based on training principles
- Selecting appropriate music and creating a playlist
- Physically testing for effectiveness
- Perfecting form demonstration
- Planning modifications and alternate choices
- Scripting and planning cues
- Practicing the class in its entirety

Instructors are then responsible for putting this all together seamlessly to teach a polished and professional group fitness class. See **Figure 2.1** for an example of how your time may be spent as a professional Group Fitness Instructor.

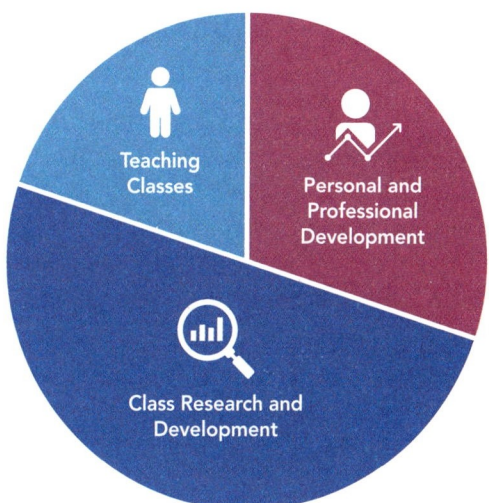

FIGURE 2.1 Example Distribution of Professional Time

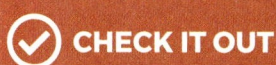 **CHECK IT OUT**

Class Prep: Perception Versus Reality

What people think instructors do to get ready for a class:

- Listen to music before class and then randomly put moves together in class

What instructors actually do to get ready for a class:

- Research exercises for class format
- Go to other instructors' classes for inspiration and tips
- Listen to hours of music and map playlists to movements
- Sequence exercises
- Practice in the mirror to check for proper form
- Script cues
- Practice the entire workout to ensure it is doable

Expectations as an Employee

Fitness facilities offer group fitness for several reasons: as a service for members, as a revenue center, or as a retention tool, to name a few. Regardless of the reason, there are commonalities that all employers expect from their Group Fitness Instructors. First, as an employee, you will be expected to demonstrate a standard level of professionalism. This includes being on time, being prepared, having open and honest communication, and acting within an instructor's scope of practice. You will also be expected to maintain or be working toward relevant credentials. Certifications vary from one employer to the next and can vary based on format. All fitness facilities will require a CPR/AED (and possibly first aid) certification for an instructor to teach classes. As an employee, you will also be expected to learn how to use the equipment provided by the facility for your classes. This includes fitness modalities as well as audiovisual equipment. Finally, understanding customer service will be expected because you will be building relationships and offering a service to the participants of your facility.

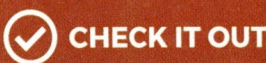

CHECK IT OUT

Different types of facilities have different focuses for their group fitness departments. The following are some examples:

- **Large-chain gyms:** Group fitness as an amenity and retention tool
- **Medium to small gyms:** Group fitness as a community builder and feeder into small group training or personal training
- **Boutique studios:** Classes as a revenue builder

Although each business will have a different focus, the common thread that pulls all group fitness classes together is a focus on the participants and providing them with the best experience possible.

Participants' Expectations

Participants come to class to fill a need that they cannot get from working out on their own. People seek out group fitness for the following reasons:

- They do not know what to do and need help from an expert.
- They feel intimidated by the gym floor.
- They want to try different types of exercise.
- They want to belong to a community.
- They want accountability and structure in their fitness schedule.
- They want movement to be fun.
- They want exercise to have a social component.

Group fitness can fill many or all of these needs for many people at the same time. As the instructor, participants are looking to you as the expert. They will expect you to have the knowledge behind the workout, including benefits and modifications. Participants will expect that you will deliver a class that is authentic to the format and delivers on the expectations that are set out in the class description, whether that description comes from you at the beginning of class or is described in the group fitness schedule. Participants are also expecting connection, whether it is to the workout, the music, the other participants, or you as the instructor. As the leader of your class, being available to connect with your participants will help you better understand their expectations and meet their needs.

Lesson 2: Class Types, Delivery Mediums, and Formats

Class Types and the Roles They Play in Your Instructor Development

When stepping into the role of a Group Fitness Instructor, it is important to look at the different class types to understand how classes are put together. Learning about the different class types will also highlight what tools are available to you within the industry when you are starting out. The three class types are **PRE-CHOREOGRAPHED**, **PRE-DESIGNED**, and **FREESTYLE** (**Figure 2.2**). Each type has benefits and limitations. Understanding how and why instructors and facilities use these class types will allow you to decide which class type is best for you.

Over the course of a career, an instructor will more than likely teach more than one class type, if not all of them. Learning and teaching different class types can be used as a tool for growth as an instructor. Because each class type has a different focus, it gives you an opportunity to master different components of teaching. Teaching a class is like getting your own home. Whether you purchase a home that is ready to be lived in or that you are building from the ground up, the end result is the same. You have a space that is yours, that is safe, and that you can invite your people to.

Pre-Choreographed

Although choreography is often associated with dance, in group fitness it refers to a sequence of exercises or moves that are planned or controlled. Often, instructors will refer to the movement plan of their class as the choreography. In a pre-choreographed class type, all the exercises are planned and set to specific music by a group fitness class production company. These classes are available in different formats from several different trademarked brands. If teaching a pre-choreographed format, an instructor is required to attend an **INITIAL TRAINING**. They will learn the principles behind the formatting along with other fundamentals that prepare them for an assessment review for final certification. After receiving certification, instructors are required to purchase monthly or quarterly (depending on the organization) educational material containing new choreography, music, and updated research relevant to the specific pre-choreographed format. These regular distributions of choreography and music may also be called releases. The instructor is responsible for learning, memorizing, and delivering the material each month/quarter in their classes.

A pre-choreographed class requires a large amount of research and planning before it is ready for instructors to teach it. The sequencing of the movement is developed ahead of time

PRE-CHOREOGRAPHED

All components of a class are created by a single person, business, or organization with a connected theme, brand, or experience.

PRE-DESIGNED

A template that provides an overall class direction, theme, or experience that allows instructors to control other variables.

FREESTYLE

Method of choreography based on the instructor's personal preference, skill set, and knowledge.

INITIAL TRAINING

Education taken to qualify to teach a specific group exercise format designed by a particular brand or organization.

TEACHING METHODS

Pre-Choreographed

Pre-choreographed classes offer instant credibility with participants because of brand or format consistency. Therefore, it is important to maintain a uniform experience throughout class planning and execution, which will require time to learn, rehearse, and master choreography with recommended cues.

- Time for initial learning, rehearsing, and memorization
- A schedule to learn and execute new choreography (e.g., 4 hours, once per month)
- All experience components (e.g., music, moves, equipment, cueing style)

Pre-Designed

An initial time investment is needed to know and practice the pre-designed class structure, as typically seen in the form of an additional qualification. Then the instructor creates interchangeable modules to bring variety and progression, while still maintaining continuity to the pre-designed structure.

- An initial time and financial investment
- Ongoing time to update movement toolkit
- Only a few new moves introduced each class

Freestyle

An instructor designs and plans every aspect of a freestyle class which, despite its name, should have a concise structure centered around a meaningful class vision.

- Design of a class vision to ensure a connected and effective experience
- Use of movement patterns that have been previously taught with success
- Extra time needed for creating entirely new class experiences
- Creativity used sparingly to avoid overwhelming a group

FIGURE 2.2 Class Types

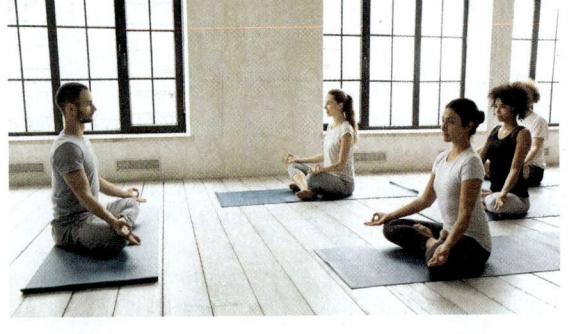
© Fizkes/Shutterstock

and the music has already been selected. This type of class can be helpful for new instructors who are still learning how to put a class together or for those who feel that formatting is not their strength. It can allow instructors to focus on other aspects of teaching, such as technique, cues, and coaching. Additionally, it can take the pressure off trying to create a great workout and help instructors build confidence and find their voice when teaching in front of participants. Pre-choreographed classes give participants a sense of consistency and credibility. They can be sure of the workout even if they do not know the instructor.

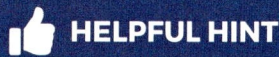

If a pre-choreographed class was your house, it would be a house that was already built, with the walls painted and the furniture already in place. It would be ready for you to live in and entertain your friends.

Pre-Designed Classes

Pre-choreographed classes are a great tool for someone who needs or wants rigid structure for their classes or wants to focus on aspects of group fitness other than class planning. A pre-designed group fitness class can be a bridge between a fully pre-choreographed class and a freestyle class. In a pre-designed program, an instructor is given a set of rules or a blueprint to follow for their class plan. Instructors select exercises and music that fit into this blueprint. For this class type, the instructor is required to attend an initial training to learn the class format and blueprint. After the initial training, instructors have the ability to teach that class format, use branding, and create their own versions as long as the class follows the requirements in the blueprint. Many large-chain fitness facilities will have their own pre-designed classes in addition to well-recognized independent brands.

Pre-designed classes provide structure and guidance to an instructor who wants some creative control but does not want to build a brand or format from the ground up. This type of class can help an instructor master selecting exercises and music and developing sequencing within a framework that will give participants confidence as to what their experience should be.

If a pre-designed class was your home, you would build your house within the guidelines of a homeowners association (HOA) or corporate home builder. All of the houses in your neighborhood would have a similar look and feel, but they would have variations and modifications based on what each homeowner wanted. Once you built your home within the rules of the HOA, it would be ready for the you to live in and entertain guests.

Freestyle Classes

Although freestyle classes are often thought of as classes where the instructor makes up a workout on the spot, the reality is that even freestyle classes are planned, researched, and memorized. A freestyle class is instructor planned in every area of the class design, including exercises, music, and format. In order to teach a freestyle class, an instructor is usually required to obtain a Group Fitness Instructor credential or certification and is expected to keep it current through continuing education units. After an instructor obtains their Group Fitness Instructor credential, they are fully qualified to design a class any way they choose as long as they follow the basic safety guidelines set out in their certification or credential.

With freestyle programming, instructors have full creative control of their classes. They can decide to create classes that follow a general format, such as dance, high-intensity interval training (HIIT), or step, or they can create a format that is unique to them. The possibilities are endless. A freestyle instructor has the ability to market and promote their classes any way they choose as well as build their own brand.

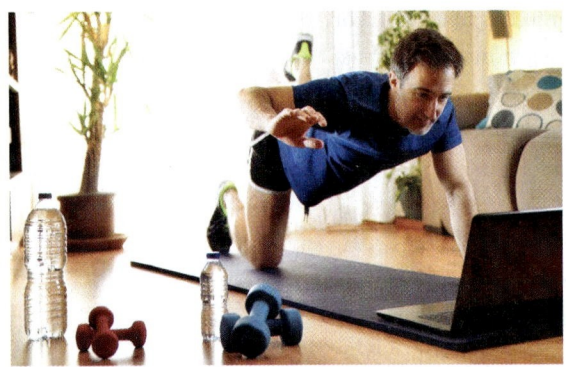

© Davrizo Photography/Shutterstock

Class Delivery Mediums

For a long time, the traditional method of delivering group fitness was in person within the confines of a fitness facility. As technology and opportunity evolve, the possibilities for how classes can be delivered have grown. In-person classes have expanded, providing more opportunities outside of the gym. Instructors have moved online to teach in the virtual space. Instructors now have more control over their audience and a greater opportunity to grow their brand. Classes delivered in person or virtually have their own unique benefits and opportunities.

In-Person Classes

Teaching in-person classes creates fitness experiences that participants cannot get on their own. The energy when the entire class is working together can create a bond between the instructor and the participants that builds community and that keeps people coming back. In-person classes have a number of advantages. Your connection with participants becomes more personal as you spend more time with them. One way to foster this connection is to be available for questions and conversation before and after class. Coaching is more personalized for the participants in your class. You are able to correct form and technique for individual participants because you can see their movement clearly and in real time. You can also see if your cueing is moving the participants in the right way or if you need to adjust and try additional cues. Another advantage is the ability to control the class's energy through the volume of the music in the room. Teaching in-person classes does have challenges, however, including the potential for negative interactions with participants and class disruptions. In-person classes also require more adjusting and thinking on the spot to accommodate the needs of different class participants.

Virtual Classes

As teaching virtually has increased over the last few years, so has the technology that allows instructors to use virtual classes to generate income. Virtual instruction allows you to reach more people than in-person classes allow for. Virtual teaching also allows you to teach a class that is more uniform and scripted than an in-person class that might need to be tailored to coaching specific participants. In some cases, platforms that offer virtual group fitness classes utilize metrics (e.g., heart rate) that are shown to the instructor in real time as a means of connection between the instructor and the participants. This allows the instructor to praise and motivate participants according to the metrics of their workout.

Livestreamed classes can be taught on a subscription-based fitness platform or can be personally hosted by an instrutor. One of the challenges of teaching on a group fitness platform is that you might need to film in studios located in specific corporate locations. Classes can also be hosted personally through a social media platform or through a web meeting tool. You may experience some challenges when hosting your own livestream classes, such as managing filming equipment and technology, participants, music licensing, and payment.

It is also possible to teach classes that are available through on-demand streaming services. With on-demand classes, participants log on to a website and take a class based on their schedule. This allows anyone with an Internet connection to take a class at any time of the day. As with livestreaming, you may be limited to specific filming locations based on the corporate fitness platform. The fitness platform will organize the filming process and load your classes to their website. Another option is to film your classes yourself and upload them to your own website or video-sharing platform. The challenges for on-demand platforms are the same as with livestreaming: managing filming equipment and technology, participants, music licensing, and payment.

As delivery methods evolve, instructors and businesses offering group fitness classes have become more creative in how they reach participants. When circumstances arise that make it challenging for instructors to teach in-person classes, many fitness instructors have found it essential to move into virtual group fitness to replace or supplement their income from in-person classes.

Class Formats

Although there are many group formats to choose from when deciding on a class to teach, many elements of group fitness flow through all of them. These include the following:

- Fundamentals of exercise science and the human movement system
- Principles of integrated fitness
- Equipment use
- Communication methods
- Learning styles
- Class engagement
- Program design
- Safety considerations

Each format uses these elements in unique ways. For example, a high-energy cardio class would use music to motivate participants, whereas a restorative yoga class would use music to promote relaxation and a gentle flow. However, in both settings the instructor is matching movement to music. Another example would be a dumbbell strength-based class and a cardio dance–based class both incorporating balance training. Understanding these commonalties will help you move from one format to another without having to start over each time.

Safety in All Formats

Keeping participants safe in group fitness classes is your primary objective. The focus on safety is important to class design, equipment use, room setup, modification choices, and in all of the components of the workout. Safety elements range from things that you cannot control, such as the fitness level of participants, previous injuries, and the type of footwear a participant wears to class, to things you can control, such as the temperature of the room, safe placement of equipment, and safe exercise selection. Abiding by general safety considerations to control the controllable and offering guidance to make modifications for things you cannot control will help keep participants safe across all formats.

The AFAA 5 Questions™

AFAA 5 QUESTIONS

A series of considerations to aid in evaluating the safety, efficacy, and appropriateness of exercise selection.

In an effort to maximize safety within classes, the Athletics and Fitness Association of America (AFAA) has long used a system for the evaluation of exercise. This system is called the **AFAA 5 QUESTIONS**. The system can be applied to any format and can be used to guide modifications and cueing for a class (**Figure 2.3**).

These questions address the core concept of creating a safe and effective class. Evaluating exercises through the AFAA 5 Questions can identify potential risks to participants and help you decide if an exercise is appropriate for your participants. It is important to note where in the workout they are going to be placed (i.e., movement prep, body of workout, or transition), as this may have an effect on the outcome.

Start with identifying the purpose of an exercise in Question 1. Understanding the purpose of the exercise will help you determine if it is appropriate for the format. In Question 2, evaluating the effectiveness of how participants are doing the exercise will allow you to create cues and

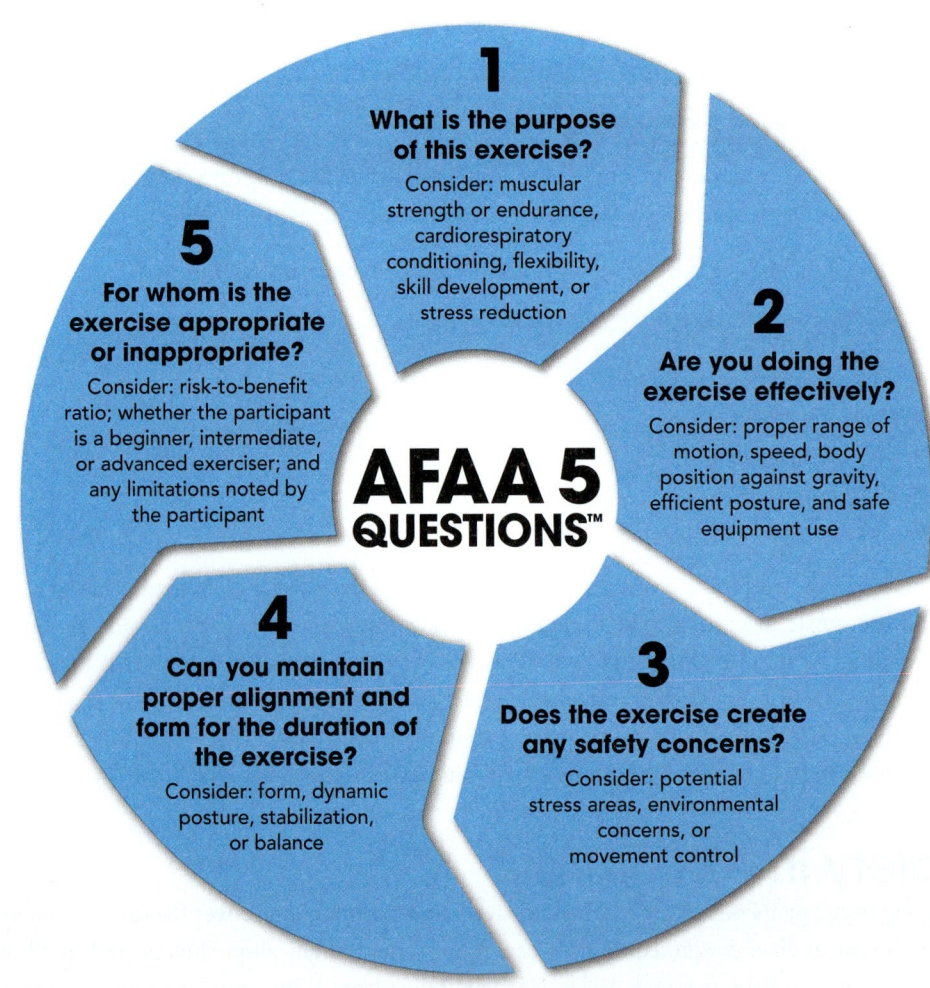

1
What is the purpose of this exercise?
Consider: muscular strength or endurance, cardiorespiratory conditioning, flexibility, skill development, or stress reduction

2
Are you doing the exercise effectively?
Consider: proper range of motion, speed, body position against gravity, efficient posture, and safe equipment use

3
Does the exercise create any safety concerns?
Consider: potential stress areas, environmental concerns, or movement control

4
Can you maintain proper alignment and form for the duration of the exercise?
Consider: form, dynamic posture, stabilization, or balance

5
For whom is the exercise appropriate or inappropriate?
Consider: risk-to-benefit ratio; whether the participant is a beginner, intermediate, or advanced exerciser; and any limitations noted by the participant

AFAA 5 QUESTIONS™

FIGURE 2.3 The AFAA 5 Questions™

coaching that can help you better describe a particular exercise or motivate participants in the most effective way. It is important to understand that exercises are performed in specific ways for specific results. Question 3 starts to evaluate safety concerns that might be present (i.e., Is there a possibility of injury from the exercise itself, the equipment being used, or the space in which it is performed?). If there is a safety concern, the exercise is not appropriate for use in a group fitness setting. Addressing proper alignment and form in Question 4 highlights opportunities for modification and coaching. Finally, Question 5 focuses on whether the exercise is appropriate for the participants in your class.

 HELPFUL HINT

Understanding the format and the population that will be attending your class will ensure that your workouts are appropriate for them. Creating a thorough and honest class description as well as having discussions with your participants regarding their needs and wants will help you recommend classes that are a great fit for them.

Strength-Based Formats

Strength-based formats are classes that incorporate the use of resistance training to achieve a wide range of results. These classes use an array of equipment. They can be choreographed to music or music can be used to motivate without being synchronized to the movement. Strength-based formats have many benefits for participants who attend on a regular basis. Physical benefits from strength training include the following:

- Increased metabolic rate
- Improved body composition
- Improved movement and postural control
- Increased bone mineral density

Strength training has also been shown to benefit mental health and cognitive ability and promote positive changes in self-esteem. Expected results from a strength-based class include increased strength, endurance, and power (Westcott, 2012). Additional benefits include aesthetic changes, improved body composition, general health benefits, or a combination of any of these.

Cardio-Based Formats

Cardio-based formats include a variety of class types. Some of these include dance, cycle, kickboxing, HIIT, step, and interval-based classes. These classes may or may not use equipment and can be choreographed to music or use music to motivate without being synchronized to the movement. The following are benefits of cardio-based classes:

- Improved blood flow
- Lower blood pressure
- Efficient calorie expenditure
- Weight management (Donnelly et al., 2013)

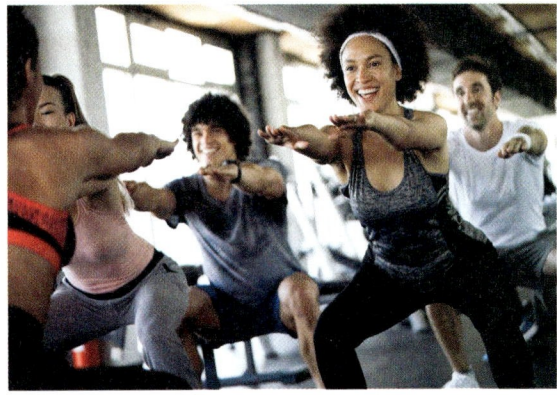

© NDAB Creativity/Shutterstock

Expected results include improved endurance, conditioning, and body composition as well as general health benefits.

5 COMPONENTS OF A WORKOUT

The five essential elements that provide a scientifically sound and holistic group exercise experience: intro, movement prep, body of the workout, transition, and outro.

Mind–Body-Based Formats

Mind–body-based formats include classes such as yoga, tai chi, and Pilates. These formats can use equipment and music in a manner similar to cardio- and strength-based formats, but they can also use ambiance and nature to connect to the workout. The benefits of mind–body-based formats include the following:

- Stress reduction
- Increased flexibility
- Reduced risk of heart disease (Granath et al., 2006)
- Reduced cortisol levels (Katuri et al., 2016)

Expected results from mind–body-based formats include increased flexibility, improvement in mood, increased strength, and general health benefits.

INTRO

Instructor engagement with participants and an explanation of the workout and class expectations.

Fusion-Based Formats

Fusion-based formats offer classes that combine two or more formats to give participants benefits from both formats in a shorter amount of time. These classes may or may not use equipment and can be choreographed to music or use music to motivate without being synchronized to the movement. Fusion-based class benefits include the following:

- Improved blood flow
- Improved body composition
- Efficient use of time

Fusion-based formats can also be a means of adding a new level of excitement or challenge for participants who may be tired of their current class routine. Anticipated results for a fusion class may include increased calorie expenditure and a favorable influence on body composition.

MOVEMENT PREP

Exercises to increase body temperature and blood flow and prime the body for the workout demands.

Lesson 3: Expectations of a Workout

Expectations of a Workout

Participants come to your class for a variety of reasons. Most likely, it is a goal that you may not be familiar with. Goals might include weight and health management or increased strength or flexibility. Although you will connect with many participants and learn some of their goals, it is not possible to know the goals of everyone who comes into your class. By considering the following questions, you can design a class plan that meets participants where they are without requiring specific, personal information from each participant:

- Can I create an experience for the participants that matches the class description?
- Is the class physically attainable while still being challenging?
- Is the class scalable/repeatable?

BODY OF THE WORKOUT

Majority of the fitness class; exercises with a singular or integrated focus on cardiorespiratory fitness, muscular endurance, flexibility, mindfulness, or fun.

Participants' Expectations of a Workout

Whether you design the class yourself or teach a pre-designed or a pre-choreographed class, class descriptions are important to a participant's first impression of a class. Participants might choose your class based on the class description for a variety of reasons. They might have prior knowledge of the format or a new interest in it. They might have an expected result in mind that matches the description. Whatever the reason, if they come to a cardio kickboxing class and there is not a single punch thrown, they are going to be confused, discouraged, and probably frustrated. The first step in building trust with your participants is aligning the description and the essence of the class.

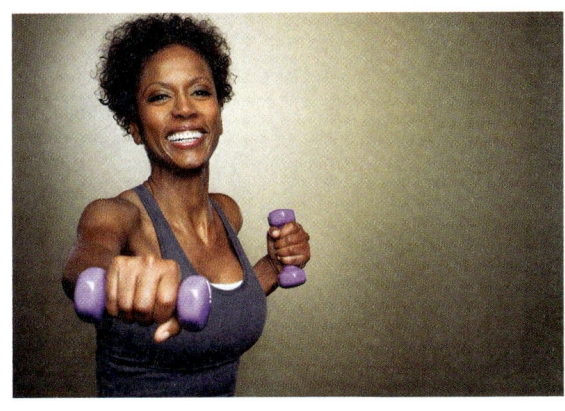

© Pixelheadphoto digitalskillet/Shutterstock

When designing or teaching your class, it is important to keep the people who will be taking the class in mind and adjust accordingly. If a class is pre-choreographed, it has probably been tested on a wide group of people to make sure the class is doable, but if you are creating your own pre-designed or freestyle class, testing the workout on yourself or a group of friends is a good place to start. Also, you should build in some options for your workout to increase or decrease the intensity if you notice it is not quite right for your class.

Creating a scalable workout gives your participants a place to grow as they improve. The intensity of a workout can be increased by increasing weights, intensity, difficulty, or duration. Creating options to make your workout more scalable not only encourages participants' growth but also increases the life of a workout by creating the extra levels.

5 Components of a Workout

Across all formats, the need to create safe and effective classes is always a high priority. The foundation for how a class is designed starts the planning process to correctly ensure that. AFAA uses the **5 COMPONENTS OF A WORKOUT** to ensure that all classes have this solid foundation. The components align with the principles of exercise science and allow for personal connection to the workout and to the participants. The components are the **INTRO**, **MOVEMENT PREP**, **BODY OF THE WORKOUT**, **TRANSITION**, and **OUTRO** (**Infographic 2.1**). Each of these components delivers important information for the workout as a whole. Understanding the importance and use of each component can help you guide your class design or recognize and coach the elements when teaching a pre-choreographed or pre-designed class.

WORKOUT DESIGN CONSIDERATIONS

1 Intro

The intro should be succinct, yet informative, to capture the attention of the participant. A good intro should be no more than 60 seconds and include:

- **A warm welcome**
- **The instructor's name and class title**
- **An overview of the workout and equipment**
- **A motivating segue into a movement prep**

INFOGRAPHIC 2.1 Workout Design Considerations

TRANSITION

A series of movements and exercises meant to guide the body back to a resting state, often while gently moving and stretching the muscles and joints that were heavily used during the body of the workout.

OUTRO

Final class segment to conclude the class, praise participants' effort, and invite participants back to the next class.

(continues)

WORKOUT DESIGN CONSIDERATIONS

2 Movement Prep

To reduce the risk of injury, preview upcoming movements, and move participants from resting to steady state, movement prep should be applied after the class introduction. This also might be called warm-up. Efficient movement prep should:

• Increase the core body temperature
• Increase blood flow and breathing rate
• Prime the body for the class movements

3 Body of the Workout

The focus of the class format occurs during the body of the workout. At this point, exercises and combinations can be executed at full intensity. The workout body should be designed with a specific population or goal in mind but must also be adjusted to meet the needs of the actual participants. Because the body of the workout takes up the majority of time, it takes the most effort in planning. The body of the workout may be focused on a single outcome or a combination of outcomes, such as:

• Achieving or maintaining a certain heart rate or rating of perceived exertion (RPE) level
• Completing a specific choreography pattern
• Performing a certain number or sets, reps, or intervals
• Burning an approximate number of calories
• Dissipating stress or anxiety
• Practicing athletic skills

4 Transition

The transition component of the class offers a steady, gradual change in intensity. The transition is focused on a downward trajectory, and it is sometimes referred to as cool-down. Flexibility is a common component in the transition section of class. Group Fitness Instructors should include static or SMR-based movements to improve joint range of motion, increase muscle length, and promote relaxation and recovery. The overall objectives of the transition are:

• Reduce workout intensity to pre-workout levels
• Complete the experience (start-to-finish connectivity)

5 Outro

The outro only takes moments and should leave an impression on participants. Exercise is not easy for most people and time is valuable, so participants in a class deserve praise. A few words at the end can shape a positive view of exercise and fitness. The outro should be brief (about the same time as the intro) and cover the following points:

• Confirmation the workout is complete
• Compliments or positive statements on effort in class
• Invitation to come back
• Request for participants to provide feedback and ask questions

INFOGRAPHIC 2.1 (continued)

THE 5 COMPONENTS IN DIFFERENT FORMATS

The 5 components of a workout are consistent through all formats; however, the use of each will vary depending on the format. The intro will contain information specific to the format, such as equipment or information that might need to be explained in depth prior to starting any movement. Movement prep should be tailored to the format by including movements and flexibility techniques (e.g., active stretching) that prepare for the specific exercises in the body of the workout. The body of the workout will be planned specifically to align with the format as described in the class description. Similar to the movement prep, the transition should include stretches and exercises that match up with the work done in the body of the workout, but at a declining intensity to prepare the body to return to baseline. **Table 2.1** provides an example of how the 5 components may be applied to different formats.

TABLE 2.1 5 Components in Different Settings

Strength Format	Cardio Format
Intro	
Hi Team! Welcome to Simply Strength. My name is Sam. Today we'll be focusing on total body strength, so you will need a selection of weights and enough room for your mat.	Hi Team! Welcome to Athletic Cardio. My name is Sam. Today in class we'll be focusing on speed and agility. No equipment needed; you just need about arm's length room around you for when we are moving side to side.
Movement Prep	
Exercises for strength-based movement prep: ■ Dynamic stretches ■ Deadlifts ■ Overhead press ■ Squats ■ Bent over row Performed with a smaller range of motion and lighter weights than the body of the workout.	Exercises for cardio-based movement prep: ■ Dynamic stretches ■ Light jog ■ Jumping jacks ■ Planks ■ Stepping lunges ■ Push-ups Performed at a low intensity (low to moderate speed).
Body of the Workout	
■ Deadlifts ■ Upright rows ■ Overhead press ■ Clean and press ■ Kettlebell swings ■ Chest presses ■ Triceps press ■ Lunges ■ Squats ■ Bicep curls Performed with full range of motion and challenging weight selection.	■ High-knee runs ■ Jumping jacks ■ Mountain climbers ■ Jumping lunges ■ Burpees ■ Push-ups ■ Tuck jumps ■ Speed skaters Performed at a high intensity (as fast as can be controlled with proper form).

(continues)

TABLE 2.1 5 Components in Different Settings *(continued)*

Strength Format	Cardio Format
Transition	
■ Hip flexor stretch ■ Lying glute stretch ■ Lower trunk rotation ■ Shoulder stretch ■ Tricep stretch ■ Standing quad stretch ■ Upper back stretch ■ Chest stretch	■ Hip flexor stretch ■ Lying glute stretch ■ Lower trunk rotation ■ Adductor stretch ■ Standing calf stretch ■ Standing quad stretch ■ Standing IT band stretch ■ Upper back stretch ■ Chest stretch
Outro	
Awesome work today, Rockstars! Were those kettlebell swings challenging or what! Thank you so much for coming today. Monday we'll be focusing on lower body, so be ready. Make sure to wipe down and put away your equipment. I'll be waiting by the door if you have any questions. Have an awesome day!	Awesome work today, Rockstars! Were those tuck jumps challenging or what! Thank you so much for coming today. Monday we'll be doing a HIIT workout, so be ready. Don't forget to grab your water bottles. I'll be waiting by the door if you have any questions. Have an awesome day!

Understanding and Applying the 5 Components

Having a deep knowledge of what is included in each component and why classes are structured around them provides a basic framework for you to effectively deliver your class. Applying that knowledge will start the process of creating safe and successful classes.

INTRO

The intro, while being clear and concise, sets the tone for the entire class and allows you, as the instructor, to take command of the room. The following information should be included:

- A brief welcome to class
- Personal introduction
- Required equipment
- Safety information
- Exercises that might need a little more explanation

A strong intro should only take about 1 to 2 minutes. The purpose of the intro is to set expectations, build trust, grab the participants' attention, and get them excited about the work ahead.

MOVEMENT PREP

Movement prep takes the participant from a resting state to a working state. This will set them up correctly for the work ahead and can help to reduce injury risk. Moving from a resting state, the movement prep will raise core body temperature, increase blood flow and breathing rate, and lubricate the joints. An effective movement prep should be based on the total time of the class, taking up 10–15% of class time.

Starting with dynamic stretching, the intensity of movement should be increased slowly to move participants into the body of the workout without causing them to fatigue too early. Oftentimes, this entails a combination of general and format-specific movements that will lead into the body of the workout. Ideally, the movement prep will include movements of similar biomechanics to those in the body of the workout. Executing basic versions of the exercises to come is one way to do this. For example, perform a stationary lunge in movement prep to get ready for walking lunges in the body of the workout. The goal is to prepare participants' sense of form and otherwise "warm them up." At the end of the movement prep, your participants should be mentally and physically ready to move to the body of the workout.

 INSTRUCTOR TIP

Using the Movement Prep as a Teaching Tool

During movement prep, you should begin to connect with your class and start to watch how they move. This is a great time to coach proper form and look for participant form that might need a little extra coaching as the movements get more complex. If possible, make a mental note of your participants who might need a little extra coaching later in class and plan to revisit them at that time.

BODY OF THE WORKOUT

The body of the workout is the core of the class and what participants are coming for. All other components should be planned around this component. At this point in the class, participants should be able to work at the desired intensity level required by the format. The movement planned in the body of the workout should reflect the format and objectives that have been selected for that class. These objectives should also align with the format and benefits of that format.

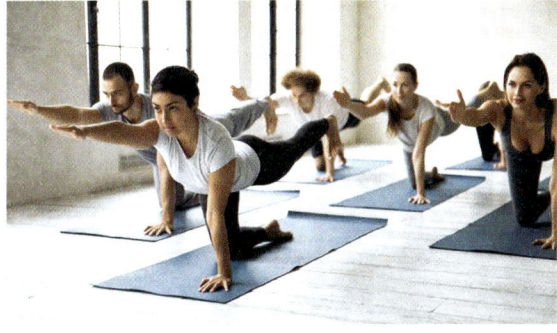

© Fizkes/Shutterstock

When creating the body of the workout, consider that this is where the majority of time will be spent. The first step is to select a format. Develop your objectives from there and select exercises that support them. Finally, sequence the exercises to your selected music. As you go through this process, keep your participants in mind. Their understanding of the class will be set in your class description, and they will look for those benefits accordingly.

TRANSITION

The transition brings your participants from the working state back into a pre-workout state. It is not wise to slam on the brakes to bring your car to a stop. You want to take your foot off the gas and allow your vehicle to slow down. Similarly, the exercises selected in the transition should be based on the movements in the body of the workout. Flexibility plays a big role in the transition, using dynamic and static stretching to slow down the body. Inform participants as to why it is important to transition from a working to a resting state by sharing the purpose and benefits of recovery time. The transition should take approximately the same about of time as the movement prep to allow for optimal recovery.

OUTRO

Just like the intro, an outro should be clear and concise, giving participants any additional information they need to know before they leave the class. A strong outro will include recognition for the work done in class, a thank you for attending, any information a person should know about the next class, and an invitation for questions. This is your last chance to connect with your entire class and make them feel successful about their experience. The entire outro should take 30–90 seconds.

INTEGRATION AND SEPARATION OF GROUP FITNESS ELEMENTS

Each workout component serves its own purpose, but how you develop each one is part of a holistic picture that aligns to the class goals and vision. Developing each part with the whole class in mind will help build a class that not only gets the desired results but also flows smoothly from one segment to the next. It will create purpose for the movement and allow the participant to evolve in their own ability. This will create a stronger bond between the participants, the workout, and you.

Lesson 4: Music and Instructor Oversights

Music

Music is a driving element in group fitness and has many functions in a class. Many factors should be considered when selecting music that go far beyond than just liking a song. Music is one of the biggest multifunctional and motivational tools available to you as a Group Fitness Instructor. It supports the movement, mood, format, and structure of a class. Mastering the use of music can take a good class and make it an amazing experience that people keep coming back for.

The Role of Music and Its Importance to Movement/Exercise

Although motivation is a big factor in using music in a group fitness class, music plays a much bigger role than just getting people excited. Using music as a tool starts with understanding how to attach movement to music and creating an emotional and physical journey attached to the tempos in the music. This will not only drive the tempo and energy of the movement but also create an emotional experience, taking the focus off the work itself.

Attaching movement to exercise starts by understanding tempo and being able to move through the desired ranges of motion within often one to two beats. This is done by using **BEATS PER MINUTE (BPM)** and utilizing movement on beat and at half time. Although exercises in different formats move at different speeds, there are some basic recommendations for BPM that allow for full ranges of motion (**Table 2.2**).

When you understand how to attach the correct exercises to music, you can allow the music to do the work for you. If you set up your participants correctly to the beat of the music, they should stay in that movement pattern without you having to say anything else until you cue a movement change. This allows them not only to focus on doing the exercise correctly but also provides time to enjoy the music.

> **BEATS PER MINUTE (BPM)**
>
> A musical term that refers to measurement of the tempo (speed) of music.

TABLE 2.2 Recommended Music Tempo (BPM) for Common Formats

Class Format	Recommended BPM Range
Resistance training	125–135
High-intensity intervals	150–160
Boot camp	130–140
Step	128–132
Barre, Pilates	124–128
Kickboxing	140–150
Aqua/water/active aging	122–128

The Role of Music to the Structure of a Workout

Music is essential to the structure of a workout when you know how to appropriately utilize track time, repetitions, and workout segments. Musical structure, such as 32-count phrasing and song components, can be a roadmap to how you plan your class. Phrasing is important, and **32-COUNT PHRASING** creates blocks of music that sound the same before switching to a different part in the song. Group fitness music is created this way to allow an instructor to fit in a number of repetitions (or *reps*) before switching to a different exercise or combination. Generally, each of these phrases is about 15 seconds long. Understanding this allows an instructor to plan out exercises in well-timed intervals without using a timer.

Similarly, song components can help to plan reps and work blocks. The components of a song often include the intro, verse, chorus, bridge, and outro. Just like with 32-count blocks, an instructor can use these components for different changes, exercises, tempos, or combinations. This can also create an emotional journey with the song as different intensities can be used in each component.

32-COUNT PHRASING

A common musical structure used in group fitness where musical sections are arranged in 32-count blocks to create choreography that can easily be broken down into exercise sequences.

Music Basics That Apply to All Formats

How deeply you will need to understand music will have to do with what formats you want to teach, but some basics are necessary across all formats. Whether you attach your music to the movement and structure or are using it as background to assist in motivation, there are a few things to consider. Understanding what style and tempo of music supports the formats and intensity of the work will create a better experience for participants. It is also important to consider your participants' preferences. It is easy to pick songs you love but adding some that will appeal and engage other participants will only add to the experience.

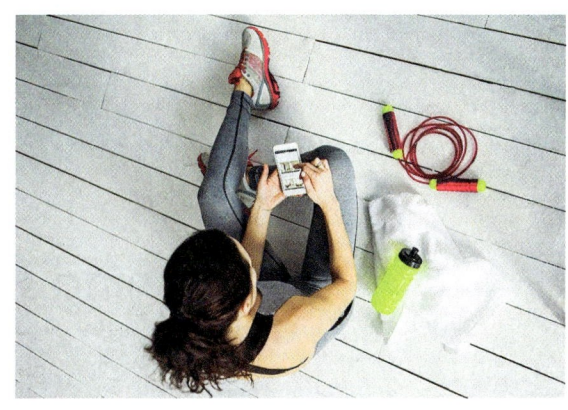

© Daria Grebenchuk/Shutterstock

Instructor Oversights

Being an instructor is an amazing career that allows you to incorporate your love of fitness with improving the health and wellness of others. Although being an instructor can be rewarding and provides a multitude of ways to connect with people, sometimes oversights may occur that could alienate participants and make it hard for you to evolve as an instructor. It often takes feedback or self-reflection to see opportunities missed or bias that may be present. However, when we step outside of ourselves and try to look through the eyes of our participants, we can begin to address any bias we may have.

Instructor Bias

A bias is an outlook, inclination, or judgment toward something or someone (*Psychology Today*, n.d.). Note that we all have biases because we are all the result of our own unique experiences. This does not make us unkind people. In fact, many biases may be unconscious. When teaching to a group, there are bound to be some biases that emerge, and it is your job to identify and adjust your approach, as necessary. As a Group Fitness Instructor, you should embrace the entire group and do your best to make everyone feel welcome and included. That includes taking time to show modifications and treat everyone who attends your class with respect, no matter their fitness level, gender, race, sexuality, or disability. If you think you might have a bias toward participants, ask a manager or another instructor to assess your class and ask for feedback.

✓ CHECK IT OUT

"Hey guys!" is an easy thing to say to your class, but it might make some individuals feel uncomfortable. Using gender-neutral language to address your class is one way to ensure that everyone feels comfortable, and it can help to cultivate a sense of community. Here are some examples of ways to address your class:

- Hey class!
- Hi everyone!
- Friends
- Team
- Yogis
- Crew
- Dancers
- Party people

Once you get to know your community, you will probably be able to come up with additional inclusive terms.

Aligning with Participant Goals

Chances are that if you are on the path to become a Group Fitness Instructor you are passionate about fitness and you might have some experience with your own fitness journey. As you begin your instructor journey, it is very easy to impose your own personal goals onto your class. This mentality can be harmful when building your community as not all participants will have the same goals, preferences, and experience as you. As much as you love the format or program that you plan on teaching, the class truly belongs to your participants. You are there to serve, engage, and encourage them. It is important to remember that your class is not your workout. As a professional fitness instructor, your job is to create a class for your participants' workout.

The first step is placing your participants at the forefront of how you develop and teach your class. Being able to discover and recognize what they want and need is a skill that is developed over time. You should work to build relationships and discuss your participants' goals, what they liked and disliked from your workout, and any concerns they might have. It is important to remember that because their goals are different from yours their feedback applies to what they want. It is not a criticism of your ability to create or teach a good class. Taking notes of their comments and looking for ways to apply it to your next workout will make them feel seen and heard.

Observing participants as they take part in your class is another tool for discovering their needs. In the beginning of your career, this might be a challenge as you will still be mastering the basics of teaching. With time and experience, it will become a natural part of your skill set. Skillful observation requires that you be mentally present and concerned with the needs of your participants. To practice, start by observing one or two participants during a class and see if you can adjust for them in the next class. Write down your observations as soon as you finish teaching, so you do not forget what you saw. As you get better at this, you will be able to adjust on the spot and cater to their needs in real time.

Assessing your own preferences for movement can also help you identify areas of oversight in this area. Reviewing class plans or recording your classes can help you to spot exercises that you use repeatedly. Once you have identified them, observe your class when you use those movements in the future. If your participants love them, that is great. Keep these as fan favorites for future classes. If they are not right for your participants, you will be able to observe their reactions during class. They may never directly tell you that some exercises do not work for them, but as you begin to form relationships with them you will be able to ask for honest feedback.

Participant-centered focus is creating, modifying, and teaching workouts based on your participants' needs and goals. This can be applied to all formats and class types. Applying this focus to the design of your class influences music selection, exercise selection, and specific modifications that all have the goal of serving your unique community. Applying it to pre-choreographed classes might look like teaching at the level that is best for your participants, even if it results in a high volume of modifications. Participants notice when instructors pay attention to their needs and not their own. Your genuine care for participants creates the ultimate trust. Using participant-centered focus will make your participants feel valued and heard.

SUMMARY

Breaking down the components of what a Group Fitness Instructor does and the expectations of the job will help you transition from learning about group fitness to actually teaching it. Clear expectations create a roadmap of what you do, how you do it, and for whom you do it. When you start to apply these concepts in a class, it creates the best experience for both you and your participants.

REFERENCES

Donnelly, J. E., Honas, J. J., Smith, B. K., Mayo, M. S., Gibson, C. A., Sullivan, D. K., Lee, J., Herrmann, S. D., Lambourne, K., & Washburn, R. A. (2013). Aerobic exercise alone results in clinically significant weight loss for men and women: Midwest exercise trial 2. *Obesity, 21*(3), E219–E228. https://doi.org/10.1002/oby.20145

Granath, J., Ingvarsson, S., von Thiele, U., & Lundberg, U. (2006). Stress management: A randomized study of cognitive behavioural therapy and yoga. *Cognitive Behaviour Therapy, 35*(1), 3–10. https://doi.org/10.1080/16506070500401292

Katuri, K. K., Dasari, A. B., Kurapati, S., Vinnakota, N. R., Bollepalli, A. C., & Dhulipalla, R. (2016). Association of yoga practice and serum cortisol levels in chronic periodontitis patients with stress-related anxiety and depression. *Journal of International Society of Preventive & Community Dentistry, 6*(1), 7–14. https://doi.org/10.4103/2231-0762.175404

Psychology Today. (n.d.). Bias. https://www.psychologytoday.com/us/basics/bias

Westcott, W. L. (2012, July–Aug.). Resistance training is medicine: Effects of strength training on health. *Current Sports Medicine Reports, 11*(4), 209–216. https://doi.org/10.1249/JSR.0b013e31825dabb8

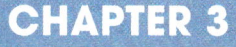

CHAPTER 3

CAREER DEVELOPMENT

LEARNING OBJECTIVES

The intent of this chapter is to identify various employment possibilities and to discuss how developing a personal brand supports your journey as a Group Fitness Instructor. The chapter will also present career development opportunities and self-care tactics to help keep you a top instructor.

After reading this content, students should be able to demonstrate the following objectives:

- **Identify** common group fitness employment venues or opportunities.
- **Describe** personal branding and its relevance to the Group Fitness Instructor.
- **Identify** key marketing and customer retention strategies for Group Fitness Instructors.
- **Identify** continuing education opportunities and their benefits.

Lesson 1: Common Employment Venues and Opportunities

Introduction

When starting as a Group Fitness Instructor, understanding the various possibilities for employment will help you shape your career. Within these possibilities, learning how to build your personal brand will also open opportunities for employment and beyond. In this chapter, you will learn about common employment venues, and how to thrive in each of them, as well as other group fitness career opportunities.

Common Employment Venues and Opportunities

Wherever you are teaching, group fitness as a modality is defined the same way. Differences in the types of employment venues and opportunities, however, may affect how it is offered and how you approach your classes and community. Some venues use **GROUP FITNESS AS A SERVICE** and as a **RETENTION TOOL**; in others, group fitness classes can be used to drive revenue as well as retention. Some venues would like to see classes with 100 participants in attendance, whereas others limit their classes to smaller numbers. Understanding the differences among these venues and their unique opportunities will allow you to make the best decisions when deciding on where and how you would like to teach.

Large-Chain Gyms

One of the most common venues is the big box, or large-chain, gym. These facilities usually have multiple locations and are often large buildings with one or more group fitness studios dedicated to specific formats (e.g., cycling or yoga) along with the typical, multipurpose cardio/strength space. Within this category, membership pricing tiers often affect how group fitness and other amenities and programs are offered. Luxury, mid-tier, and high-value/low-price are common categories in the health club space. Generally, large-chain gyms offer group fitness as a service at all membership pricing levels.

Teaching at large-chain gyms has a number of benefits:

- Multiple locations
- Multiple studios
- Extended hours
- Large group fitness class schedules
- Increased opportunity to get classes and keep a full teaching schedule
- Variety of formats and the opportunity to cross-train in different formats
- Potential to move between locations
- A large team of instructors who can act as mentors or assist with subbing classes
- Teams to maintain exercise and audiovisual equipment
- Potential for employment benefits, such as education reimbursement, insurance, or paid time off

Large-chain gyms have challenges to consider as well:

- Difficulty getting prime class slots due to a larger pool of Group Fitness Instructors
  - More challenging to differentiate yourself from the other instructors
  - Possible requirements to teach only particular formats
  - Potential regulations against teaching with other instructors

Large-chain gyms look for instructors to create a full and diverse class schedule in the pursuit of serving their members. They expect their instructors to foster relationships with their members to build the community. They also expect their instructors to act professionally and remain current with credentials and trends in group fitness.

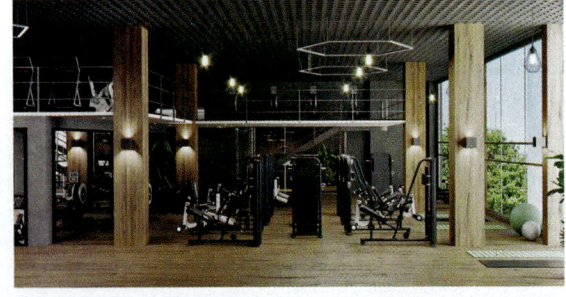

© Shcherban Oleksandr/Shutterstock

Small-Chain and Single-Location Gyms

Small-chain gyms have a handful of locations, and single-location gyms have just one location. Generally, they are still larger-sized facilities equipped with a main gym floor, a main group fitness studio, and, occasionally, a secondary studio for cycling or yoga. They mainly offer group fitness as a service but may have a few classes that are revenue generating. Gyms may charge a fee for their most popular classes or ones that might have limited spaces available, such as an indoor cycling class. In these facilities, group fitness is often measured as a retention tool, meaning it is viewed as a method to keep members connected with the gym. As a retention tool, instructors are generally paid a flat rate per class. When teaching a revenue-generating class, it is possible to be paid an amount per person who attends.

Teaching at small-chain or single-location gyms has a number of benefits:

- Can have large group fitness schedules
- Large group of instructors
- Tend to have a built-in community due to their family atmosphere
- Potential for stronger relationships with your participants
- Potential to host instructor training courses to accrue continuing education credits

Small-chain and single-location gyms have challenges to consider as well, including:

- Heavy focus on class attendance and growth of classes and schedule
- Limited class availability due to the small number of locations
- Less of a focus to grow with new technology and innovation due to budget constraints

Small-chain and single-location gyms, similar to large chains, build their class schedule with a variety of formats to attract new members and keep existing members engaged. They are interested in hiring instructors to build community and offer safe and effective classes. Their Group Fitness Instructors are expected to stay current with credentials, fitness trends, and advancements while always acting in a professional manner.

Boutiques and Studio-Only Facilities

Boutiques and studio-only facilities are smaller locations that offer group fitness classes only. These can include unbranded and branded formats. Single-location studios may offer one format or a variety of formats, including yoga, cycling, Pilates, rowing, and dance studios. These studios are driven by revenue, usually via a pay-per-class, class package, or recurring membership model. Often, instructors are paid relative to attendance (usually a higher flat rate or an amount per person) to reward them for building bigger class numbers. Instructors may also be paid a commission for participants that purchase memberships.

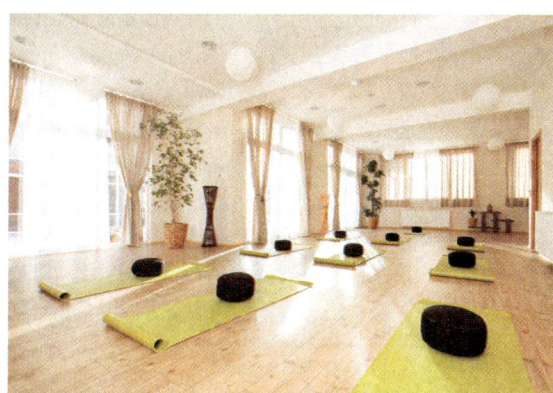

Branded studios provide extensive training for their specific format. They can also offer a high volume of coaching and educational support, allowing instructors to develop and sharpen their skill sets. These additional opportunities may come at no additional cost to the instructor. Branded studios are widely recognized and drive a lot of participants into classes, creating an exciting and energetic environment to teach in. These studios can be a great place to work on your personal branding as an instructor because of the heavy focus on using and building your social media to promote classes. Unbranded

© Project1photography/Shutterstock

studio locations can offer instructors a lot of freedom in format and how they can market their classes. In some cases, unbranded studios allow you to charge the participants directly for a class, allowing you to earn more income per class.

One challenge associated with small studios is a limited class schedule. This can make it difficult to obtain classes. Branded studios sometimes have very rigid class expectations and policies that make it challenging to be creative in class. Unbranded studios rely heavily on instructors' creativity, knowledge, and personality to draw participants into their classes (and keep them coming back), which can be challenging when an instructor is starting out and may not have the confidence and community that an experienced instructor might have.

Boutiques and small studios are looking for instructors to promote their brand and/or drive people into classes. Group fitness classes are what bring most of the revenue to their businesses, so those businesses seek instructors to promote classes and brand themselves in the best interest of the studio. They expect their instructors to always have current credentials and act in a professional manner.

Other Group Fitness Venues

Outside of the traditional facilities, a number of additional opportunities are available for instructors to pursue. Hotels and resorts often have fitness centers that offer group fitness classes. Facilities such as these may offer vacation teaching, where instructors receive a complimentary (or discounted) rate for accommodations at the resort in exchange for teaching scheduled classes offered to their guests. Apartment fitness centers, homeowners associations, and country clubs may offer opportunities to teach classes as well. Athleticwear stores, sporting goods stores, and shopping centers may have events in which local instructors are asked to teach classes. Corporate fitness companies may hire Group Fitness Instructors to teach classes for corporate wellness programs.

Lesson 2: Personal Branding and Customer Service

Personal Branding

As a Group Fitness Instructor, it is typical to teach at multiple venues. Understanding personal branding and implementing a strategy to market what you offer provides additional teaching and networking opportunities. How you present yourself to the public is important to your work with employment venues, as a freelancer, or as a business owner. A strong personal brand creates loyalty and trust with class participants, and they will be a continuous source of support throughout your career.

What Is Personal Branding?

PERSONAL BRANDING is the outward display of your vision, values, talents, expertise, and beliefs. It is the actions taken with a conscious effort to communicate who you are and your purpose to your audience. This includes interactions you have outside of class, during class, and on social media.

PERSONAL BRANDING

Efforts made through interpersonal interaction and online presentation that communicate your vision, values, talents, expertise, and beliefs.

Cultivating a personal brand is important because it can create a bridge between you and your participants. This gives your participants a clear idea of your purpose, who you are, and what you are an expert in. It provides an additional point of alignment between you and your participants beyond the context of the studio. If your personal brand is authentic to who you are, it creates trust with your audience and gives them a depth of knowledge about you that makes them feel like they know you personally. Personal branding can raise your position as an expert in your field and expand your reach to more people.

© ImageFlow/Shutterstock

Establishing Your Brand and Philosophy

Establishing your brand starts with having base knowledge (credentials and education) and a skill set (the ability to present group fitness classes). From this point on, as an instructor, you will need to self-assess what you are doing, why you are doing it, and for whom. Once you perform this self-assessment, you can create and implement a plan for personal branding.

Completing a self-assessment can assist you in making decisions about your career that are authentic to who you are. Authenticity is being true to who you are in all aspects of your life, including teaching group fitness. It is allowing your genuine self to show so your participants can connect with the real you. You can show your authentic self through the formats you are teaching by focusing on what you love to teach. You can also convey authenticity in how you deliver workouts, by adding education, different styles of coaching, or humor. It will show in the way you personally connect with your participants one-on-one by building relationships. Remaining authentic in your role as a Group Fitness Instructor will create trust with your participants because they will really know you.

In the beginning stages of a Group Fitness Instructor's career, it is not uncommon to have the desire to teach every format and engage with every type of participant. This is even more true when working in a facility that offers many classes and has the expectation that instructors will teach as many different formats as possible. It is not sustainable to teach every format and to all audiences for an entire career, nor is it feasible to become an expert or authority in every area of group fitness. Pressure to do it all can come from the fear of missing out, your employer, or participants. Trying to be everything for everyone can take the joy out of teaching and creates an unclear or unfocused personal brand. As an instructor, you will never be able to make everyone happy or reach every single person. However, defining your personal brand, and having your professional interests guide you, will develop your **NICHE**.

If you have conducted a personal branding self-assessment (**Table 3.1**), you will notice that some themes are connected. For example, if you love group fitness because of the intense

NICHE

A specific area of expertise that is focused for a specific audience.

TABLE 3.1 Personal Branding Self-Assessment

Answer these questions to start defining your personal brand:

1. What made you decide to become a Group Fitness Instructor?
2. What are your goals as a Group Fitness Instructor?
3. What area(s) of group fitness do you feel most confident in?
4. What area or format makes you the happiest?
5. What differentiates you from other Group Fitness Instructors?
6. Who are you trying to reach (can include in person and virtually)?

workouts and the high energy that comes from everyone in the room, you would be interested in formats and groups of people that support that type of experience, such as high-intensity interval training (HIIT), interval, or indoor cycling classes. Teaching these types of classes and focusing your brand to attract these types of people would feel more authentic and natural. In contrast, teaching a yin yoga class to older adults would not feel aligned with your brand.

Aligning Your Presentation with Your Brand

As you gain experience teaching, your personal brand will develop. Over time, your brand will align with how you present yourself in classes. At the beginning of your teaching career, the focus is on teaching safely and efficiently. Once you feel confident in that, consider evaluating your teaching style and look for ways to strengthen your personal brand and your connection with your participants. For example, if you love learning the *how* and *why* behind exercises, start scripting educational nuggets to share during the workout. Being prepared and finding opportunities to interject elements of your personal brand is going to help your participants see what you have to offer.

Personal Branding and Your Employer

As a new Group Fitness Instructor, look for any opportunity to gain experience from your employer. As you start to polish who you are as an instructor, it becomes more important to find employers that fit your brand or to evaluate if your personal brand is in alignment with your current employer's. Ideally, your vision for your teaching style will fall in line with the vision your employer has for their facility. If your brands align, their target audience will reach the people in your target audience. If your brand and your employer's do not align, it can create challenges in building the audience that you can best serve.

Marketing and Presenting Your Brand

Once you start to understand the components and nuances that make up your personal brand, the next step is communicating with and marketing to your current and target audiences. Many opportunities are available for you to present and market yourself in person and online. Creating a consistent marketing plan is key for this communication. The plan does not have to be complex, but it does need to stay consistent with timing and messaging.

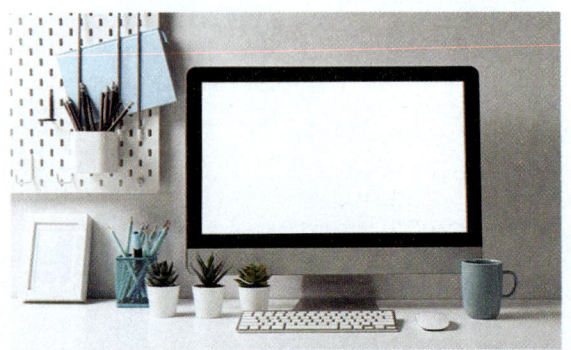

Know Your Audience

To effectively communicate and market your brand, you need to know your audience. Your audience will be made up of the people who enjoy or connect with your expertise, personality, and/or values. Understanding these three components, as well as the demographics of the participants in your class, will reveal the type of people who you are trying to reach. Your format may help you to learn more about your audience as well.

One of the best ways to understand your audience is to connect with them one-on-one. Taking some time before and after class to

INSTRUCTOR TIP

When trying to learn about your audience, ask yourself these questions:

1. Who would benefit from my expertise?
2. What personality type enjoys my class format?
3. What motivates the people in my class?
4. Who are the people in my area that come to my classes?
5. What questions do your participants ask you before and after class?

talk to your participants can offer insight as to why they are attending your classes and how you can serve them better with your brand. Do not be afraid to ask for feedback as well. It could alert you to an area in which you might expand.

INSTRUCTOR TIP

Asking for feedback from participants is a useful tool to help you learn how you can connect with and serve your participants better. Often, if you ask your participants to give you honest feedback in class, they will tell you what they love about class, but they might not mention things that they worry will insult your teaching. Here are a few ways to get honest feedback from your participants:

- Ask a participant that you know will not have a problem providing critical feedback. As you start to build relationships with your participants, you will have some that you know will be honest with you.
- Create a way for participants to give you anonymous feedback. Have comment cards that they can leave at the front desk or in a box by the door of the studio.
- Create a survey either on paper or online with prompts, such as what they like about your class or what they feel might be missing from your class.

Once you receive the feedback, review it, and see if there are areas where you can improve. Your participants will appreciate the effort and notice when you make a change based on their feedback.

Potential Employers

Having a developed brand (and knowing how to market it) can be appealing to the right employer. It shows that you take the initiative and have a full understanding of what you are delivering in and out of the studio. Building your own strong brand will also add value to your employer's presence in the marketplace, cultivating credibility for everyone involved. Being clear about who you are will also eliminate any employment opportunities that are not a right fit for you.

Potential Clients

Knowing how to market yourself through your brand can build trust between you and your audience. Once you have their trust, they will be eager to not only participate in classes but also follow you should you decide to change locations. You can earn this trust by continuously giving valuable information and content through your branding while expecting nothing in return. If potential clients witness this and feel a connection with your brand, you will have created rapport, even without having met them personally. Positioning yourself as an expert demonstrates to potential clients a reason to work with you. Sharing your knowledge freely by creating content to educate your audience is an effective way to demonstrate your expertise.

Customer Service Strategies

Building your personal brand is about creating credibility and building relationships. Begin with serving your customers. Anyone can deliver a great class, but service is what keeps participants engaged and willing to follow you from class to class over the course of an entire career. This starts in every class by building out a thoughtful, well-planned, scripted experience. Being prepared and putting in the time to offer the best workout experience possible can elevate you from being a great instructor to an exceptional one. Add in being available for your participants, learning names, building personal relationships, and using inspiring moments when possible. This is the difference between exceptional and extraordinary. Consider including the following strategies:

- Create special workouts to celebrate holidays or events.
- Organize events outside of the class.
- Set up the necessary equipment before class.
- Provide useful education for your participants.
- Build a community within your class between members.

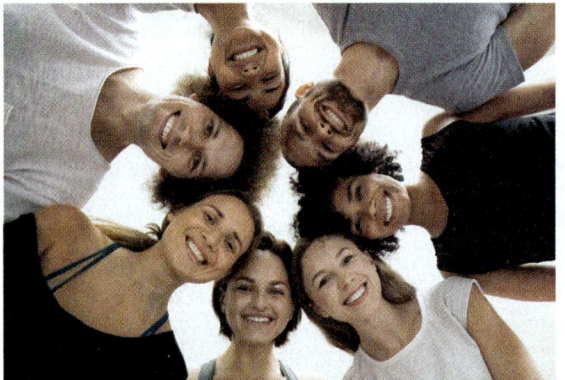

© Fizkes/Shutterstock

These customer service strategies keep your participants loyal to you no matter where you go and can help your employer retain members, making you an even more valuable part of their team. If you have created a community within your classes, your presence at a facility will have a monetary value that your employer may recognize, especially if they are using group fitness as a retention tool. Understanding the value of your brand and communicating it can be an attractive trait to many employers.

Social Media

Having a social media presence that fully displays your personal brand offers a number of benefits. The primary benefit is that it can increase the number of people who follow you as an instructor. In addition, many facilities highly encourage or require the use of social media as part of employment. Understanding how to brand yourself using social media can expand your reach to more people and create opportunities to offer classes on your own either in person or in a virtual setting.

As you build your social media presence, consider what will serve your group fitness career. Understand what the purpose of social media is for your brand and business. Note that there is a difference between a personal social media account and a branded or professional one. If you have a personal social media account, you should consider having a separate account for your brand or business. Of course, there will be some overlap because your personal audience will likely want to support your brand, but it may show deference if you have a private account for your personal audience and a public account for your professional one. If you decide to split

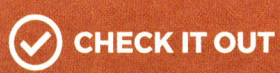

Using Different Posting Mediums

When creating social media posts, how you use images, video, and text matters and can help better express your idea(s). Using images, video, text, or a combination of these can increase the impact of your post if used correctly. Consider the following tips for how to use different elements for your social media posts:

- Images are great for grabbing a person's attention as well as showing something that happens in a single moment. Use images to tell your audience something important, encourage interactions on social media, or display a comparison (such as a before/after image).
- Video is great for expressing more complex ideas fast. Use this method to demonstrate movements, explain a new technique, or create excitement.
- Text is great for exploring ideas or asking your audience to participate in some way. Use text to elaborate on a subject your audience has been asking about. You can also invite your audience to a class, inform them of a sub, or capture information as to what they want to see more of.
- Infographics can be a great bridge between images and text by delivering information in quick and memorable snapshots. Use infographics for tips or quick recommendations.

your accounts, your professional account should include content that will benefit your professional audience, such as:

- Educational topics related to fitness or attending classes, which might include form and technique, types of classes and their benefits, and different types of training and their benefits
- Recommendations for items that relate to group fitness or working out, such as athleticwear, shoes, or music
- Entertainment that relates to group fitness such as behind-the-scenes content, funny things that happen in class, or fun things that you do (remember to ask for permission whenever posting content that involves a participant)
- Inspirational and motivational posts related to fitness, health, and wellness

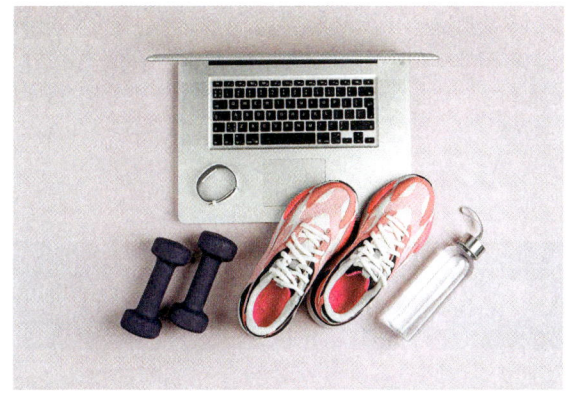

© Igisheva Maria/Shutterstock

If you decide to manage an account that includes both personal and professional content, it is best to stay away from topics that are controversial or that are overly personal. These types of topics can alienate members of your audience and cause arguments not only with your audience but among them. Such conflicts can take away from the brand you are trying to portray. Know that your participants and employers will be looking for you on social media, so you need to plan how you present yourself. Your social media content could play a large role in attracting potential job opportunities (or keeping the ones you have). It is important to be mindful of what you wish to represent.

Building your brand on social media allows you to create valuable content for your followers. They are looking for education, tips, information about you, and a peek behind the scenes. Building a social media following that will help to build your brand can be simple but it should be consistent, just like creating your personal brand. See **Table 3.2** for common and useful content categories. Using the insights from creating your personal brand, you can build a social media plan that will attract your people to you.

TABLE 3.2 Social Media Content Categories

Category	Content
Instructor life	Talk about your life as an instructor
Community	Anything that includes your participants or community
FITSPO	Fitness + Inspiration = FITSPO
Behind the scenes	Anything that is interesting about prepping for classes that your audience might not know
General fitness tips or education	Any fitness tips that could be helpful
Transformation	Participant transformations (not restricted to just the physical)
Format insights or tips	Anything related to your format
Shareable	Anything where you might ask your followers to help you out and share their thoughts in the comments
Call to action	Invite people to your class
Your interests	A personal post so your followers can connect with you as a person (keep it noncontroversial)

🤖 GETTING TECHNICAL

Building a social media plan can be intimidating, especially with regard to thinking about what you should post. Breaking down your personal brand can give you a blueprint of ideas to choose from. If you build out your topics this way, you can cycle through them as your social media plan.

Using a color-coded calendar to break down the components of your personal brand, color-code your weekly posting plan based on the topics.

Here is an example of a week of posts:

Monday—*Transformation:* Share a story about a participant who has experienced a positive change from group fitness. Detail their journey and how group fitness played a role in that journey. (Remember to always get permission from participants before posting information about them.)

Tuesday—*General Fitness Tip:* Share the benefits of rest and recovery in a training plan in an infographic or in the text of a post.

Wednesday—*Your Interests:* Share a "get to know me" post and include five fun facts about you that your participants might find interesting.

Thursday—*Behind-the-Scenes:* Share an image of how you collaborate with other instructors, perhaps a practice session or sharing music or exercise ideas.

Friday—*Call to Action:* Share an image or video of your class and invite your audience to attend a class on the weekend.

Saturday—*Community:* Share an image or video of you and your participants after class.

Sunday—*Instructor Life:* Share about how you rest when you are not teaching classes.

Lesson 3: Self-Care and Continued Development

Self-Care

A career in group fitness is physically demanding and places a large amount of stress on the body, especially over time. As a Group Fitness Instructor, practicing self-care from the beginning of your career can extend its longevity and help reduce chronic injuries. In addition to being physically stressful, teaching can require a lot of emotional energy. It is just as important to take care of yourself emotionally as it is physically.

Protecting Your Voice

Whether you are participating in the entire class or only coaching throughout, your voice will be one of the main tools you use for class. Studies have shown that over 50% of Group Fitness Instructors report vocal problems over their career and less than 40% report receiving any guidance in vocal care (Fontan et al., 2017). Overuse of your voice may create strain and long-lasting injuries. Chronic laryngitis and vocal nodules are the most common complaints (Fontan et al., 2017). Treatment is available for vocal distress, but proper prevention will reduce the risk of injury.

Some techniques for protecting your voice include the following:

- Use a microphone correctly and ideally every time you teach.
- Use visual or nonverbal cues whenever possible.
- Do a vocal warm-up.
- Keep your vocal cords hydrated by drinking water before and during class.
- Do not teach when sick.
- Schedule time in between classes rather than teaching back-to-back classes, if feasible.
- Protect your voice outside of class by minimizing shouting and allowing your voice to rest when possible.

Managing Overtraining

Teaching group fitness classes is physical work no matter how fit you are. Although you should not view your class as your own workout, you should be mindful of how many classes you are teaching and the intensity of movement you endure over your weekly class schedule. It is not uncommon for a full-time instructor to teach 15 or more classes per week. If you are teaching more than 15 classes per week, participating for the entire class could lead to **OVERTRAINING**. Balancing movement demonstration, coaching (verbal and nonverbal), and form correction will allow you to teach at a higher volume while still protecting your body.

Increasing Resistance to Injury

Although not every type of injury is preventable, optimizing your resistance to injury relies heavily on applying knowledge of common misalignments, overactive and underactive muscles, and prevention through proper technique and recovery inside and outside of class. Taking extra time to evaluate your own form in a mirror, with a fellow instructor, or recording a video of yourself, will help you address any misalignments that could lead to injury. Consider resting

OVERTRAINING

Condition in which the individual trains too much, which results in a decrease in function and performance.

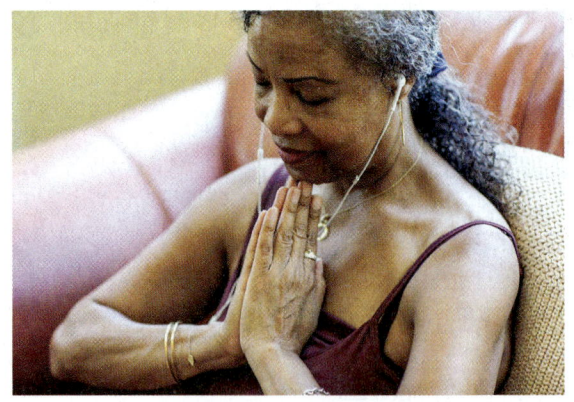

© Deborah Kolb/Shutterstock

when scheduling your classes and training so your body has adequate time to recover between workouts. This will not only help you perform better but also reduce the risk of improper form due to fatigue.

Preventing Burnout

Teaching group fitness classes can be an incredibly fulfilling career, especially when you are able to experience the changes in your participants. However, instructors are not immune to physical, mental, and emotional burnout. Constantly moving, motivating, and maintaining the energy that motivates your audience, regardless of what is happening in your personal life, can eventually wear you out. Being able to recognize the signs of burnout will signal you to step back and rest so you can continue doing what you love. Most instructors experience burnout at one time or another over the course of their career, especially in the case that it is a long one.

EMOTIONAL BURNOUT

Emotional burnout can be brought on by prolonged periods of stress and can be associated with depression and anxiety. It can also cause a person to withdraw, especially in their work environment (Koutsimani et al., 2019). Signs of emotional burnout can include feelings of being overwhelmed, helplessness, decreased motivation, and loss of joy in teaching. If these feelings arise, it is important to discuss them with your employer and ask if there are options for taking some time to rest and focus on sleep and recovery. Look for inspiration in a new format or another instructor's class. Lean on your support systems such as your family, friends, and fellow instructors; they have most likely experienced similar feelings. Protecting your mental and emotional health can help in ensuring longevity and the love you have for your career.

PHYSICAL BURNOUT

Physical burnout can be associated with emotional burnout, but it can also result from overtraining or teaching too many classes without adequate rest. Instructors often teach multiple classes per week and then perform additional training outside of class, which can lead to a high risk for overtraining syndrome. Recognizing the signs of physical burnout is critical to addressing it. Signs of overtraining include increased muscle soreness, decreased performance, sleep troubles, constant fatigue, and decreased ability to fight off illness (Roy, 2015). Should these symptoms arise, discuss them with your doctor and explore options for taking some time to rest with your employer.

The following are some ways to prevent overtraining:

- Be mindful of how your body is feeling and take extra recovery time if needed.
- Use **PERIODIZATION** in your classes and in your personal workout plan.
- Stay hydrated and fuel your body based on the volume of your training.
- Focus on getting good sleep (7 or more hours per night).

PERIODIZATION

Division of a training program into smaller progressive steps with built-in recovery phases.

Hydration and Pre- and Post-Workout Nutrition for Instructors

Hydration is a key factor in performance for anyone engaging in physical activity. A decrease in exercise performance and endurance can occur with a loss of just 2–3% of a person's total mass in water (Kraft et al., 2012). However, simply drinking a large amount of water before teaching a class is not going to help an instructor stay hydrated. Focus on staying consistently hydrated, consuming 14–20 ounces of water 2 hours before teaching and another 16 ounces after class. Additionally, instructors should drink 16–24 ounces for every pound lost during exercise (Roy, 2013).

As a Group Fitness Instructor, it is important to consider nutrition for optimal performance in class. Eating a pre-exercise meal higher in carbohydrates, moderate lean protein, and low in fat 3–4 hours before class will supply optimal energy with enough time to digest properly. If that timing does not work for your schedule or you are teaching an early morning class, consider eating a small meal or snack higher in carbohydrates so your stomach is not so full. This will give you the energy you need for class. Post-exercise fuel is just as important. Consuming a meal 30–45 minutes after exercise that is a 3:1 ratio of carbs to protein can reduce muscle breakdown, replenish glycogen stores, and rebuild muscle (American Dietetic Association et al., 2009).

Continuing Education: Development Beyond the Credential

Completing your credential is the first step on your journey to becoming a Group Fitness Instructor. However, education does not stop there. As exercise science, fitness trends, and teaching methods continue to evolve, it is important to continue learning through your entire career. Continuing your education keeps you relevant as an instructor and helps keep you engaged. Additionally, most credentialing associations require an instructor to participate in regular continuing education to remain certified.

Recertification/Renewal

RECERTIFICATION/RENEWAL ensures that instructors stay current with improvements and changes in the fitness industry. AFAA requires instructors to seek out education in the form of workshops, education courses, and format specializations every 2 years by submitting proof of completion. This will keep your AFAA credential current and promotes a habit of continued learning. The benefits, however, go beyond staying current. Your credential maintains your relevance in an industry that is highly competitive and always changing. Being up-to-date with your knowledge and skill set allows you to better serve your participants. Keeping your credential current also ensures that you are providing current evidence-based practices that will help your participants gain the greatest benefits from their workouts.

> **RECERTIFICATION/RENEWAL**
>
> Continuing group fitness education to remain in good standing as an AFAA instructor.

Continuing to learn will only sharpen your skills and help to refine your personal brand even more. AFAA offers additional education that furthers your expertise and can be applied to continuing education requirements. Additionally, many major group fitness brands offer education and/or industry conferences.

Teacher Training

Instructor training is designed with the objective of fine-tuning existing teaching skills. You can look for available training courses offered by your facility or research other respected group fitness brands offering training courses/workshops at different locations. These courses

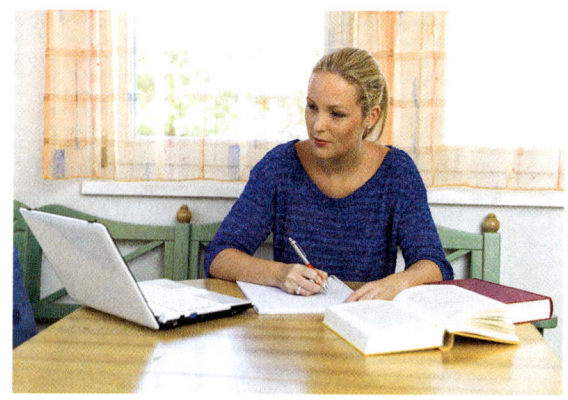
© Lisa-S/Shutterstock

usually include a combined exploration of coaching, motivation, and improved class planning. By helping you develop well-rounded skills, they can provide a more holistic approach to how you teach your class. Additionally, they offer opportunities to learn alongside other instructors and to develop networking and professional relationships. Valuable best practices are often provided around how to design and sequence your class, select music, promote participant engagement, and create effective class objectives. Attending a teacher training can elevate the experiences that you provide to your participants.

Conferences

Group fitness conferences are another way to accrue continuing education credits, and they can be lots of fun. Instructors from all over the world gather to learn immediately actionable concepts and new innovations in the industry. Conferences provide opportunities to network with peers while providing a variety of training options offered by a variety of experts in group fitness. This is a great time to explore other specialties if anything outside your current class schedule piques your interest. Asking peers or your group fitness manager for recommendations can help identify a conference that is the right personal fit. Additionally, search large industry brands online to find events they host or participate in.

Specializations

Group fitness specializations provide a chance to hone skills in specific group fitness formats or brands. The Group Fitness Instructor (GFI) credential is intentionally designed to give a broad scope of group fitness. However, attending specialization workshops to focus on technique, exercise selection, coaching, and authenticity for a particular format will only elevate your knowledge. These workshops are designed to provide in-depth knowledge of unique and specific formats to enable you to lead your class as an expert. AFAA offers a range of different specializations that will also offer usable continuing education credits. Discussing specializations with your group fitness manager or researching industry leaders in your desired format can also help you find specialized instructor training courses.

SUMMARY

When you are ready to start teaching, understanding the different class settings can help you thrive in an environment that best suits your career needs. If you know what to look for, and what your personal needs are, different employment venues will provide support, creative freedom, education, and/or communities that fit those needs. Once you have gained teaching experience, you can then apply the concepts of personal branding to further your career or branch out on your own. Regardless of your employment venue, continuous learning and specialization will make you a valuable and trusted resource to your participants and an asset to your employers. Additionally, applying the concepts of instructor self-care can help you have a long career in the group fitness industry.

REFERENCES

American Dietetic Association, Dietitians of Canada, & American College of Sports Medicine. (2009). Nutrition and athletic performance. *Medicine & Science in Sports & Exercise, 41*(3), 709–731. https://doi.org/10.1249/MSS.0b013e31890eb86

Fontan, L., Fraval, M., Michon, A., Déjean, S., & Welby-Gieusse, M. (2017). Vocal problems in sports and fitness instructors: A study of prevalence, risk factors, and need for prevention in France. *Journal of Voice, 31*(2), 261.e33–261.e38. https://doi.org/10.1016/j.jvoice.2016.04.014

Koutsimani, P., Montgomery, A., & Georganta, K. (2019). The relationship between burnout, depression, and anxiety: A systematic review and meta-analysis. *Frontiers in Psychology, 10*, 284. https://doi.org/10.3389/fpsyg.2019.00284

Kraft, J. A., Green, J. M., Bishop, P. A., Richardson, M. T., Neggers, Y. H., & Leeper, J. D. (2012). The influence of hydration on anaerobic performance: A review. *Research Quarterly for Exercise and Sport, 83*(2), 282–292. https://doi.org/10.1080/02701367.2012.10599859

Roy, B. A. (2013). Exercise and fluid replacement. *ACSM's Health & Fitness Journal, 17*(4), 3. https://doi.org/10.1249/FIT.0b013e318296bc4b

Roy, B. A. (2015). Overreaching/overtraining: More is not always better. *ACSM's Health & Fitness Journal, 19*(2), 4–5. https://doi.org/10.1249/FIT.0000000000000100

CHAPTER 4

LEGAL AND ETHICAL RESPONSIBILITIES

LEARNING OBJECTIVES

The intent of this chapter is to identify your scope of practice as a Group Fitness Instructor and to ensure that you stay within your legal and ethical boundaries as a fitness professional, both in person and virtually. It will provide information about safety responsibilities, emergency protocols, insurance considerations, and music licensing.

After reading this content, students should be able to demonstrate the following objectives:

- **Define** *scope of practice* for the Group Fitness Instructor.

- **Describe** legal and ethical responsibilities and practices for Group Fitness Instructors.

- **Identify** safety considerations and emergency response protocols for Group Fitness Instructors.

- **Explain** considerations for professional behaviors in a virtual space.

Lesson 1: Scope of Practice

Introduction

Whether you are employed with a specific organization or fitness facility or self-employed as a fitness professional, the way you carry yourself, conduct yourself, and relate to others has an enormous influence on the relationships you will build with participants, employers, peers, and coworkers. Professionalism starts with practicing basic principles of customer service, including arriving on time; communicating in a friendly, professional manner; and setting appropriate boundaries for contact with others in your place of work. As with any job that involves frequent and direct interaction with the public, instructors must be aware of the influence their attitudes, behaviors, and communication styles can have. To earn respect and trust, as well as to maintain the integrity of the profession, instructors should strive to act responsibly and professionally at

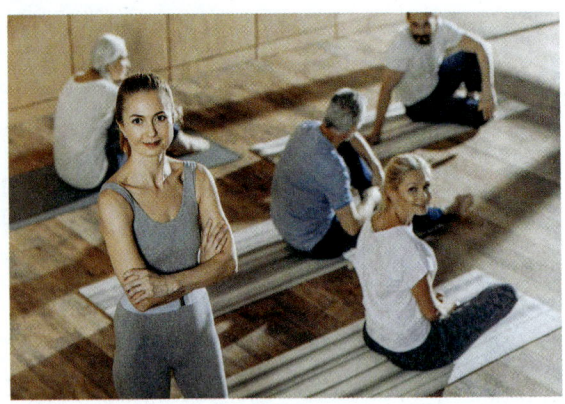

© LightField Studios/Shutterstock

all times. As such, it is important to understand the factors that can influence the impression you will leave on your participants as well as your ethical and legal responsibilities as a Group Fitness Instructor.

Scope of Practice and Professional Limitations

Health professionals in all settings—from hospitals to rehabilitation centers, to clinics and fitness facilities—focus on one area of practice and work within guidelines and expectations that have been standardized and legally defined by national and state agencies.

In the group fitness setting, scope of practice refers to what an instructor can legally and ethically do in their professional practice. It includes the knowledge, skills, abilities, processes, services, and limitations for which an instructor should be held accountable. It helps instructors know where their responsibilities begin and end. For this reason, AFAA has defined the tasks and responsibilities that make up a Group Fitness Instructor's scope of practice:

- Prepare and deliver evidence-based exercise content for groups of individuals with varying fitness needs and capabilities.
- Dynamically react to group or individual needs by providing modifications and alternatives based on fitness level and ability.
- Lead participants with energy, enthusiasm, and optimism to create positive associations with exercise.
- Understand how to use various types of fitness equipment, particularly equipment relevant to the specific format being taught.
- Be able to work independently and require minimal supervision.
- Maintain CPR/AED certification to properly respond to emergencies that may occur before, during, or after class.
- Answer questions related to the workout, such as how to do specific moves, why they are beneficial, or how one might modify or progress movements.
- Avoid one-on-one recommendations regarding health conditions, injuries, nutrition, and remedies for pain. However, pre-class assessments of participants (including observational, postural, and movement assessments) are appropriate for recommending modifications to class movements.
- Refer personal health questions to appropriate health professionals.

The fitness professional's standard can be summarized as: All questions outside of the Group Fitness Instructor's scope of practice should be referred to qualified professionals with appropriate training.

When teaching, instructors must demonstrate sufficient knowledge of exercise science and an ability to provide safe and progressive exercise programming (Abbott, 2012). Participants expect that their workouts will bring about positive change and that their instructors have a sufficient grasp of anatomy, physiology, and exercise science to ensure safe and effective workouts (Abbott, 2012). Given that assumption, participants may also presume Group Fitness Instructors have more in-depth medical knowledge or credentials than they do and thus may pose questions instructors are neither qualified nor licensed to answer.

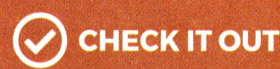

Group Fitness and Personal Training

An instructor does not know each participant's health history or goals. They simply know that a participant attends a certain class in order to experience the stated objective of the class (as indicated by class title, description, and content).

A Personal Trainer is trained and qualified to work with individuals. They collect relevant personal health information, exercise history, and detailed client goals and develop personalized (often long-term) programs to help clients achieve their health and fitness objectives.

An instructor who is asked to provide individualized programs in order to achieve specific fitness goals should refer those individuals to a credentialed Personal Trainer. It is advisable that Personal Trainers and Group Fitness Instructors communicate with each other when an exerciser is both a training client and class participant. Individual and group exercise can complement and support each other as the client works toward their goals. Likewise, it is also important that the exerciser is not overtraining.

Scope of practice refers to the limitations imposed by law on different vocational pursuits—pursuits that require specific education, experience, or skills, as well as demonstrated competency. Scope of practice is used by national and state licensing boards, as well as various professions, to determine the procedures, actions, or processes permitted by a licensee or practitioner (Abbott, 2012). When an individual who is not licensed engages in the practices of a licensed profession, they are violating the scope of practice. Simply put, this means an instructor must understand what they are and are not qualified to do or say when working with participants; operating outside of those boundaries can constitute a violation of the law.

Instructors must be especially cautious to not go beyond the scope of practice in areas such as postural assessment, diagnosis or treatment of an injury, nutritional recommendations, and psychological advice (Abbott, 2012). The instructor should develop a network of trusted, qualified healthcare providers and refer clients to them accordingly.

Diagnosing and Prescribing

Diagnosing involves a comprehensive review and understanding of an individual's health history, current medical conditions, current symptoms, and then—after a complete review—determining a specific condition or disease. Prescribing involves providing specific treatment plans in the form of exercise, dietary counseling, nutritional supplementation, meal planning, home remedies, therapeutic aids, or prescription drugs in order to treat a certain condition or disease.

Group Fitness Instructors should politely refer participants to other appropriate licensed professionals for questions such as (but not limited to) the following:

- "I'm experiencing knee pain. Can you tell me what it is?"
- "I have high blood pressure and high cholesterol—what's the best workout program for me?"

However, Group Fitness Instructors should be ready and willing to answer questions about the workout or class being taught. The following types of questions are within the scope of practice of a Group Fitness Instructor:

- How to perform movement patterns: "Hey, can you show me again how to do that squat exercise?"
- How to modify movement patterns: "My knees are uncomfortable when I squat. How can I modify them?"

> ### ⚠ CRITICAL
>
> Under no circumstances is it appropriate for a Group Fitness Instructor to diagnose health conditions or prescribe treatments for individuals. This includes exercises, diets, or supplements to treat health conditions.

NUTRITION

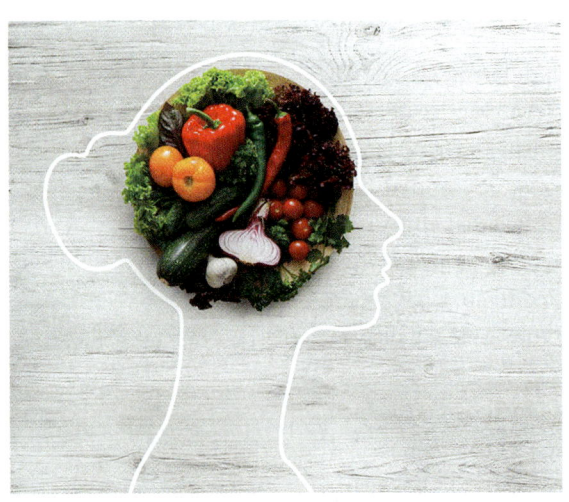

© Prostock-studio/Shutterstock

Nutrition is founded in disciplines such as biochemistry, physiology, psychology, and food science. Research is sometimes misinterpreted, leading to confusion and misinformation. It is important to rely on licensed professionals, such as registered dietitians, to interpret the science. In most states, only licensed or registered dietitians can provide nutritional counseling and diet prescription. Participants might ask questions about the latest nutritional trends, so it is critical for instructors to stay current but within their scope of practice. Additionally, networking and maintaining relationships with registered dietitians will ensure a go-to source when making referrals. In general, Group Fitness Instructors should avoid making specific nutritional recommendations to participants, especially in relation to health conditions (e.g., diabetes).

Referring Participants

When participants ask questions or make requests that fall outside the scope of practice for a Group Fitness Instructor, it is important to direct participants to other professionals or organizations that may be able to help. The following are some examples:

- If participants are asking questions about a personalized training program, they should be referred to a National Academy of Sports Medicine (NASM) Personal Trainer.
- If participants are asking health- or disease-related questions, they should be referred to their medical doctor for clearance and specific recommendations.
- If participants are asking questions about pain during movement, they can be referred to a physical therapist or medical doctor.
- If participants are asking about other training modalities for which the current instructor is not qualified, they should be referred to certified or trained instructors in that **MODALITY**, such as kettlebells or yoga.

MODALITY

Form or mode of exercise that presents a specific stress to the body.

Referring a participant to another expert is not a sign an instructor is uneducated or unqualified in their area of study. In fact, knowing when and who to refer participants to is a sign of proper education, confidence, and loyalty to your practice, as well as a sign of respect for the participant's time, money, and personal health.

Lesson 2: Legal and Ethical Responsibilities

Legal Responsibilities

Exercise programs, by nature, can result in injuries, from minor incidents to life-threatening events. The Group Fitness Instructor must not only have a working knowledge of legal and risk management concepts, but must also adhere to ethical practices to avoid legal consequences (Eickhoff-Shemek, 2013).

In addition to operating within the scope of practice, instructors should also be aware of other legal liability exposures and risk management strategies. Incidents or injuries due to negligence (carelessness) can result in costly litigation for both the facility and the instructor (Eickhoff-Shemek, 2013).

These claims may include the following:

- Failing to provide a qualified instructor with sufficient knowledge, training, and experience to safely instruct participants
- Failing to supervise or improperly instruct a participant
- Failing to have or to properly execute a written emergency plan and procedure

Risk management strategies for the Group Fitness Instructor include the following (Eickhoff-Shemek, 2013):

- Maintaining current Group Fitness Instructor and CPR/AED certification at all times
- Adhering to industry standards and guidelines for safety and efficacy when teaching group exercise
- Obtaining necessary training for all formats instructed and equipment used
- Operating within scope of practice
- Understanding and being able to execute emergency action plans
- Being familiar with and acting within all facility policies and procedures
- Completing incident reports properly and in a timely manner

Insurance

Group Fitness Instructors must be familiar with liability insurance and maintain those requirements as well as participant liability waivers to minimize risk for themselves and the organization. There are two types of liability insurance: general liability and professional liability. General liability insurance protects the insured from ordinary negligence (Eickhoff-Shemek, 2003). This refers to public liability and, in the case of a fitness facility, covers the premises and all equipment therein (Riley, 2005). Professional liability insurance covers professional negligence, which may be cited when a participant sustains a loss as a result of an instructor's negligent actions or behaviors (such as unsafe exercise or equipment misuse) (Riley, 2005). Professional liability insurance is recommended for all fitness professionals (Riley, 2005).

The instructor can minimize risk by practicing common sense when dealing with participants, watching for potential problems, and making corrections before an accident happens. If an injury or incident should occur, the actions of the instructor immediately following can go a long way to mitigate the risk of negligence; it is important to promptly contact emergency or medical personnel and take detailed notes to provide to the insurer (Riley, 2005).

INSTRUCTOR TIP

Professional liability insurance can be obtained through a number of credible organizations. Instructors should carefully evaluate their coverage needs and liability risk when determining which type of professional liability insurance to purchase.

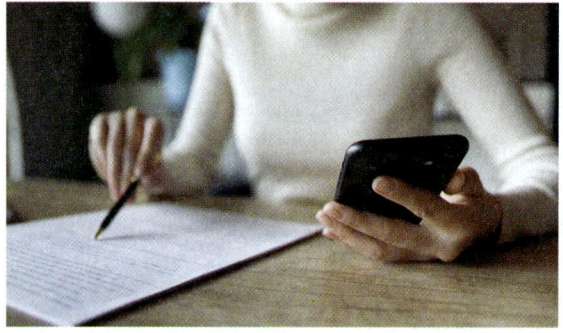

© Fizkes/Shutterstock

Confidentiality

Group Fitness Instructors should always maintain confidentiality and avoid discussing a participant's personal information with others. In the case of health-related matters, sharing personal information could result in liability for both the instructor and the facility. Although Group Fitness Instructors may not keep detailed records of the participants who attend their in-person classes, it is important that you consider carefully before sharing information that might be told in confidence between participant and instructor, employer and employee, or among coworkers with an awareness of the full scope of potential ramifications or loss of trust. Additionally, if you are privy to personal files or information, it is important to maintain that information in a place that is secure and inaccessible to those prohibited from viewing the material. Most organizations will have instructions for standards of practice, but, in lieu of that information, defer to state standards or best practices for record keeping.

⚠ CRITICAL

If you discover or someone discloses information that indicates someone may be at risk for injury, you must immediately report that to the appropriate authorities. You should also report any illegal activities as quickly as possible to both the appropriate authorities and in accordance with your organization's code of conduct.

 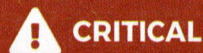

Certification and Credentialing

Throughout the course of their careers, Group Fitness Instructors affect the lives of countless individuals. Participants trust instructors to have the knowledge, skills, and abilities to lead safe, effective workouts. Instructors must strive to provide the best possible information, methodology, and experience to their groups. Obtaining an AFAA credential is a critical first step, but ongoing professional development is equally important to keep pace with changes in the fitness industry as exercise science and technology advance. For career development, an instructor should explore options to gain experience, seek feedback and evaluation, stay current with research and trends, and investigate specializations.

Continued educational development is essential for instructors to provide up-to-date, accurate information and techniques. Numerous resources and organizations are dedicated to providing instructors with the best new research and methods available.

CONTINUING EDUCATION

Continuing education refers to lectures, courses, webinars, and other programs designed to educate individuals and provide additional skills or knowledge. Continuing education may consist of workshops, trainings, assigned readings and quizzes, or online courses presented by an approved continuing education provider. It is important to verify the course has been preapproved or is eligible to be petitioned for credit as not all available continuing education options have been approved by AFAA.

Obtaining a specified number of approved continuing education units is required during each certification period to maintain the credential or as part of recurrent recertification.

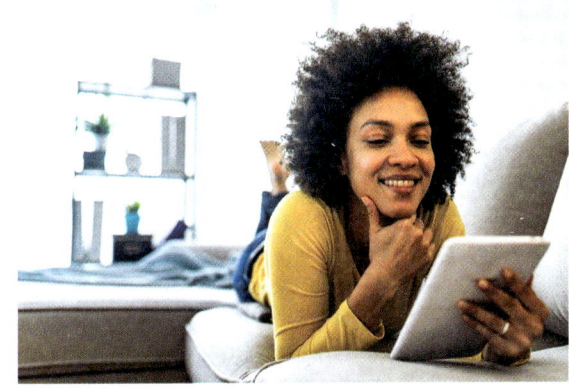

© Dragana Gordic/Shutterstock

 CHECK IT OUT

Regardless of whether an instructor decides to be trained and participate in a format-specific program, maintaining your credential as an AFAA Group Fitness Instructor is important. Most specialty programs do not comprehensively cover the fundamental information provided by the primary certification or credential and, as a result, development, growth, and employment opportunities may be limited if your AFAA credential is not current.

RECERTIFICATION

Recertification or renewal ensures that instructors stay current in information and approach as the industry evolves, preventing the instructor's knowledge and skills from stagnating. When instructors fail to seek new sources of continuing education, they limit their development and do a disservice to their participants, their fellow instructors, and the industry at large. Visit www.AFAA.com and review the information for the most up-to-date requirements and options for recertification.

SPECIALTY COURSES

Because of the intentionally broad focus of the AFAA Group Fitness Instructor program, additional specific training is required to teach popular classes such as indoor cycling, mind–body formats, cardio kickboxing, dance-based formats, water-based formats, and others specific to

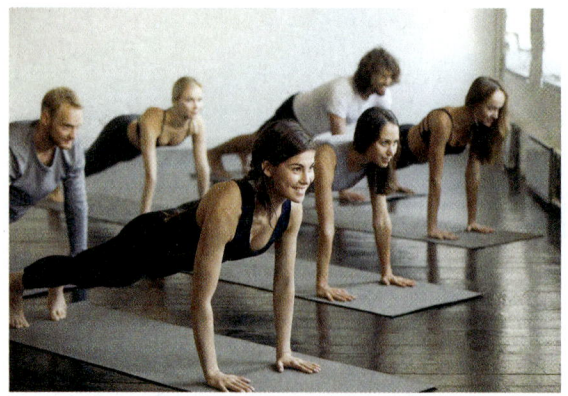
© Fizkes/Shutterstock

various populations such as youth, older adult, or pre- and post-natal fitness. Many different courses and format trainings feature specialized equipment, pre-designed branded formats, or advanced instructor skills. Specialty courses enhance the skills, interests, and abilities of the instructor and also broaden their opportunities for employment.

WORKSHOPS AND LIVE EVENTS

Workshops delivered by a qualified provider can range from a few hours to a few days. Live, multi-day events and conferences offer the opportunity to attend various sessions on a variety of topics and formats from diverse educators. Each can be valuable to the instructor, not only to earn requisite credits to maintain credential or certification status, but also for exposure to new areas of interest and specialization.

✓ CHECK IT OUT

Once you have determined that you are ready to attend a live, multi-session event, here are some tips to help make the most of it:

- **Go with a game plan.** Decide on your primary focus of the conference and use that to guide your session choices.
- **Plan your sessions for success.** Carefully read the session descriptions and the presenters' bios to determine which are most interesting and relevant for your current needs.
- **Do not leave out the lectures.** The information obtained in lectures can often help you to design your own classes more effectively.
- **Consider the keynote.** Often, these are inspiring and influential individuals who provide insight and motivation.
- **Make time for rest.** Try to set aside time to rest before, after, and during the event when possible.

Licensing

Fitness professionals have access to a number of resources that may help increase participant engagement or facilitate in designing or offering specific workouts (such as music tracks, branded formats, and pre-designed workouts). Many of these resources are proprietary (exclusive and copyrighted/trademarked) in nature, and therefore require the health club or fitness professional to license the material. Because licensing varies by material and provider, it is important to understand some general information as well as to defer to the specific licensing organization.

MUSIC

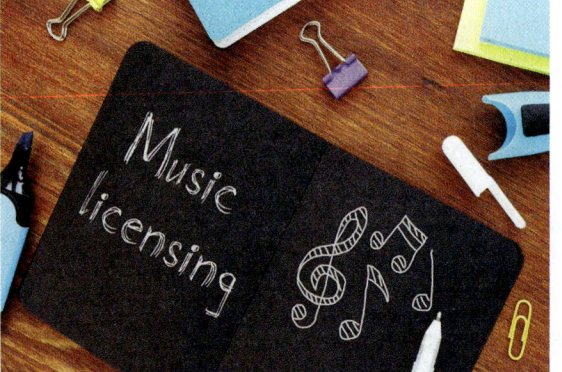
© Jack_the_sparow/Shutterstock

Teaching in a public place in front of groups of people and in a commercial setting requires a commercial music license. For music to be legal, two groups of contributors must be compensated:

- Publishers and songwriters
- Record labels and artists

Both parties contribute to a complete sound recording, but they are separate entities, and each deserves fair compensation. According to the U.S. Copyright Office (2015), publishers and songwriters create and manage the musical compositions and record labels and artists record and provide the sound equipment and vocal talent to make the recordings, and therefore own the actual recording. Legal music pays royalties to both parties.

Group Fitness Instructors who want an easy, legal music option should use music from a fitness music company, as these companies produce and own their own recordings and provide proper master recording licenses for commercial use. You can also defer to your health club or employing fitness organization for any existing contracts they may have.

PROGRAMMING

Branded formats for group fitness offer specific programming that must be licensed in order to make use of and market the provided materials and/or the brand. Some of these organizations provide training for their programs and additional support with their licensing plans. Self-employed Group Fitness Instructors can seek out the education and license as needed. For Group Fitness Instructors who are employed by a health club or boutique, these licenses may have been acquired already. Regardless of the nature of the relationship with the specific licensing brand, it is important to be aware of the licensing status to ensure that you are in compliance.

Ethical Responsibilities

To be in alignment with ethical standards, Group Fitness Instructors commit to always act in the best interest of participants by maintaining the necessary education and knowledge, operating within their scope of practice, and behaving in a consistently positive, constructive, and professional manner (International Dance Exercise Association, 2016).

The following are some of the most important ethical considerations for instructors (International Dance Exercise Association, 2016):

- Prioritize safety.
- Teach class with the best interests of the group in mind, while still acknowledging individual needs.
- Adhere to guidelines for proper music speed and volume.
- Obtain and maintain necessary training and education for all formats instructed.
- Work within your scope of practice.
- Be guided by truth, fairness, and integrity.
- Respect professional boundaries.
- Always uphold a professional image.

Code of Conduct

AFAA Group Fitness Instructors are also expected to adhere to AFAA's Code of Professional Conduct (Appendix), conducting themselves in a manner that merits the respect of the public and other colleagues.

Credible Sources of Information

Credible resources are supported by evidence-based, peer-reviewed research from respected organizations, groups, and individuals. When evaluating new information, instructors should consider the source and context before using it to influence their class design or cues (Infographic 4.1). When in doubt, seek out established industry associations and businesses and the works of the groups and individuals who contribute to them.

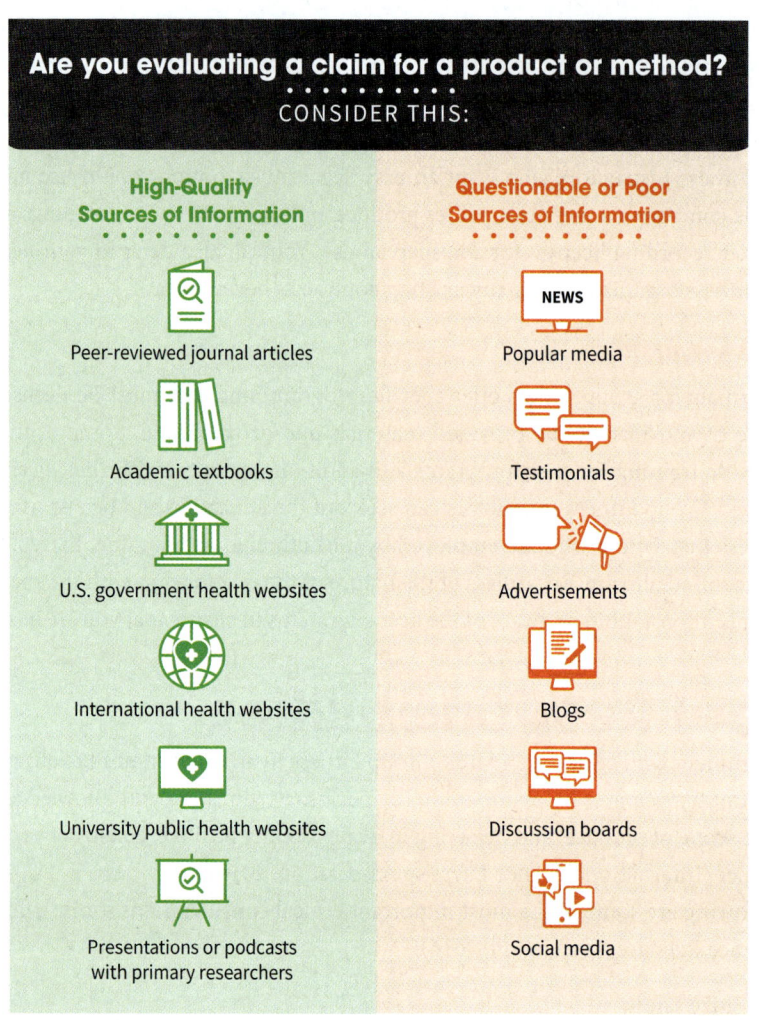

Are you evaluating a claim for a product or method?
CONSIDER THIS:

High-Quality Sources of Information	Questionable or Poor Sources of Information
Peer-reviewed journal articles	Popular media
Academic textbooks	Testimonials
U.S. government health websites	Advertisements
International health websites	Blogs
University public health websites	Discussion boards
Presentations or podcasts with primary researchers	Social media

INFOGRAPHIC 4.1 Evaluating Sources

Instructor–Participant Relationships

The relationships instructors and participants create together are the core of group fitness. Because these relationships are so important, they must also be built on trust and mutual respect. Reciprocal respect and trust are fostered through professional behaviors from all parties as well as inclusive language and behaviors, but they are also rooted in cultivating boundaries from which the relationship functions. This means that both participants and instructors are respectful of the nature of the relationship. Inclusive in these boundaries is physical touch. Due to the physical nature of teaching group fitness, it is important for the instructor to maintain appropriate professional boundaries with regard to contact. If a participant agrees to physical contact, it should always be done with care and sensitivity for the individual. If a participant displays any sign of discomfort, contact should be immediately discontinued. Physical contact should always be appropriate to the task at hand (such as helping adjust positioning) and never in sensitive areas.

Inclusive Teaching

Approaching your role as an instructor as inclusively as possible through language, modifications, and general engagement with participants is a fundamental part of your work. It is also important from an ethical perspective. As one of AFAA's Group Fitness Instructors, the expectation is that you will act justly and inclusively toward participants, members, peers, and employers. The rule is not to treat others as you wish to be treated, but rather to treat them as *they* wish to be treated. It is your ethical responsibility to act fairly and inclusively at all times.

Interpersonal Skills and General Professionalism

In forming relationships with participants and peers, it is also important that you do so with effective communication and personal presentation (i.e., the way you present yourself). Instructors should communicate in a manner that is friendly, considerate, and inclusive. Vocal tone, choice of words, rate of speech, eye contact, and body language all contribute to professionalism or lack thereof (Russell, 2011). These are all key factors in relating to others that affect the way you are perceived.

Another factor that is crucial to the way you present yourself is simply how you appear to those around you. This is your personal presentation, and it includes the following:

- **Punctuality:** Every effort should be made to start and end class at the scheduled time.
- **Attire:** The instructor should dress in a manner that facilitates required movements without distracting participants or making them feel uncomfortable.
- **Language:** In general, profanity or explicit language is best left out of the teaching environment.

These are just a few factors, but they contribute to the professional impression you leave. First, punctuality is important for building trust with participants and peers and shows that you honor the time participants have dedicated to spending with you and that you respect those with whom you work. Next, although group fitness leaves a lot of room for creativity and self-expression through clothing, being well-groomed and dressed appropriately for the workouts you instruct will show others that you hold respect for yourself and for the career you have chosen. This does not mean you cannot have fun with your attire (say, a 1980s-themed bike ride), but it does mean that you should consider the impression you are making as well as alignment to your employer's dress code where applicable. Finally, the way you speak communicates a lot about your values and personal brand. Those can be strengths and ways to be authentically you, but when you use exclusive, offensive, or explicit language it can detract from the trust that is necessary for engaging with and motivating participants, as well as relating to peers. So, be cognizant of the words you choose to ensure they best represent who you are and who you want to be. This can also apply to the music you select for your classes.

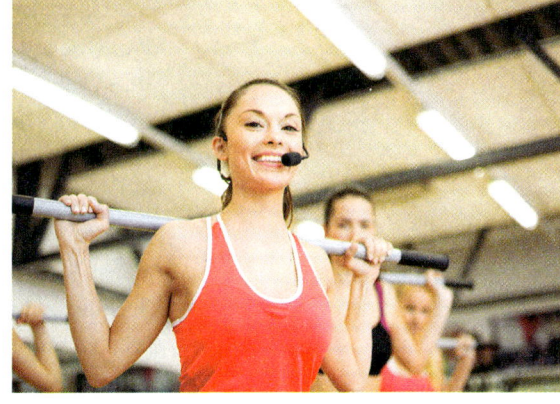

© Ground Picture/Shutterstock

Safety Responsibilities

It is the instructor's responsibility to make the workout environment and the exercises as safe as possible to prevent injury. The following issues fall under an instructor's safety responsibilities:

- **Equipment safety:** A participant using equipment inappropriately could be at risk of injuring themselves or another participant. This might include improper bike fit, incorrect form when using weights, poorly stacked step platforms, or incorrectly fastened straps.

- **Overexertion:** Overexertion can be dangerous. Stopping the class, attending to the participant, and referring them for medical attention is a priority (La Forge, 2003). Some signs a participant could be at risk include the following:
  - Abnormally rapid heart rate
  - Fever
  - Nausea and vomiting
  - Disorientation or confusion
- **Dehydration:** An instructor should seek help for a participant immediately if they show the following signs of dehydration (Mayo Clinic, 2021):
  - Confusion
  - Rapid heart rate
  - Rapid breathing
  - Passing out
  - Lack of sweating
  - Extreme thirst
- **Excessive fatigue:** If a participant shows the following signs, the instructor should halt the class and seek medical help for the participant immediately (Mayo Clinic, 2020):
  - Shortness of breath
  - Chest pain
  - Irregular or rapid heartbeat
  - Dizziness or feeling lightheaded
  - Severe abdominal, pelvic, or back pain
- **Temperature:** The recommended temperature for a fitness facility is 68–72°F (20–22°C). Some specialty formats are performed in a heated environment and require additional instructor education and qualifications.
- **Sound volume:** Sound/noise levels are measured in decibels (dB). The permissible exposure is 85 dB averaged over an 8-hour period (Occupational Safety and Health Administration, n.d.). Instructors will want to balance the volume of the music with the volume of their voice to avoid yelling and possibly damaging their voice permanently. If participants are having trouble following the music, consider turning up the bass so they can feel the beat while still hearing instructor cues.
- **Clothing and footwear:** Instructors usually cannot advise participants prior to the first class, but they can discuss the best options in class and offer modifications for next time.
- **Flooring:** Wood flooring is soft enough for impact and smooth enough for movement. Some locations have other types of flooring such as carpeting, rubber, or concrete, which make movements more difficult and increase the risk of injury. Flooring should be taken into consideration when selecting exercises.
- **Contraindicated exercises:** Some exercises are not recommended in a group setting because of an increased injury risk in the general population or the required technique requires more individualized coaching than is possible in a group:
  - Straight-leg (locked-knee) deadlifts
  - Hurdler stretch
  - Straight-leg sit ups
  - Overhead kettlebell swings
  - Good mornings
  - Exercises not recommended for those with special considerations

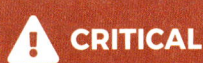

The louder the music, the shorter amount of time it takes for noise-induced hearing loss to occur. Make sure you know your decibels and consider the long-term hearing health of yourself and your participants before you crank up the volume.

Safe Movement: The AFAA 5 Questions

Risk of an injury or other emergency in the group fitness classroom can never be fully avoided; however, a number of best practices and training techniques can be implemented to ensure that participants are exercising in the safest environment possible.

Participants can be safeguarded from harm when instructors design classes that minimize injury risk. Revisit the AFAA 5 Questions in **Figure 4.1**.

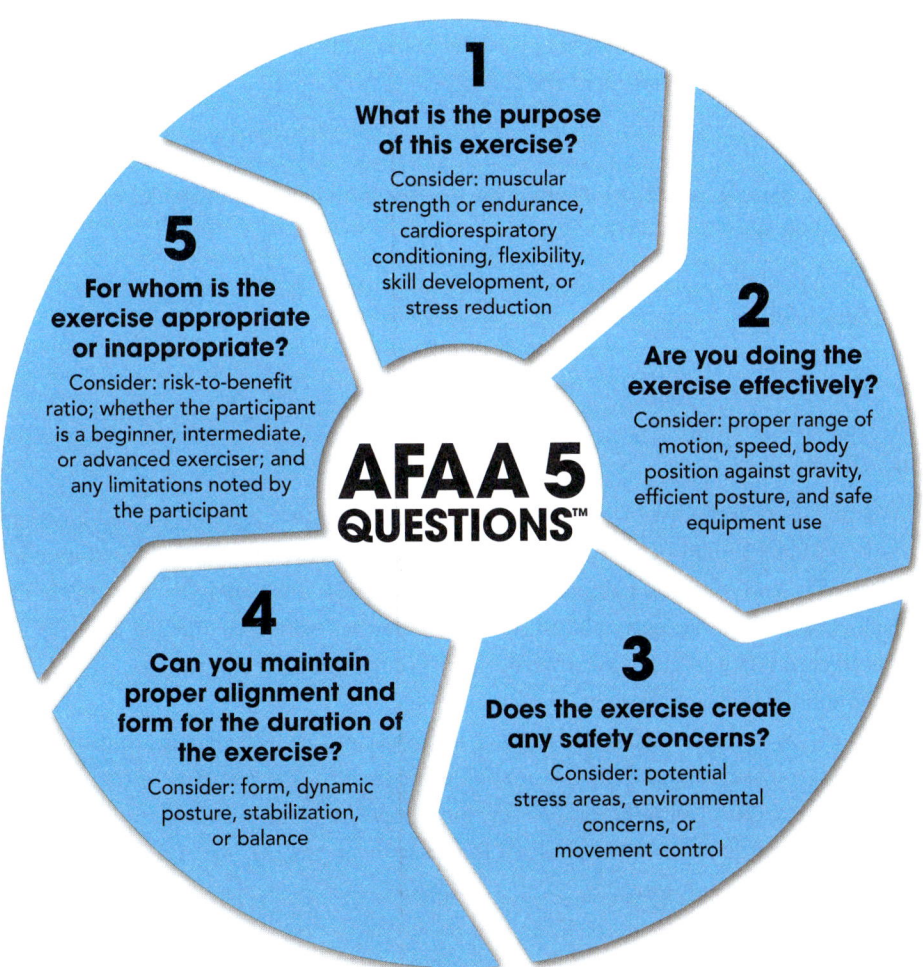

FIGURE 4.1 The AFAA 5 Questions™

INTEGRATED FITNESS

Comprehensive approach combining all exercise components to help a participant achieve higher levels of function.

Injury risk can be reduced through the progressive application of **INTEGRATED FITNESS**, specifically during the movement preparation segment of a class. Strains, sprains, and other noncontact injuries can be further reduced by matching the movement prep to the higher-intensity body of the workout to ensure that the body will be ready.

Emergency Situations and Response

The content that follows is for reference and review purposes only because instructors must remain within their scope of practice. It is the instructor's responsibility to react correctly and efficiently when waiting for emergency services to arrive.

Group Fitness Instructors need to be competent in emergency response protocol for participants. This is accomplished through training and certification in cardiopulmonary resuscitation (CPR) and operation of the automated external defibrillator (AED) device.

Group Fitness Instructors should be familiar in emergency response topics, including the following:

- Recognizing an emergency
- Disease and injury prevention
- CPR/AED/first aid
- Blood-borne pathogen training
- Emergency preparedness

RECOGNIZING AND RESPONDING TO AN EMERGENCY

The most important step in minimizing the effect of a medical emergency is recognizing it as early as possible. An initial survey of the area gives the responder an idea of the circumstances and potential conditions of individuals, as well as the hazards to anyone in the immediate area, including yourself.

Next, look for any signs that may indicate that the individual is in trouble, which may include the following:

- Position of the individual (standing, seated, crouching, doubled over, or supine)
- Skin color
- Bleeding
- Level of consciousness
- Pain or discomfort
- Distress

As soon as both the individual and the situation have been surveyed and assessed, emergency medical personnel should be notified by calling emergency services. If the affected individual is unresponsive and there is an absence of breathing or pulse, the responder must begin CPR/AED efforts while another party places the call (if no other person is available, the responder should call emergency services first, then begin resuscitation). Even in situations where a pulse and respiration are present, emergency services should be contacted.

In situations where the individual has not lost consciousness yet remains in distress, after calling emergency services the instructor should progress to the next part of the assessment phase: communication. Communication is the most important phase in assessing an individual's condition and will direct the next phase of the assessment process. Ask a few concise, direct questions, such as the following:

- What happened?
- How are you feeling?
- Where is the pain?

If the individual's health history is unknown, ask if they have any medical conditions that may exacerbate the emergency.

Each fitness facility should have a prearranged emergency response activation plan; employees should familiarize themselves with these protocols. First responders may be responsible for calling emergency services, providing details on the injury or illness, and directing emergency services to the scene while also diverting bystanders away from the area. Each facility may have protocols in place for recording and reporting situational details after the event for liability purposes.

 CRITICAL

A participant in distress cannot stop you from calling emergency medical services (EMS), even if they insist. If you feel EMS must be activated due to the nature of the emergency, you are within your rights, and it is your responsibility to do so. Although the participant may refuse care directly from the medical personnel that arrive on scene, you do not have to forgo calling EMS as an instructor.

SUMMARY

In the current health and fitness industry, Group Fitness Instructors have a responsibility not only to themselves, but also to participants, peers, employers, and the industry at large to pursue ongoing development, obtain continuing education, operate within their scope of practice, and adhere to ethical practices. With the influx of new information, trends, and social influences, instructors must constantly seek to learn, grow, and adapt in the dynamic fitness environment. To endure, they must also be open to feedback and be diligent about legal, ethical, and safety responsibilities. By being aware of and utilizing the many resources available for support and continued development, the Group Fitness Instructor can look forward to a long, healthy, and rewarding career.

REFERENCES

Abbott, A. A. (2012). The legal aspects: Scope of practice. *ACSM Health Fitness Journal, 16*(1), 31–34. https://doi.org/10.1249/FIT.0b013e31823d0452

Eickhoff-Shemek, J. (2003). Distinguishing "general" and "professional" liability insurance. *ACSM Health Fitness Journal, 7*(1), 28–30.

Eickhoff-Shemek, J. M. (2013). Minimizing legal liability for the exercise professional: Strategies that work! *ACSM's Certified News, 23*(4).

International Dance Exercise Association. (2016). *IDEA codes of ethics for fitness professionals.* https://www.ideafit.com/fitness-library/idea-codes-of-ethics-for-fitness-professionals

La Forge, R. (2003). *Overexertion can cause serious harm.* IDEA Health & Fitness Source. https://www.ideafit.com/uncategorized/exercise-overexertion/

Mayo Clinic. (2020). *Symptoms: Fatigue: When to see a doctor.* http://www.mayoclinic.org/symptoms/fatigue/basics/when-to-see-doctor/sym-20050894

Mayo Clinic. (2021). *Diseases and conditions: Dehydration.* http://www.mayoclinic.org/diseases-conditions/dehydration /basics/symptoms/con-20030056

Occupational Safety and Health Administration. (n.d.). *Occupational noise exposure.* https://www.osha.gov/SLTC /noisehearingconservation/

Riley, S. (2005). *Liability insurance: Accidents happen regardless of how diligent and professional you are. Protect yourself.* IDEA Trainer Success. http://www.ideafit.com/fitness-library/liability-insuranceaccidents-happen-regardless -of-how-diligent-and-professional-you-are-protect-yourself

Russell, J. E. A. (2011, February 4). Career coach: The wrong tone can spoil the message. *The Washington Post.* http:// www.washingtonpost.com/wp-dyn/content/article/2011/02/04/AR2011020406095.html

United States Copyright Office. (2015). *Copyright and the music marketplace: A report of the register of copyrights.* Copyright.gov. https://www.copyright.gov/policy/musiclicensingstudy/copyright-and-the-music-marketplace.pdf

SECTION 2

FUNDAMENTALS OF EXERCISE SCIENCE

CHAPTER 5

HUMAN MOVEMENT SCIENCE AND EXERCISE

LEARNING OBJECTIVES

The intent of this chapter is to review the benefits of exercise and connect them to applied human movement and exercise science. This chapter will go over the major systems of the body, planes of motion, and other exercise science topics as they relate to movement and bioenergetics.

After reading this content, students should be able to demonstrate the following objectives:

- **Identify** the benefits of exercise for group fitness participants.

- **Describe** fundamental principles related to human movement.

- **Describe** foundational principles of exercise metabolism.

Lesson 1: Benefits of Exercise

Introduction

Exercise is awesome! Making the decision to become a Group Fitness Instructor shows that you know how great group fitness can be for mental and physical health, and you want to share it with others. In this chapter, you will learn about the benefits of exercise and the body systems involved. Knowledge of the science behind exercise will allow you to fully appreciate how the human body works and enable you to design effective programs that will keep your participants coming back for more.

Benefits of Exercise

The benefits of participation in regular **EXERCISE** and **PHYSICAL ACTIVITY** have been well established, and most people know that exercise is part of a healthy lifestyle. Exercise

EXERCISE

Physical activity that is usually planned, structured, generally repetitive in nature, and intended to induce some level of overload on the body's physiological systems.

and physical activity provide numerous benefits, including improved **HEALTH**, functionality, **FITNESS**, and improved body composition. Despite these well-known benefits, most people still fall short of meeting the minimum guidelines for exercise and physical activity. As a Group Fitness Instructor, you can help make exercise fun and approachable to get people moving.

Delivering effective, results-oriented group fitness classes begins with a fundamental knowledge of what is happening in the body during movement. Instructors rely on scientific principles to provide classes that are planned, structured, and progressive to optimize the benefits of physical activity. Some benefits, such as reduced stress, improved mood, and better sleep, begin with just a single bout of exercise. Other benefits are gained over time as the individual adheres to an exercise program.

Considering the diversity of participant goals, it is likely you will be asked questions ranging from "What is the best way to burn fat?" to "What are the benefits of high-intensity interval training?" to "Will this class help me to build muscle?" Equipped with an understanding of how the body works during exercise, as well as the variables that most influence adaptations in the categories of health, fitness, and performance, you can design classes that best meet the participants' needs and feel confident answering many of their questions regarding how to best achieve their goals. It will also allow you to communicate these benefits to participants in a way that will increase motivation for and connection with their group fitness classes.

📋 INSTRUCTOR TIP

Many benefits from exercise can be experienced directly after a group fitness class. Communicating these benefits to your participants will increase their awareness of the psychological and physical improvements they are feeling. As they develop positive associations with exercise, they are more likely to form healthy habits and increase their chance of experiencing real behavior change.

Here are some examples of how to include positive associations in classes:

- Can you feel that energy flowing through you right now?
- How great do you feel now?
- You are going to sleep so great tonight!
- Breathe slowly to let your heart rate recover and feel how great your body feels after that amazing workout.
- Isn't it amazing how great you feel while walking out of here?

What other ways can you think of to increase positive associations with physical activity?

Improved Mood

Anyone who has completed a workout can report the immediate effect it has on mood. **MOOD** is the emotional state of the individual, and it can have a dramatic influence on how an individual feels about their environment. In other words, mood can directly influence how a person perceives the world (Zadra & Clore, 2011). Being in a good mood can help improve a person's overall sense of well-being and give feelings of lightness and positivity.

Exercise aids in the release of hormones such as serotonin, which is associated with mood regulation, and decreases cortisol levels, which are associated with stress, and thus can improve both brain health and a person's emotional state (Esch & Stefano, 2010a). The incorporation of social interactions can also help to decrease feelings of isolation and loneliness (Holt-Lunstad et al., 2015). Exercise, like group fitness classes, can be used as an intervention for anxiety and depression in both clinical and non-clinical settings, possibly serving as an alternative to pharmacological methods. In addition, research has demonstrated that individuals who are more physically active report fewer poor mental health days (Chekroud et al., 2018). Note, however, that it is outside of a fitness professional's scope of practice to treat diagnosed mental health disorders. Although exercise has been shown to improve mental health, long-term and chronic mood disorders require professional care.

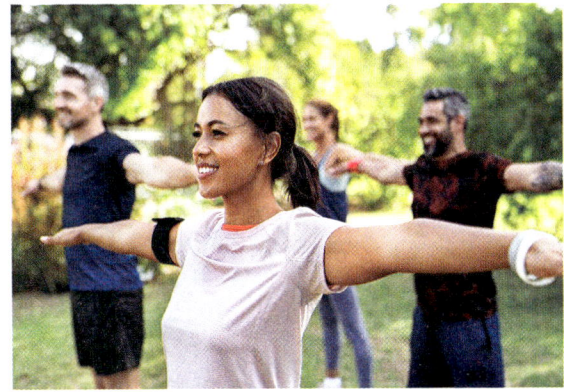

© Rido/Shutterstock

Improved Sleep Quality

Sleep is an important aspect of overall health and is necessary for both physical and mental health. Sleep plays a vital role in restoring the nervous, immune, skeletal, and muscular systems, helping to repair any damage that has been accumulated throughout the day (Luyster et al., 2012). Sleep status affects immune function by influencing the body's ability to respond to infection and heal wounds (Besedovsky et al., 2012; Bryant et al., 2004). Most people can relate to the foggy feeling created by lack of sleep and can attest to the impaired cognitive function that comes with it. This can be attributed to the important role that sleep plays in neural development, removal of waste products from the brain, and memory consolidation (Eugene & Masiak, 2015). It is no surprise that a lack of sleep often is compared with feelings of intoxication (Williamson & Feyer, 2000). Sleep-related cognitive impairments are both short term, affecting day-to-day function, and long term, amplifying age-related cognitive decline (Cochrane et al., 2012).

The National Sleep Foundation recommends that adults sleep 7–9 hours per night, yet most people struggle to get this (Hirshkowitz et al., 2015). It is also true that as we age we experience a decrease in sleep quality and quantity, causing people to feel fatigued throughout the day and decreasing cognitive performance. Furthermore, sleep disorders, such as insomnia, lead to reduced physical and mental health and decreased quality of life.

Given the important role that sleep plays, it is not surprising that those who do not get enough sleep often experience decreased physical and mental health. Specifically, not getting enough sleep has been shown to increase the incidence of depression, anxiety, cardiovascular disease, stroke, cancer, type 2 diabetes, and overall mortality (Laksono et al., 2022; Li et al., 2022; Luyster et al., 2012; Wang et al., 2021). Inadequate sleep can lead to impaired metabolic and immune system function. This can make it difficult for people to improve their body composition if they desire to do so. Worse, decreased sleep has been found to alter metabolic rate, increase appetite, and decrease insulin sensitivity (Bryant et al., 2004; Spiegel et al., 2005; Schmid et al., 2008). Conversely, sleep quantity and quality are positively associated with physical activity levels during the day. Individuals who get more quality sleep feel more energized during the day, which can help increase the likelihood of participating in physical activity (Kline, 2014).

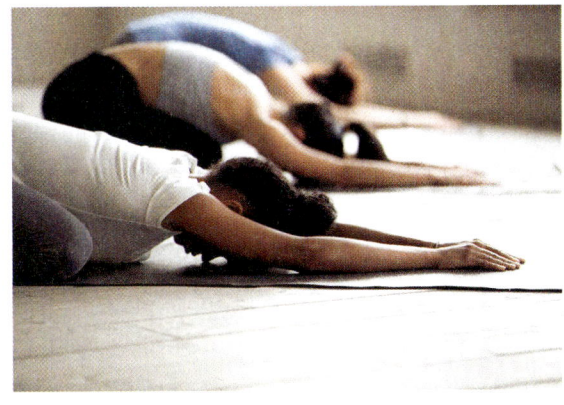

The good news is that exercise can help improve sleep quality and quantity, helping individuals fall asleep faster and awaken less frequently after falling asleep (Yang et al., 2012). The quality of sleep improves due to an increase in the amount of deep sleep, which is a restorative stage of sleep, and rapid eye movement (REM) sleep, which has been associated with memory processing and learning. Group

© Fizkes/Shutterstock

fitness participants can benefit from these improvements in sleep from their first workout and from regular exercise participation. Exercise shows promise in improving sleep in a wide range of populations (Kredlow et al., 2015). Other methods of improving sleep often include the use of medications. Exercise is a non-pharmacological method for improving sleep, providing physical and mental health benefits without the potential negative side effects associated with medication.

Stress Management

Exercise is one of the best ways to help manage and relieve stress from daily life (Esch & Stefano, 2010a; Esch & Stephano, 2010b). **STRESS** is the body's physiological response to a stressor, often an event or condition, which can be either positive (**EUSTRESS**) or negative (**DISTRESS**). It is important to remember that not all stress is bad, and it is indeed necessary to grow and improve. Thoughtfully planned exercise is a form of eustress. As the body experiences the stress of workouts, it (ideally) will recover from them better off than it was before by responding with physiological adaptations over time, such as becoming stronger, better conditioned, and so on. Stress becomes problematic when it is chronic or exceeds our ability to recover and adapt to it. Everyone will experience stress in their life, be it with work, relationships, money, or their environment.

The basic stress response starts in the brain when a threat is perceived. This starts a cascade of events that results in a coordinated response from the whole body. The body responds by releasing adrenaline and cortisol, affecting various organs to prime the body to either stay and fight the threat or run away from it. Muscles become tense and ready for action, glucose is released into the bloodstream, heart rate increases, blood pressure spikes, and the body is ready for combat! This is referred to as a **SYMPATHETIC NERVOUS SYSTEM** response, also known as fight-or-flight response.

This full-body effort is appropriate if the threat is a matter of life or death, say, if you were to come into contact with a predator. However, this stress response is problematic when the body is continually in this heightened state, constantly releasing hormones that are not needed, if you are just sitting at a desk. In our modern world with high-stress jobs, the stress response can lead to tense muscles and trouble sleeping as well as development of chronic health conditions such as hypertension, type 2 diabetes, and heart disease (Harris et al., 2017; Yaribeygi et al., 2017).

Any type of exercise can help with stress management by simply serving as a break from common stressors, such as work or school (Breus & O'Connor, 1998). Taking the time to work out can reduce our focus on the everyday problems that create anxiety and tension. Exercise can be an effective tool to help manage stress in a healthy way, improving how the body copes with stress, and additionally giving the individual a sense of gratification (Esch & Stefano, 2010a, 2010b). Participation in aerobic and moderate exercise has been shown to improve the stress response immediately following exercise as well as over the long term and can mitigate the risk of developing heart disease (Spalding et al., 2004). Regular exercisers show more stress resilience and are not as negatively affected by a stressful situation (Childs & de Wit, 2014). Mind–body exercises such as yoga and tai chi may also help decrease stress and anxiety by decreasing sympathetic nervous system activity. These benefits have been shown to last for several hours post workout (Li & Goldsmith, 2012; Wang et al., 2014). Group fitness also fosters a sense of social support, which has been linked to a reduction in stress hormone responses (Elsenberger et al., 2007).

Note that stress management is different for everyone and that there is no single program that will work for all populations. However, Group Fitness Instructors can create fun and engaging classes that provide a break from life's everyday stressors and a supportive community to help participants cope with stress effectively.

Mind–Body Connection

The negative effects of stress highlight the importance of the mind–body connection. Having a beneficial **MIND–BODY CONNECTION** means that an individual is in touch with their physical sensations and can recognize how the mind and the body are interconnected. The mind controls the movement of the body, and the movement of the body can affect our mental state. Mind–body exercises combine low-intensity physical exercise with breathing and mindful movement, usually done at a slower pace to allow a heightened focus on the present state.

Instructors can improve the mind–body connection by teaching participants to listen to their body and then provide them with various techniques to modulate their physiological state. Some examples of this in a group exercise setting would be completing a yoga flow while moving in tandem with the breath, taking time to meditate at the end of a workout, or focusing on the breath during a portion of the workout.

In several populations, mind–body exercise has been shown to result in structural and functional changes in the brain that can improve both physical and mental health (Zhang et al., 2021). Mind–body exercise has also been shown to decrease cardiovascular disease risk by enhancing stress management and improving stress-related cardiovascular responses, such as lowering blood pressure (Yang et al., 2021). Making the most of the mind–body connection can help individuals consciously harness the power of the mind to influence the state of the body, sensing when there is heightened stress or pain and understanding how to deal with it in a healthy way. In a group fitness class, instructors can use various techniques, including progressive relaxation, breathwork, meditation, focus, and movement flow, to help participants be aware of the connection that their mind has to their body and the present state. These techniques often are used in formats that are considered mind–body classes but they can also be incorporated into the transition phase of any style of workout.

Increased Energy

Exercise and physical activity increase feelings of energy and decrease feelings of fatigue. On the cellular level, regular exercise will improve cardiovascular system function, which makes it easier for the body to produce and distribute energy to the cells throughout the body. Individuals who engage in regular exercise have more mitochondria in their cells and increased oxygen circulation, both of which play a key role in supplying readily available energy to all the cells in the body. Exercise has also been found to increase **ENDORPHINS** as the sympathetic nervous system adapts to meet the needs of the exercise session. These endorphins increase the body's available energy and contribute to the post-workout mood boost that many people experience. In fact, getting the body moving has been shown to help increase energy levels, even in those who report chronic levels of fatigue (Puetz et al., 2006).

All types of exercise can help to facilitate these improvements in energy, benefitting a variety of populations. A dose–response relationship has been shown between physical activity and feelings of energy and fatigue, with those reporting more physical activity in a week expressing more feelings of being energetic (O'Connor & Puetz, 2005). In extreme cases, such as with athletes or sometimes Group Fitness Instructors who teach too many classes, too much exercise can lead to overtraining. Chronic fatigue is one symptom of overtraining, and the Group Fitness Instructor should keep in mind that they, too, need balance when it comes to frequency of training.

MIND–BODY CONNECTION

The relationship between the brain and the physical body whereby a person's thoughts, emotions, beliefs, and attitudes can affect their physical functioning and performance.

ENDORPHINS

Chemicals produced by the nervous system to cope with stress.

Preventing Chronic Disease

Chronic diseases account for the majority of the top causes of mortality in the United States (Centers for Disease Control and Prevention, 2022). These diseases are significantly affected by lifestyle choices, such as diet, physical activity levels, and other behaviors. Participation in exercise has several health benefits and may reduce the risk of several adverse health outcomes. Luckily, these benefits begin when the individual starts participation in any amount of activity, and the benefits amplify as the individual becomes more active. A moderate amount of physical activity on most days of the week has been shown to decrease the risk for several chronic diseases, including coronary heart disease, stroke, type 2 diabetes, multiple types of cancer, obesity, hypertension, and osteoporosis (Booth et al., 2012). Exercise can also help to improve cognitive function and decrease the risk for developing brain and cognitive diseases such as anxiety, depression, and Alzheimer's (Firth et al., 2020; Paillard et al., 2015; Zhao et al., 2014). These benefits can be gained with less intensity, duration, and frequency than the amount of physical activity needed for weight loss or weight maintenance. Note that some activity is better than none, with an inverse relationship existing between physical activity and chronic disease risk (Miller et al., 2016).

Both aerobic and resistance training exercises have been found to be beneficial to health and should be encouraged (Miller et al., 2016). According to the *2018 Physical Activity Guidelines Advisory Committee Scientific Report* (U. S. Department of Health and Human Services, 2018), substantial health benefits can be gained with 150–300 minutes per week of moderate-intensity aerobic activity or 75–150 minutes per week of vigorous-intensity aerobic activity as well as 2 days of muscle-strengthening activities. This could be achieved with consistent participation in group fitness classes designed for both aerobic and muscle-strengthening purposes. Group Fitness Instructors can share the importance of consistency with class participants to help them benefit from exercise participation in a fun and social environment.

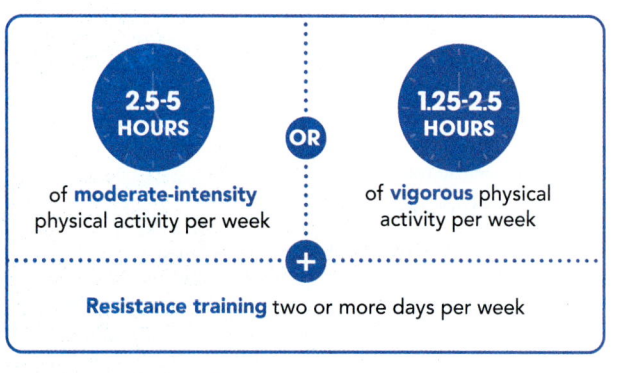

U.S. Department of Health and Human Services. (2019). *Move your way: What's your move?* https://health.gov/sites/default/files/2019-11/PAG_MYW_Adult_FS.pdf

Improved Body Composition

Many group fitness participants will come to classes with body composition goals. These may be expressed as generic goals such as "I want to lose weight," "I want to get in shape," or "I want to tone my muscles." A fitness professional can recognize these goals as changes in body composition and direct participants to the appropriate classes for their goals. Participants' goals can also help instructors design classes that help their participants get the results they are looking for.

So, what exactly is body composition? **BODY COMPOSITION** is the relative proportion of fat mass and fat-free mass in the body. How much of each component comprises total body weight? Fat-free mass includes bone, muscle tissue, connective tissue, organs, skin, interstitial fluid, hair, and any other non-fat tissue. Body composition is usually expressed in terms of percent body fat. Keep in mind that this is just a ratio or an expression of how much of a person's overall body weight is made up of body fat alone (e.g., 20% body fat).

Although a person's body weight is not synonymous with their health status, a high body fat percentage (greater than 25% for men and greater than 30% for women) has been associated with negative health outcomes, such as increased cardiometabolic risks (Kim et al., 2013) and an increased risk for all-cause mortality (Padwal et al., 2016). Exercise can influence body composition in two primary ways: (1) by increasing total caloric expenditure and (2) by increasing

BODY COMPOSITION

The relative proportion of fat mass and fat-free mass in the body.

the amount and density of muscle tissue (i.e., fat-free mass). Exercise has been shown to help improve and maintain body composition as people age, helping to increase longevity and vitality and improve movement capacity and general well-being (Stehr & von Lengerke, 2012).

An understanding of how to change body composition in group fitness settings enables instructors to design classes that will best meet the needs of those with this particular fitness goal. Instructors can help by getting participants moving consistently and enjoying that movement to increase adherence. Any movement that is done to reduce sedentary time can be beneficial to health. Designing group fitness classes that involve lifting weights can help to increase the amount of muscle mass (fat-free mass), which can improve body composition by increasing the proportion of the overall weight that comes from fat-free tissue.

Relevance of Movement and Human Body Science for Class Design and Planning

The human body was made to move. Some of the benefits of movement will start with the very first group fitness class that someone takes. However, the body will adapt in very specific ways depending on the type of exercise performed. In order to design classes that are as safe and effective as possible, you must have a thorough understanding of the human movement system and knowledge of how to plan each class to contribute to participants' goals.

A well-designed group fitness program can help improve several components of fitness, including cardiorespiratory fitness, muscular strength, muscular endurance, and flexibility. The adaptations that are gained are specific to the demands of the program. The **PRINCIPLE OF SPECIFICITY** states that the body will adapt to the demands placed on it in very specific ways. When the body is consistently exposed to a stimulus, it will respond by enhancing each system to better meet the needs of the activity. However, only the muscles that are working will adapt, and they will adapt specifically to the energy system used and the particular joint actions that have been performed.

You do not need to be an expert in biomechanics or physiology to be a successful fitness professional, but a base of knowledge in each of these areas will help you understand what is going on inside the body's systems when they are challenged with exercise. This knowledge can help you organize and plan the variables to address to get the results that participants are looking for when designing a group exercise program or a single session.

PRINCIPLE OF SPECIFICITY

The type of exercise stimulus placed on the body will determine the expected physiological outcome.

Lesson 2: Kinesiology and the Human Movement System

Kinesiology for Group Fitness

The first step is learning about the basics of **KINESIOLOGY**, or the study of movement. Have you ever looked at an exercise and wondered what its purpose is? Have you ever watched an athlete complete a play and wondered how they were able to perform so well? Understanding some of the basics of the structure and function of the human body will allow you keep your participants moving safely and help you write well-balanced programs. Grasping the basics of

KINESIOLOGY

The study of human body movement.

anatomy will help you recognize what the proper form is for each exercise and provide you with options for every level of exerciser. Being comfortable with this science will prepare you to answer questions from participants such as "What muscle group does this work?" or "Where should I feel this?" The next section provides an overview of how you can objectively analyze movement and design exercise programs for real results.

Planes of Motion

The planes of motion can be used to understand how the body is moving and aid in analyzing movement (**Figure 5.1**). Movement occurs in three cardinal planes, with each plane dividing the body into two halves in a specific direction. In reality, many activities and movements take place in multiple planes simultaneously, but becoming familiar with the individual planes can help you write workouts that match your participants' needs. A common understanding of standard terminology will also help you communicate with other fitness professionals. Because everyday movement occurs in all three planes of motion, you want to make sure that you are giving your participants exercises for all three planes of movement. This well-rounded approach will aid in reducing the risk of injury while also enhancing activities of daily living. This will help you choose exercises that isolate or target goal-related body parts.

The **SAGITTAL PLANE** divides the body into right and left halves. Imagine that there is a sheet of glass that runs down the center of the body, dividing the body into left and right sides. You can move the arm straight forward or back without breaking this sheet of glass. All

SAGITTAL PLANE

Plane of motion that divides the body into right and left halves.

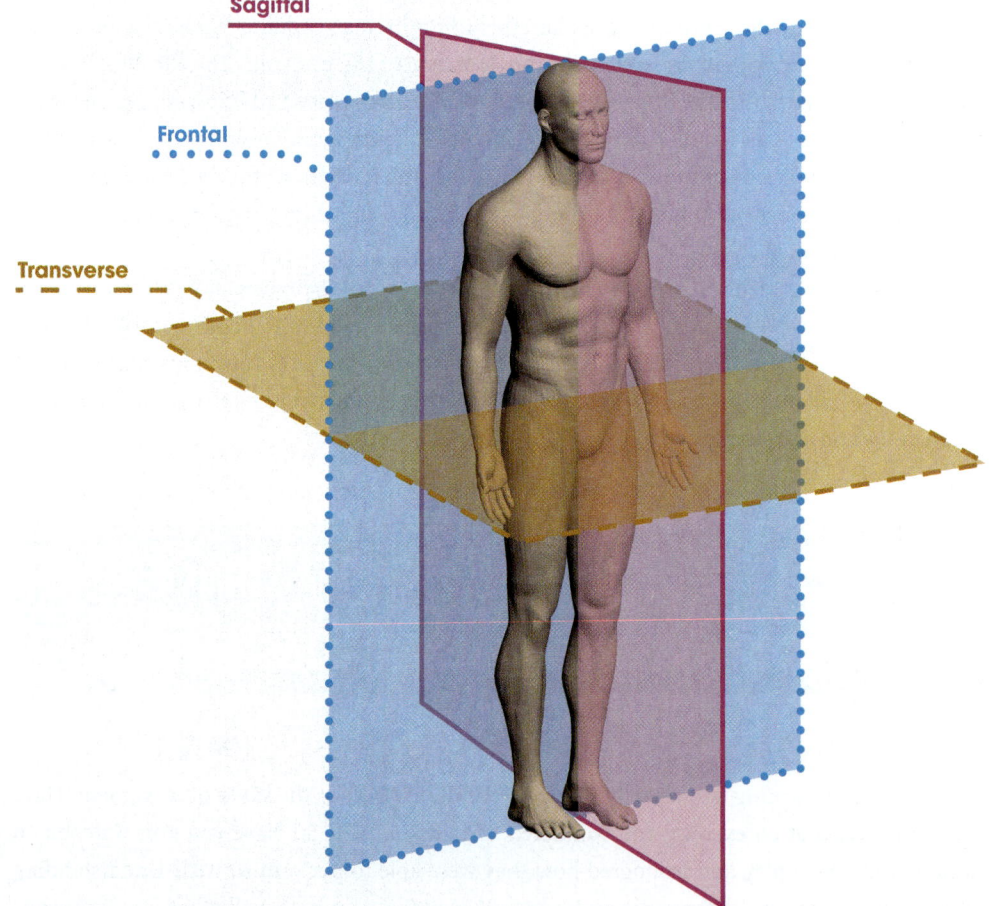

FIGURE 5.1 Planes of Motion

movements in the sagittal plane run parallel to this sheet of glass. The movements that occur in the sagittal plane move forward and backward, and they include flexion and extension. For example, knee flexion, or bending the knee, is a sagittal plane movement.

The **FRONTAL PLANE** divides the body into front and back (anterior and posterior) halves. In this example, the sheet of glass would run from right to left and divide the front and back of the body. Movements that occur in the frontal plane are side to side and usually include abduction, adduction, and lateral flexion of the spine. A great example of a frontal plane movement is a jumping jack.

The **TRANSVERSE PLANE** divides the body into top and bottom (superior and inferior) halves. The sheet of glass would be horizontal in the transverse plane. Movements that take place in the transverse plane include any type of rotation, internal/external rotation, horizontal adduction/abduction, pronation, and supination. A good example of a transverse plane movement is to turn the head to look over the shoulder. The transverse plane is also often referred to as the horizontal plane.

FRONTAL PLANE

Plane of motion that divides the body into anterior and posterior halves.

TRANSVERSE PLANE

Plane of motion that divides the body into superior and inferior halves.

ANATOMICAL POSITION

The anatomical position serves as a reference point for movement and is something most people have seen in science class (**Figure 5.2**). In the anatomical position, the individual is standing upright with the feet together, the arms resting by the sides, and the palms facing forward. When talking about joint motion or movement, one can refer to where the body part is in relation to the anatomical position. For example, if the individual has their arms lifted in front of them, then compared to the anatomical position, the shoulder joint is in shoulder flexion in the sagittal plane.

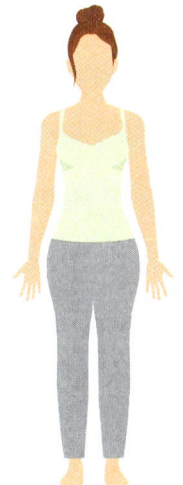

FIGURE 5.2 Anatomical Position

 INSTRUCTOR TIP

Although it is important for you to know anatomical terms, you should not use them with participants. When instructing classes and communicating with participants, you want to avoid using jargon and stick to terms that they are more familiar with.

For example, cues should be short and to the point and help participants move properly without much thought. You should keep your language concise and easy to understand. Do not make them try to translate your words while trying to move properly!

ANATOMICAL TERMINOLOGY

Do the terms *flexion* and *extension* seem overwhelming? If so, it is a good idea to spend some time learning some basic anatomical terminology (**Infographic 5.1** and **Table 5.1**). It is important to be familiar with anatomical terms so that you can learn more about movements that a muscle will produce. As fitness professionals, you need to be able to pinpoint what muscles are working during an exercise and how neighboring or distant groups may be working as well. If

Terminology to describe human movement requires the use of a consistent body position, called the **anatomical position.** Here, the body stands upright with the arms beside the trunk and the palms and head facing forward.

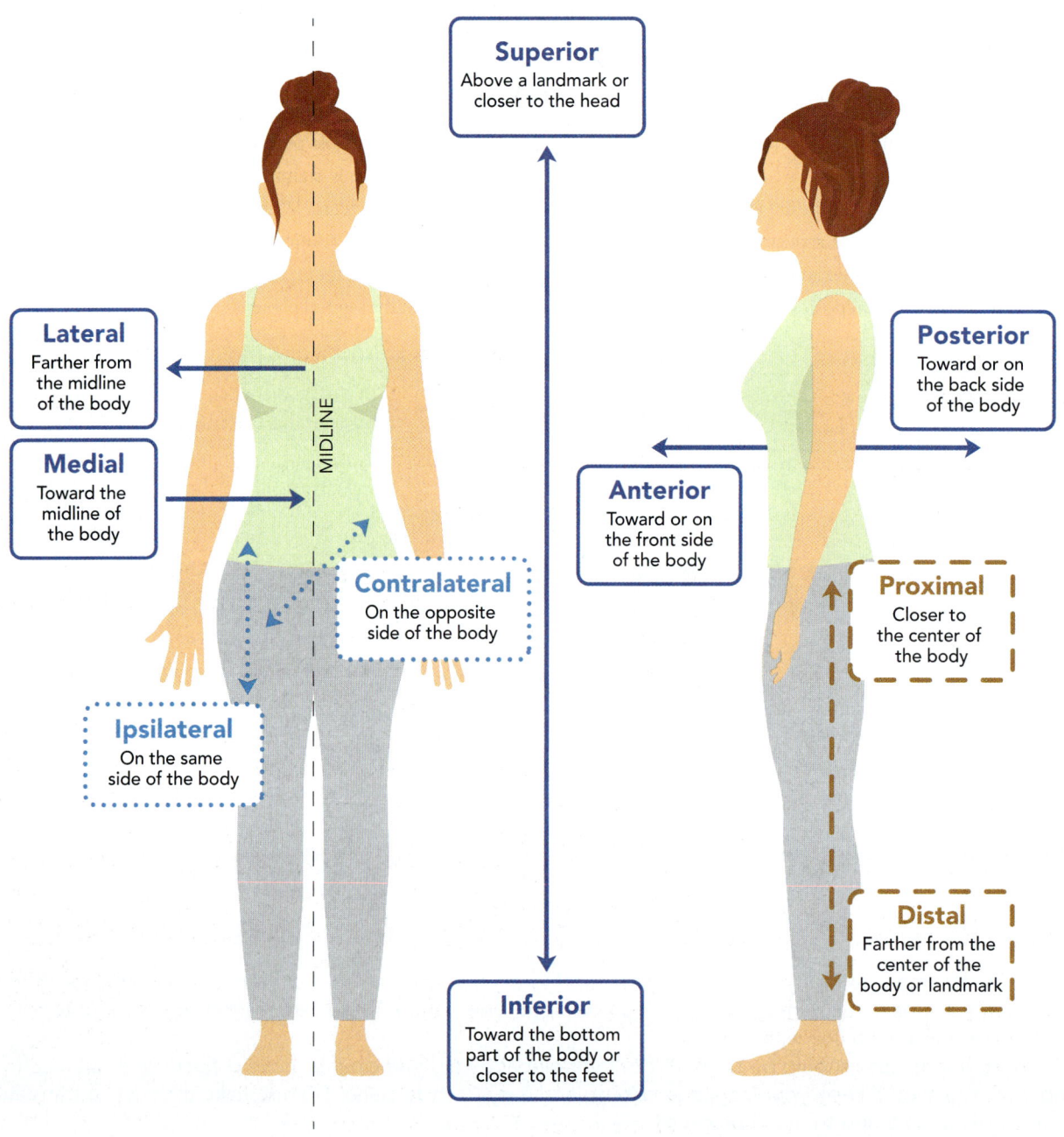

INFOGRAPHIC 5.1 Anatomical Locations

TABLE 5.1 Joint Motion Terminology

Plane	Term	Description	Example
Sagittal	Flexion	Decreases the angle of the joint	Bending the elbow
	Extension	Increases the angle of the joint	Straightening the elbow
Frontal	Abduction	Moves away from the midline of the body	Lifting arms out to the side
	Adduction	Moves toward the midline of the body	Bringing the arms back in to the body
Transverse	Internal rotation	Rotates toward the midline of the body	Rotates the shoulders forward/inwards
	External rotation	Rotates away from the midline of the body	Rotates the leg outward (turning the toes out)

you want to improve the strength of one muscle group, you can learn what movement that muscle is responsible for and then find a suitable exercise. This is how you can watch a movement or exercise and know right away that it is a great exercise. Understanding this terminology will not only allow you to learn muscle movement better, but it will also help to communicate effectively with other fitness professionals.

 HELPFUL HINT

Sometimes it can be challenging to remember the difference between *abduction* and *adduction*. Remember, ADDuction means you are *adding* something to the body, or moving a body part toward the body's midline. ABDUCTion means you are *taking away* (or abducting) a portion of the body away from its midline.

It is also helpful to remember that abduction and adduction are common, but not exclusive, to the frontal plane. For example, horizontal adduction of the humerus (upper arm bone) in the transverse plane is the overly technical description of a simple chest press.

Kinetic Chain Checkpoints

Although it is useful to learn about the human body by observing individual joints and muscles, in reality human movement typically occurs as a more fluid, multi-joint, multiplanar series of events. What happens at one joint can and will affect the joints that are above and below it. The **KINETIC CHAIN** is a concept that comes from engineering that compares the segments of the human body to the links in a chain. When one link in the chain moves, it will affect the position and the amount of tension on nearby segments. *Kinetic* refers to the force that is transferred from one portion of the system to the other. When comparing this to the human body, this theory states that the function and position of one joint can affect the joint structures above and below it. If one muscle group is overly tight, out of alignment, or not functioning properly, it will affect the joint structures above and below it, often leading to pain and dysfunction. Instead of trying to analyze every single joint angle on a participant's body, watching five key areas is the simplest way to assess movement quality. Five basic kinetic chain

KINETIC CHAIN

A concept that comes from engineering that compares the segments of the human body to the links in a chain, with each joint affecting those above and below it.

checkpoints (**Figure 5.3**) can be observed to assist the fitness professional with observing and correcting movement patterns:

1. Foot and ankle
2. Knee
3. Lumbo-pelvic-hip (LPHC) complex (i.e., lower back and hips)
4. Shoulders and thoracic spine (i.e., shoulders and mid/upper back)
5. Head and cervical spine (i.e., head and neck)

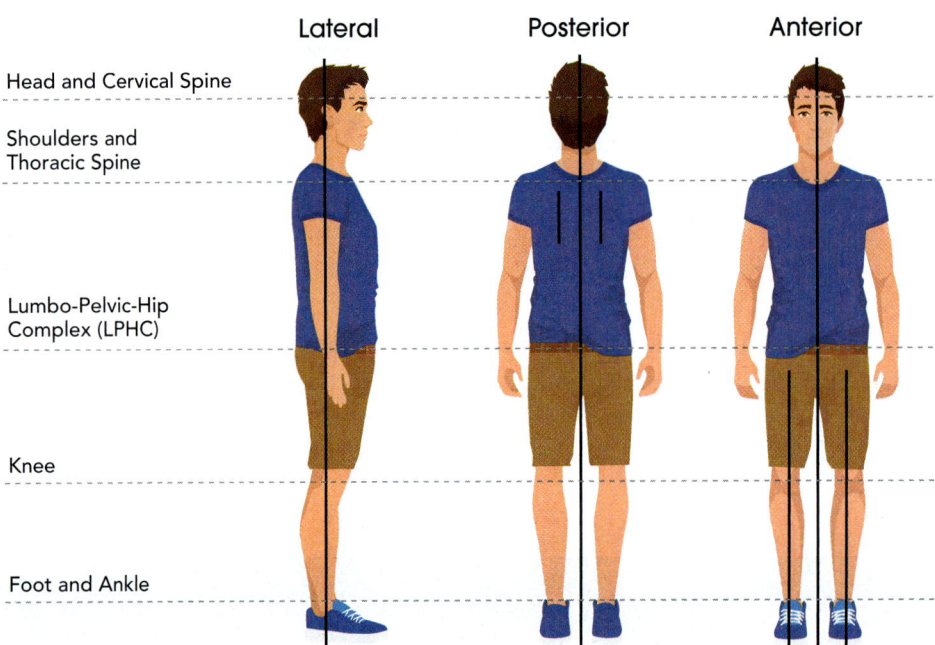

FIGURE 5.3 Kinetic Chain Checkpoints

GETTING TECHNICAL

Several movement dysfunctions in one area are a result of tight muscles or restricted joints above or below them in the kinetic chain. Here are some examples:

- The knees caving in can be due to a lack of stability in the foot or ankle.
- Excessive low back arching can be a result of tight hip flexors.
- A lack of overhead shoulder mobility can result from restriction in the thoracic spine.

It is important to be familiar with these kinetic chain checkpoints so that you can recognize correct form during workouts and give feedback to participants. Proper alignment and control of movement requires a balance of flexibility and strength between the muscles that are working together. The kinetic chain allows the movement to be looked at holistically and not limited to an isolated joint. This will help you to better serve your participants during movement and feel confident answering questions you may get in classes.

Basic Joint Motions

With this basic understanding of anatomical terminology, let us now look at some basic motions that happen at individual joints (Table 5.2; Figures 5.4 and 5.5). Joints are the portion of the skeletal system where two or more bones meet. Depending on the joint structure and the

TABLE 5.2 Basic Joint Motions

Joint and Motion	Description	Muscles Used	Example Exercises
Spine			
Flexion	Rounding the spine forward	Abdominals	Abdominal crunch
Extension	Extending the spine backward	Erector spinae muscles of the back	Back extension
Rotation	Twisting the spine in either direction	Core musculature (internal and external obliques)	Russian twist or lunge with a twist
Shoulder Joint			
Flexion	Reaching forward in sagittal plane	Deltoids (shoulders) and pectoralis major	Front raise
Extension	Bringing the arm down and back or swimming motions	Latissimus dorsi	Row
Abduction	Moving the arm away from the body in the frontal plane	Deltoids (shoulders)	Lateral raise or the upward motion of a jumping jack
Adduction	Moving the arm toward the body in the frontal plane	Latissimus dorsi	Downward motion of a jumping jack or lat pull down
Horizontal abduction	Moving the arm away from midline in the transverse plane	Rear deltoids, rhomboids, middle and lower trapezius	Wide-grip row
Horizontal adduction	Bringing the arm forward toward midline in the transverse plane	Pectoralis major (chest) and anterior deltoid (front of the shoulder)	Push-up, bench press, or chest fly
Scapular retraction	Bringing the scapula toward midline (toward spine)	Rhomboids, middle and lower trapezius	Wide-grip row
Scapular protraction	Moving the scapula away from midline (away from spine)	Serratus anterior, pectoralis major, and pectoralis minor	Chest press
Hip Joint			
Extension	Extending the leg backward in the sagittal plane	Gluteus maximus and medius and hamstrings	Upward phase of a squat or deadlift, and the propulsion phase of running or cycling

(continues)

TABLE 5.2 Basic Joint Motions (*continued*)

Joint and Motion	Description	Muscles Used	Example Exercises
Flexion	Bringing the leg forward in the sagittal plane	Hip flexors	Leg lifts or high knees
Abduction	Bringing the thigh away from midline	Gluteus medius, gluteus minimus, tensor fascia latae	Side plank with leg raises
Adduction	Bringing the thigh toward midline	Adductors	Lateral lunges
Knee Joint			
Flexion	Bending the knee	Hamstrings	Hamstring curls
Extension	Straightening the knee	Quadriceps	Upward phase of squats or lunges
Ankle Joint			
Plantar flexion	Pointing the toes	Calf complex (gastrocnemius and soleus)	Calf raise, jumping, or bouncing
Dorsiflexion	Flexing the foot	Tibialis anterior (shins)	Heel walking or toe lifts

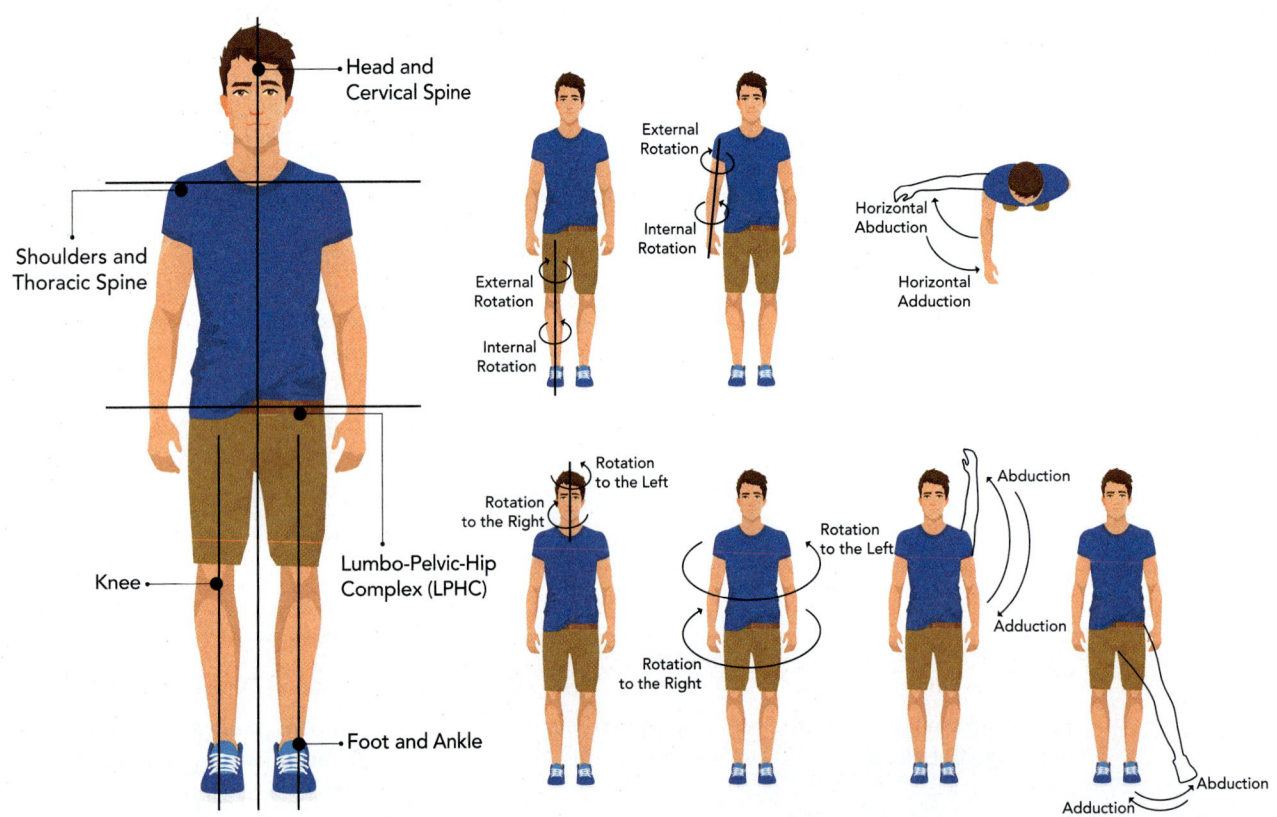

FIGURE 5.4 Joint Motions: Anterior View

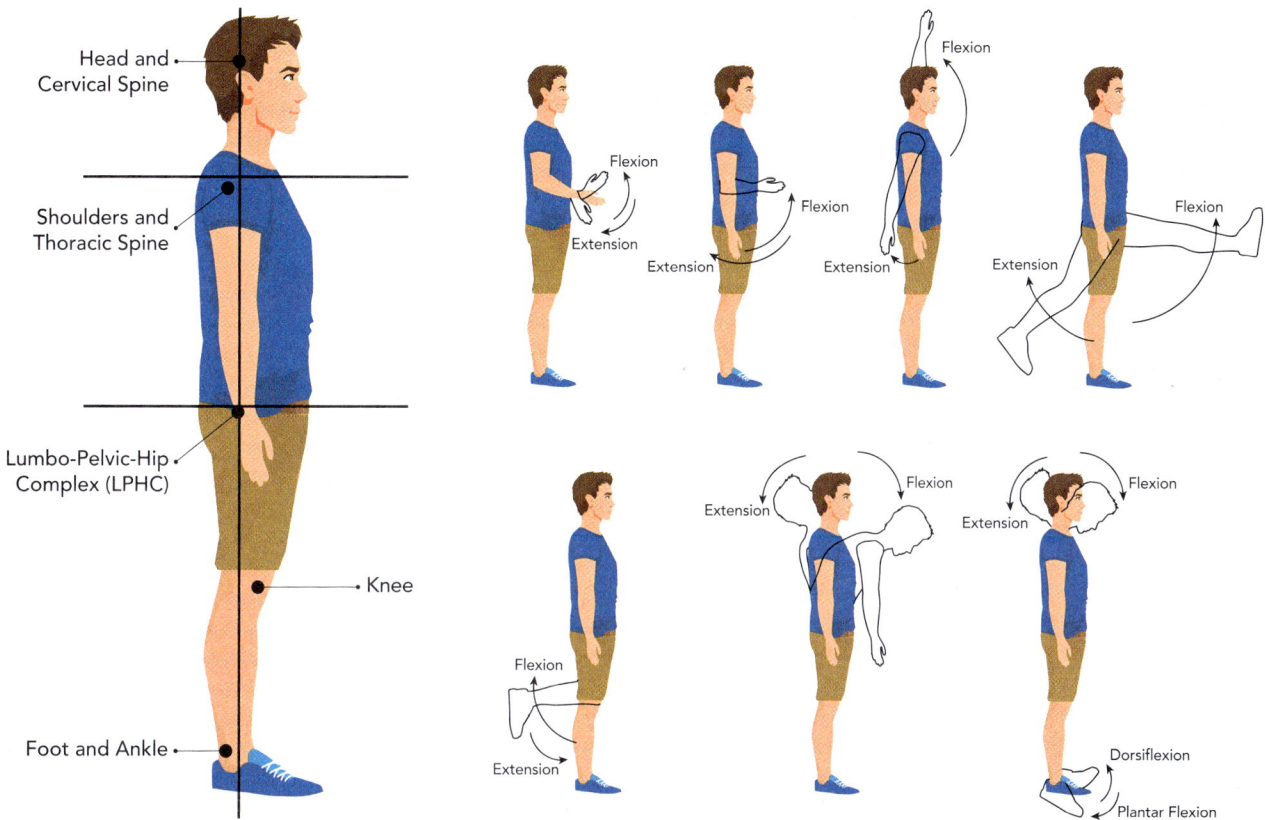

FIGURE 5.5 Joint Motions: Lateral View

muscles that surround the joint, each joint will have varied functions and mobility. Some joints, such as those in the skull, do not move and have limited function. Other joints provide a variety of movements that allow the human body to complete action in all three planes of movement. These are the joints that fitness professionals should know. For example, ball-and-socket joints such as the shoulder allow the arm to move in all three planes. This mobility helps the body to perform several tasks that require a large range of motion, such as throwing, pulling, pushing, lifting, and holding.

Once again, note that understanding these basic joint motions will help you plan effective classes. It is important to understand the role of balance between muscle groups and movement. For every flexion you want an extension, and so on. For this reason, you need to understand these basic joint motions.

The Human Movement System

Group Fitness Instructors are tasked with designing programs that engage participants and provide results. The body is able to accomplish a variety of tasks based on the coordinated efforts of the nervous, muscular, and skeletal systems (**Figure 5.6**). Because these systems work together, we are able to complete familiar activities without much thought or effort, and we are able to learn new, unfamiliar activities. This section provides a brief overview of the essential systems that make up the neuromuscular system, allowing you to design classes with movement science in mind.

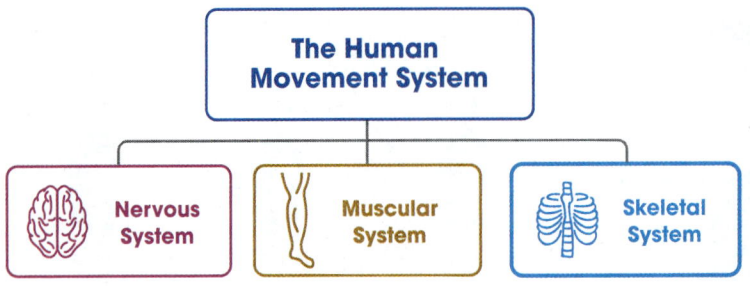

FIGURE 5.6 The Human Movement System

Nervous System

CENTRAL NERVOUS SYSTEM (CNS)

Division of the nervous system comprising the brain and the spinal cord. Its primary function is to coordinate activity of all parts of the body.

The nervous system (the brain, spinal cord, and nerves) controls, regulates, and directs everything the body does, from seemingly simple tasks such as walking, to coordinated sports performance, and everything in between (**Figure 5.7**). The **CENTRAL NERVOUS SYSTEM (CNS)** is made up of the brain, or control center, and the spinal cord, which functions as the brain's primary transmitter. The CNS gathers information from the neurons in the body, processes and integrates that information, makes a decision as to the best course of action, and then communicates this action to the proper neuron or gland.

The **PERIPHERAL NERVOUS SYSTEM (PNS)** is composed of all the neurons outside of the CNS, such as sensory neurons and motor neurons. Sensory neurons communicate what is happening in the body and in the environment to the CNS. Sensory neurons are in every muscle and joint in the body. Motor neurons control the muscles needed for movement. The CNS

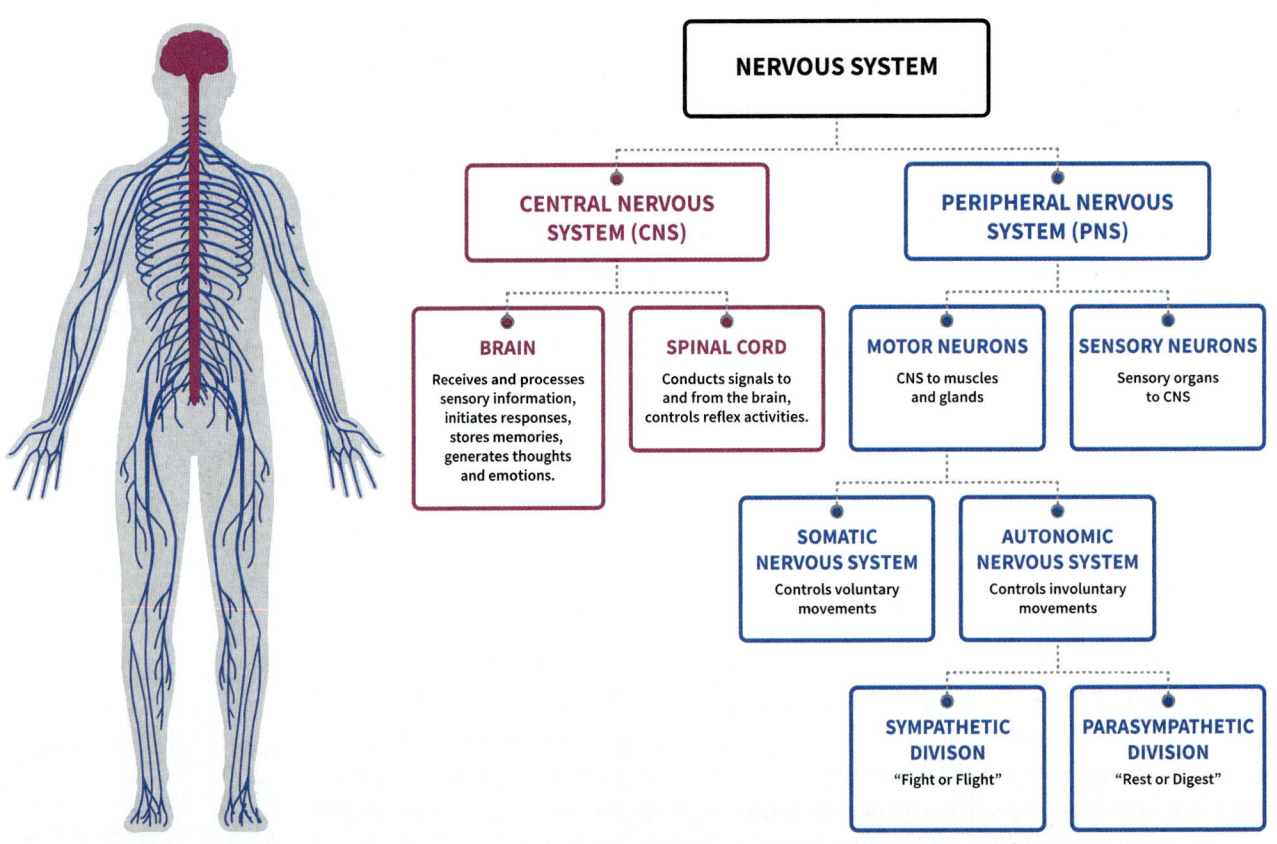

FIGURE 5.7 The Nervous System

Adapted from Piscean. (2012, October 6). Organization of the autonomic nervous system. *Pharmacology.* https://pharmacology-notes-free.blogspot.com/2012/10/organization-of-autonomic-nervous-system.html

and the PNS are in constant communication to coordinate movement. When we first learn new movements or exercises, the CNS is responsible for adjusting and refining the movements to find proper mechanics. The PNS provides several inputs to the brain about movement, the environment, and our sensations. The CNS then analyzes all that information while at the same time controlling the human movement system. Because of this, the nervous system can be trained through exercise by practicing proper movement patterns until more automatic. The PNS is critical for providing the feedback to the CNS during this process. You can see participants working through this process as they learn new exercises and moves. At this point, form and technique cues can really make a difference and help participants to develop proper movement patterns. This is also a good reminder to program enough repletion of movements to allow participants to master each move before moving forward.

Neuromuscular Control and Motor Learning

A simplified way to think about motor learning and acquiring new motor patterns is that the human movement system will get better at what it repeatedly does. The important thing to remember is that we will get better at something whether we perform it with good technique or poor technique. For example, if we repeatedly perform lunges with poor technique, we will get good at doing lunges with poor technique! This underscores the importance of coaching, feedback, and cueing to encourage participants' proper form during movement.

Have you ever noticed when learning a new exercise that it sometimes feels awkward and uncomfortable? When we are first learning an exercise, there is a lot of work being done to refine the movement. The CNS and the PNS are constantly working together to find the proper sequence of muscle firing to coordinate a movement. As we become better at that exercise, the CNS does not have to work as much as our motor neurons learn.

You will notice this in your classes as your participants get better with repetition. Keep this in mind when it comes to programming. New is not always better! If you keep some of the main exercises/moves the same, it will give your participants the opportunity to master the move. This will allow them to focus on increasing intensity instead of always working to learn a new move. This is what results-based programming is all about!

MECHANORECEPTORS

MECHANORECEPTORS are an important component of the PNS. They give the CNS information about what is happening inside the body. The three most important types of mechanoreceptors in relation to exercise are the muscle spindles, Golgi tendon organs, and joint receptors. The mechanoreceptors play a role in **PROPRIOCEPTION**, which is our sense of where our limbs are in space. Proprioception helps people learn new motor skills and refine execution of movements (Moore, 2007). You can use your understanding of mechanoreceptors when setting guidelines for static stretching and other flexibility programs. For example, the recommendation to hold a static stretch 30 seconds is because that is the approximate amount of time needed for mechanoreceptors to respond, allowing the muscle to relax and improving range of motion.

MUSCLE SPINDLES help protect the muscles by monitoring the length of the muscle fibers. Their job is to detect how quickly muscle fiber length changes. If they detect that the

PERIPHERAL NERVOUS SYSTEM (PNS)

All of the nerve fibers that branch off from the spinal cord and extend to the rest of the body.

MECHANO-RECEPTORS

Sensory receptors responsible for sensing change of position in body tissues.

PROPRIOCEPTION

The body's ability to naturally sense its general orientation and relative position of its parts.

MUSCLE SPINDLE

A receptor that senses the amount and rate of stretch in muscle tissue.

muscle is lengthening too quickly, they will relay this information to the CNS, resulting in the muscle contracting to prevent itself from tearing. Have you ever fallen asleep in class or at work? Your head falls forward as you doze off and the muscles in the back of the neck are lengthened at an alarming rate for the muscle spindles. As a result, they send an impulse to the CNS, which tells those same muscles to contract and your head snaps back up, hopefully before anyone around you has noticed! The muscle spindles also help in exercise classes. When jumping, you will naturally do a quick countermovement (like a quarter squat) before leaving the ground. This move stretches the muscle spindle and results in an automatic **MUSCLE CONTRACTION** that aids in the power produced for the jumping movement. If you were to jump without a countermove, your jump would not be nearly as high. Put simply, muscle spindles protect the muscles and also play a part in their elasticity.

The **GOLGI TENDON ORGANS (GTOS)** are located in the tendons that connect muscles to bones. The purpose of this mechanoreceptor is to sense how much tension is developed in the junction between the muscles and tendons at any given time. When too much tension is produced or develops too fast, the GTOs will cause the muscle to relax as a safety response.

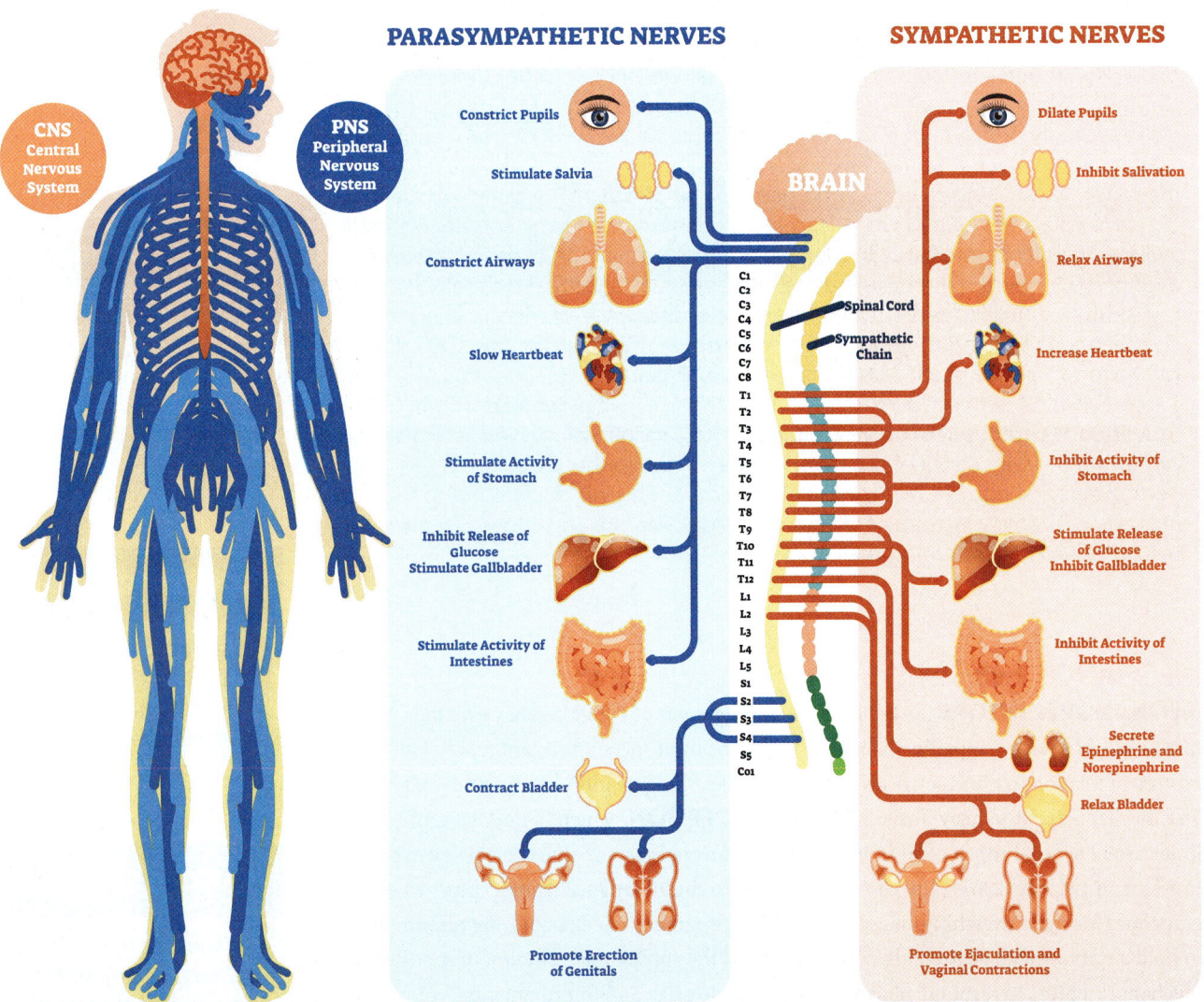

Human Nervous System
© VectorMine/Shutterstock

AUTONOMIC NERVOUS SYSTEM

The PNS is further divided into the somatic and autonomic nervous systems. The **SOMATIC NERVOUS SYSTEM** controls voluntary actions, whereas the autonomic nervous system controls involuntary actions, such as digestion, heart rate, and breathing. The movements in an exercise program involve the somatic nervous system. The autonomic nervous system will also be hard at work to adapt to the demands placed on the cardiorespiratory, skeletal, muscular, and other physiological systems of the body.

SYMPATHETIC NERVOUS SYSTEM

The sympathetic nervous system is the portion of the nervous system that activates the body's fight-or-flight response in response to a stressor. During a group exercise class, participants will experience increases in heart rate, breathing rate, and blood flow to the muscles and a decrease in non-essential functions such as digestion. The sympathetic nervous system helps to prime the body for activity and adapts as necessary to the demands of the workout.

PARASYMPATHETIC NERVOUS SYSTEM

The **PARASYMPATHETIC NERVOUS SYSTEM** helps the body return to a resting state following an increase in stress. These responses reverse all the changes from the fight-or-flight response and shifts the body into "rest and digest." Using intentional and slow breathing is one way to enhance the function of the parasympathetic nervous system and allow the body to return back to a resting state.

SOMATIC NERVOUS SYSTEM
The portion of the nervous system that is under voluntary control.

PARASYMPATHETIC NERVOUS SYSTEM
The portion of the autonomic nervous system that helps the body to return to a resting state.

🤖 GETTING TECHNICAL

The Nervous System in Group Exercise Programming
The movement prep (warm-up) allows the sympathetic nervous system to have time to adapt and prepare the body for more vigorous movement.

The transition (cool-down) will help increase the activity of the parasympathetic nervous system and allow participants to return closer to a resting level before leaving class. This is important because it prevents blood from pooling in the extremities and decreases the risk of cardiovascular events. Encourage participants to stay to get the benefits of the cool-down and do not forget to include this important component in your workout design!

Muscular System

The human body has more than 600 muscles of three primary types: smooth, cardiac, and skeletal. Group Fitness Instructors should have adequate knowledge and understanding of the larger muscle groups so that they can help others improve their strength and endurance. Muscles are responsible for producing force to create movement, maintain posture, and provide stability for activities of daily living, exercise, and physical performance. The muscles function in conjunction with the somatic nervous system that helps control and refine all of the body's actions.

MUSCLE ACTION SPECTRUM

When muscles contract, they develop internal tension to manage an external force. Muscle actions describe the direction of that tension as muscles move with or against the source of resistance. In most cases, this is gravity (as with body weight, dumbbells, kettlebells, weight stacks, medicine balls, etc.), but occasionally elastic resistance tools such as tubing or bands can be used to create a specific direction for resistance. Your understanding of muscle actions will help you communicate with other professionals about your programming variables and the different portions of an exercise. Most important, it can help you understand how muscles are working during the phases of any exercise.

The three types of muscle actions that are most relevant to group fitness are **CONCENTRIC**, **ECCENTRIC**, and **ISOMETRIC** muscle actions. A description of each follows:

- Concentric muscle action is when the muscles contract and shorten. This is what is visible during the upward phase of a bicep curl, for example. It is also associated with the acceleration of movement such as the upward portion of a jump.
- Eccentric muscle action is when the muscles lengthen when controlling or lowering resistance. The controlled downward phase of a bicep curl illustrates this. Keep in mind that as a muscle lengthens back out, the muscle proteins are still doing work! They are controlling the muscle as it returns to its resting length. It is also associated with the deceleration of movement such as the landing phase of a jump.
- Isometric muscle action occurs when tension is being produced but there is no change in the muscle length. For example, the postural muscles of the trunk work isometrically to keep you upright during a standing bicep curl.

👍 **HELPFUL HINT**

There is a simple way to discern which muscle action is taking place during any exercise. When the form of resistance is moving away from the floor (i.e., away from the force of gravity), it is the concentric phase of a movement (e.g., a person's body weight during a push-up, while standing during a lunge, or pushing the handles away on a chest press machine). In that last case, the form of resistance is the weight stack on the machine, and, as you perform the movement, the stack moves away from the floor. Conversely, when the form of resistance moves toward the floor, that is the eccentric phase of a movement.

Elastic tools create the direction of resistance within themselves. The concentric portion of a movement corresponds to when the band or tubing is lengthening and the eccentric portion to when the band or tubing is shortening.

MUSCLE ORGANIZATION

Our muscles are constantly working throughout the day. Even now, the muscles in your body are maintaining your posture, moving your eyes, and helping you turn the pages or scroll down a screen. The unique structure of muscle allows it to function like no other tissue in the body (**Figure 5.8**).

In some ways, a muscle cell is much like the other cells in the body, with a cell membrane, nuclei, specialized organelles, and cytoplasm. A skeletal muscle cell is also called a muscle fiber. These cells are multi-nucleated (i.e., have more than one nucleus) and have a threadlike appearance. What makes muscles special is that they are made up of long, thin proteins that are organized together in bundles that run parallel to each other and are surrounded by connective tissue. This allows the muscles to all work together when needed and gives our muscles properties that allow for movement.

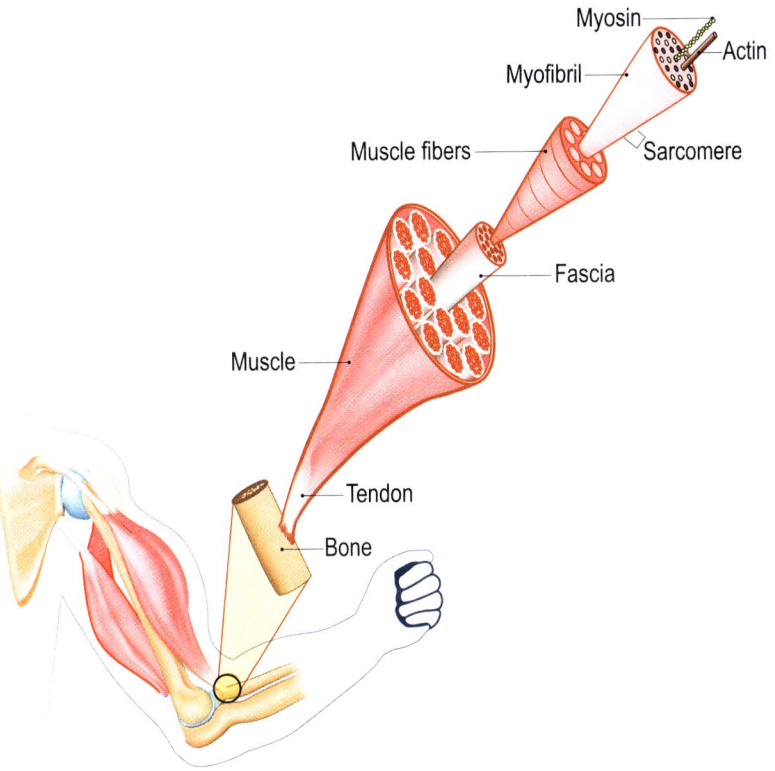

FIGURE 5.8 Skeletal Muscle
© Designua/Shutterstock

The smallest functional unit of a muscle is the **SARCOMERE**. These are made up of long proteins called actin and myosin. When the muscle receives a signal from the nervous system to contract, these two proteins interact to produce movement. The thicker myosin filaments attach to the thinner actin filaments and pull them close to the center of the sarcomere. This causes the muscle to shorten in length, producing the muscle contraction (shortening) visible with any movement. Each individual muscle cell has several sarcomeres arranged end to end for the length of the fiber. These work together when a muscle is stimulated by the nervous system.

The sheer number of muscles and the endless options for human movement might seem overwhelming to you. As a Group Fitness Instructor, you should have basic knowledge of the primary muscles used for exercise and activity so that you can plan your programs with an understanding of what muscles you will be training with each exercise and movement. The primary movers of a movement are referred to as the **AGONISTS**. Here are some examples: the biceps brachii is the agonist for a bicep curl, the pectoralis muscles are the agonists for a push-up, and the quadriceps are the agonists in a squat. The more you understand these agonists and how they function, the better you will be at designing unique and effective programs for your class. The muscles on the opposing side of the joint of movement are the **ANTAGONISTS**, and this group of muscles must relax (lengthen) to allow the agonist to contract (shorten).

Anatomy is the study of the various structures in the body, including muscles. Functional anatomy is the study of not only where the muscles are structurally, but how they work synergistically to create movement and produce, reduce, or stabilize forces in the body. Becoming more familiar with the structure and function of muscles, bones, and joints will help you develop effective and results-driven programming. If you understand how the body produces movement and how it handles external and internal forces, you can plan safe workouts that improve

SARCOMERE

Individual contractile unit of muscle made up of actin (thin) and myosin (thick) filaments.

AGONIST

Muscle that works as the prime mover of a joint exercise.

ANTAGONISTS

Muscles that oppose the prime mover.

strength, endurance, or performance. You can also effectively target muscle groups as indicated by your exercise format. It is important to understand muscle anatomy, and in particular how muscles on either side of a joint work together (i.e., opposing muscle groups). This will help you design programs that encourage muscle balance, reduce injury risk, and set the stage for long-term participation in physical activity (**Figure 5.9** and **Table 5.3**). Keep in mind that an ideal program will have equivalent demands placed on both sides of a joint over time (it does not always have to be in that same workout). Avoid focusing on the mirror muscles on the anterior side of the body and neglecting the posterior side of the body, which would result in poor posture, compromised movement quality, and increased risk for overuse injuries.

As noted earlier, the principle of specificity states that the body will adapt to training based on the specific mode and intensity used. Muscle fiber types develop in response to specific types of training. Therefore, we can train our muscles to improve very specific properties of our choosing. Understanding the muscle fiber types and how they adapt to programming can help you determine what types of exercises to do, what intensity to use with training (weight selection, speed of movement, etc.), and how long to rest.

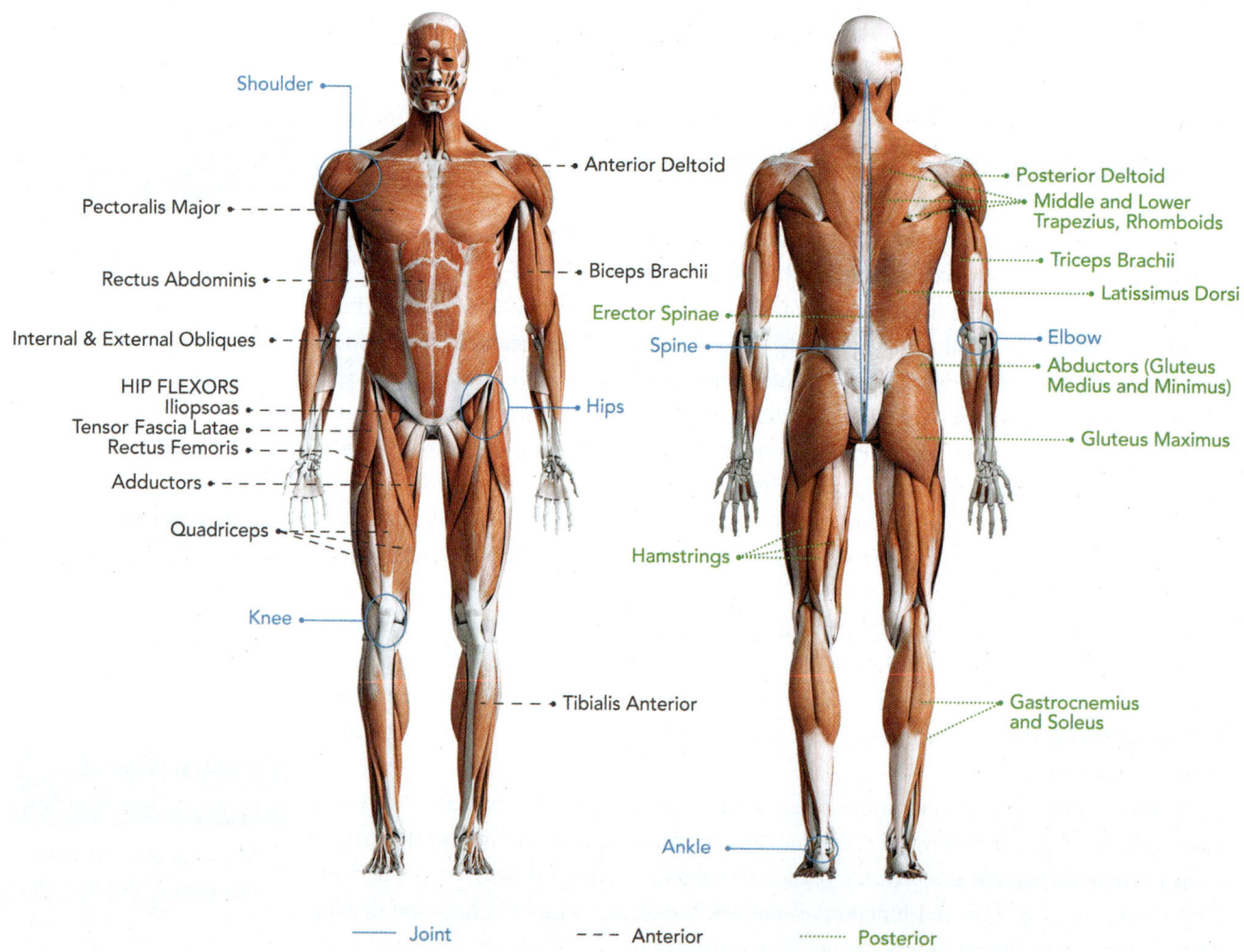

OPPOSING MUSCLE GROUPS

Shoulder

Pectoralis Major

Rectus Abdominis

Internal & External Obliques

HIP FLEXORS
Iliopsoas
Tensor Fascia Latae
Rectus Femoris

Adductors

Quadriceps

Knee

Anterior Deltoid

Biceps Brachii

Erector Spinae

Spine

Hips

Posterior Deltoid
Middle and Lower
Trapezius, Rhomboids

Triceps Brachii

Latissimus Dorsi

Elbow

Abductors (Gluteus
Medius and Minimus)

Gluteus Maximus

Hamstrings

Tibialis Anterior

Gastrocnemius
and Soleus

Ankle

—— Joint   --- Anterior   ····· Posterior

FIGURE 5.9 Muscular Anatomy

TABLE 5.3 Opposing Muscle Groups

Joint	Anterior	Posterior
Elbow joint	Biceps brachii	Triceps brachii
Shoulder joint (transverse plane)	Pectoralis major	Posterior deltoid, middle and lower trapezius, and rhomboids
Shoulder joint (sagittal plane)	Anterior deltoid	Latissimus dorsi
Spine	Rectus abdominis and internal and external obliques	Erector spinae
Hips (frontal plane)	Adductors	Abductors (gluteus medius and minimus)
Hips (sagittal plane)	Hip flexors (iliopsoas, tensor fascia latae, and rectus femoris)	Gluteus maximus and hamstrings
Knee	Quadriceps	Hamstrings
Ankle	Tibialis anterior	Gastrocnemius and soleus

 INSTRUCTOR TIP

Although a myriad of movement problems can develop, there are some patterns that are common in the general population.

The opposing muscle pairs shown in Table 5.3 work as agonist–antagonist pairs. This means that as a group of muscles contract and shorten on one side of a joint, their opposing muscles relax and lengthen in synergy to allow fluid movement. It is common for some muscle groups to be consistently tight and shortened. For example, our hip flexors are often shortened because we sit so much. This chronic overactivation and shortening is paired with chronic underactivity and lengthening of the primary opposing muscle group, the gluteus maximus. This is referred to as a muscle imbalance.

Because certain muscle groups are more likely to be tight, overactive, and shortened, you should strive to include some targeted stretches for these muscles. Stretching helps to reduce the activity of and calm overactive muscles. The following muscles are commonly tight, overactive, and shortened:

- Calves (gastrocnemius and soleus)
- Hip flexors (iliopsoas, tensor fascia latae, and rectus femoris)
- Anterior trunk and shoulder (pectoralis major, pectoralis minor, and anterior deltoid)

Muscles on the other side of those joints may be lengthened and underactive. These will benefit from isolated strengthening exercises to improve activation of underactive muscles. Common examples of such muscles include the following:

- Gluteus maximus and medius
- Upper and mid-back (middle and lower trapezius, rhomboids, and posterior deltoid)

It is common to overemphasize the muscles you see in the mirror when choosing strength exercises. Similarly, programming may overemphasize concentric muscle actions and neglect eccentric and isometric ones. It is important to train muscles through their full action spectrum: the production and acceleration of force (concentric), the reduction and deceleration of force (eccentric), and the stabilization of force (isometric). It is the equivalent of making sure your car has properly working brakes and suspension, not just acceleration. Safety and performance are both optimized when you program for balance in targeted muscle groups and muscle actions.

MUSCLE FIBER TYPES

The two primary muscle fiber types—slow-twitch (Type I) and fast-twitch (Type II) muscle fibers—are differentiated by their function and work capacity (**Table 5.4**). The term *twitch* refers to how quickly a muscle contracts when stimulated by the nervous system. All muscular contractions are fast by objective standards, but Type I fibers have a slower contraction speed compared to Type II fibers. No single muscle is Type I *or* Type II; every muscle is a mix of both fiber types. Although the proportion of muscle fiber types is largely determined at birth (you are born with a unique blend of both), most of your class participants will have roughly a 50/50 mix (Costill et al., 1976).

TABLE 5.4 Muscle Fiber Types

Characteristics	Slow Twitch	Fast Twitch	
Fiber type	Type I	Type IIa	Type IIx (also known as IIb)
Contraction speed	Slow	Fast	Fast
Fiber size	Small	Large	Large
Force production	Low	High	Very high
Fatigue resistance	Slow	Quick	Very quick
Work capacity duration	Unlimited	Approximately 2 min.	Approximately 6 sec.
Mitochondrial, capillary, and myoglobin density	High	Medium	Low
Primary energy pathway	Aerobic	Aerobic and anaerobic	Anaerobic [primarily adenosine triphosphate (ATP)]
Examples	Maintaining posture, endurance activities, and recovery during higher intensity intervals	Lifting weights and higher intensity work	Maximal effort, short sprint, and vertical jump test

Note that muscle fibers are very trainable. Certain fibers, with the right training demands, can lean toward one end of the spectrum over the other. This is how high-performing athletes can train their bodies to the point that it looks as if they were made for their sport. For example, think of the muscular composition of a fast-twitch–dominant sprinter versus a slow-twitch–dominant marathon runner. The sprinters generally carry more muscle mass than the marathon runners. This is because when Type II fibers grow larger in diameter (i.e., hypertrophy), they do so to a greater degree than Type I fibers. Indeed, training can change muscles in several ways depending on the type of activity performed. What this means to you as an instructor is that you will now have an increased awareness of how the physical demands in your class directly affect the way your participants' bodies adapt. Considering specific fiber-type characteristics will allow you to design programs that induce the specific changes that you desire from an exercise program. Is the goal to get stronger, bigger, or build endurance? Each fiber type confers different benefits to each goal.

An individual's ability to tolerate or excel at different sports and activities is related to their genetically determined muscle fiber–type distribution *and* how they train. Genetics plays a role in the types of activities our bodies naturally gravitate toward, but training variables will greatly affect how muscles respond to different types of activity. Remember the principle of specificity: how you train will determine how the muscles will adapt. In the group fitness context, think of programs as increasing the efficiency and work capacity of particular fiber types, not necessarily transforming one to another. Muscles will change the enzymes that are responsible for energy production. The following are common changes seen due to training:

- **Resistance training:** Increase in strength, power, rate of force production, and hypertrophy
- **Aerobic training:** Increase in ability to produce energy aerobically (increases in mitochondria, capillary density, and key metabolic enzymes used for energy production)

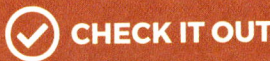 CHECK IT OUT

Type IIa fibers are also known as intermediate muscle fibers because they are a mix of Type I and Type IIx fibers. They can use both aerobic and anaerobic energy pathways.

 INSTRUCTOR TIP

Remember when you are teaching that each participant is different! Some participants will perform really well with endurance-based activities because of their genetics and training history, and they will enjoy the feelings they get, whereas others will struggle with these same exercises. Some participants will feel very uncomfortable with heavy weights or high-intensity bouts of activity. You should be aware of this so you can work to keep them engaged during these periods of discomfort. Some participants may become frustrated by this discomfort, feeling "out of shape." However, you should assure them that training is the best way to see improvements and help the body adapt to new challenges.

Skeletal System

The skeletal system provides the structure, or scaffolding, for the body (**Figure 5.10**). Bones and joints make up the skeletal system, along with ligaments, tendons, and cartilage. As the nervous system gives directions to control movement, and the muscles produce the forces that create movement, the bones of the skeletal system serve as levers that the muscles pull into action. The movement produced at any joint is dependent on the structure of that joint and the tissues that surround it.

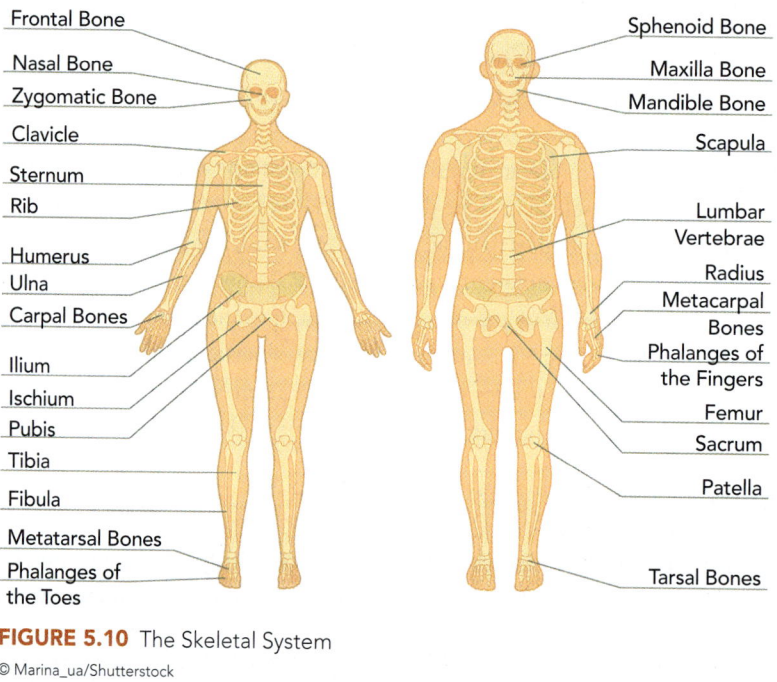

Frontal Bone
Nasal Bone
Zygomatic Bone
Clavicle
Sternum
Rib
Humerus
Ulna
Carpal Bones
Ilium
Ischium
Pubis
Tibia
Fibula
Metatarsal Bones
Phalanges of the Toes

Sphenoid Bone
Maxilla Bone
Mandible Bone
Scapula
Lumbar Vertebrae
Radius
Metacarpal Bones
Phalanges of the Fingers
Femur
Sacrum
Patella
Tarsal Bones

FIGURE 5.10 The Skeletal System
© Marina_ua/Shutterstock

The skeletal system is organized into two groups: the axial skeleton, comprising the skull, spine, and ribcage, and the appendicular skeleton, which includes the limbs, the shoulder, and the pelvic girdle. The axial skeleton is the foundation, or anchor point, for many of the large and powerful muscles in the body. It serves as a rigid structure to help with movement. The appendicular skeleton consists of the bones that get pulled into action when we are running, throwing, jumping, or dancing. The skeletal system has several key functions:

- **Movement**: Acts as levers that skeletal muscles attach to and pull to create movement
- **Support**: Provides a framework for the body
- **Protection**: Surrounds vital organs to protect them
- **Blood cell production**: Forms blood cells in the bone marrow
- **Mineral storage**: Acts as a depot for minerals such as calcium

As a Group Fitness Instructor, you will focus on the skeletal system's role in movement. You do not need to know or memorize all of the bones in the skeletal system; however, you should be familiar with the shape and location of the primary bones used in locomotion and activity. Knowing these bones will improve your understanding of various joint motions, which are dependent on the unique structure of each joint. In addition, familiarity with some of the large bones is important because you may refer to them when communicating with participants.

Cardiovascular and Respiratory Systems

Most group fitness classes will result in an increase in the eustress response from the sympathetic nervous system. Remember that this is the fight-or-flight system that results in increased heart rate, breathing rate, and blood pressure, among other changes. Because exercise and physical activity result in increased demand for oxygen and energy in the working muscles, the cardiovascular and respiratory systems must work hard to meet those needs. The cardiovascular and respiratory systems are critical for transporting oxygen, nutrients, and other important substances to the tissues in the body as needed (Table 5.5). Both systems are activated in a group fitness class as heart and breathing rates increase to meet the increased needs of muscles during movement.

TABLE 5.5 Cardiorespiratory System

System	Description
Cardiovascular	<ul><li>Includes the heart and all the blood vessels (arteries, capillaries, and veins).</li><li>Pumps blood throughout the body.</li><li>Gets rid of waste products produced as a byproduct of metabolism.</li><li>The right side of the heart pumps blood from the body to the lungs to pick up oxygen.</li><li>The left side of the heart pumps oxygenated blood from the lungs out to the body.</li><li>The arteries carry blood to the muscles.</li><li>The capillaries are small permeable blood vessels where gas exchange occurs.</li><li>The veins transport the low-oxygen blood back to the heart and lungs.</li></ul>
Respiratory	<ul><li>Includes the lungs and airways from the nose and mouth.</li><li>Inhales oxygenated air into the body.</li><li>Exhales carbon dioxide.</li></ul>

The cardiovascular and respiratory systems often are collectively referred to as the cardiorespiratory system to reflect their coordinated function (Figure 5.11). The autonomic nervous system is in control of breathing and heart rate and will adjust both as intensity changes. With regular physical activity and exercise, both of these systems will adapt in several ways to make movement more efficient and familiar.

CARDIAC OUTPUT

The average number of times the heart beats per minute is known as the **HEART RATE (HR)**, and the average resting heart rate is 70–80 beats per minute (BPM) (Brooks et al., 2004). The amount of blood pumped by the heart with each contraction is referred to as **STROKE VOLUME (SV)**. The SV multiplied by the HR, or the total volume of blood pumped out of the heart per minute, is called the **CARDIAC OUTPUT (Q̇)**:

$$SV \times HR = \dot{Q}$$

HEART RATE (HR)

Rate at which the heart pumps, usually measured in beats per minute (bpm).

STROKE VOLUME (SV)

Amount of blood pumped out of the heart with each contraction.

CARDIAC OUTPUT (Q̇)

Heart rate multiplied by stroke volume; a measure of the overall performance of the heart and the amount of blood the heart pumps over a period of time.

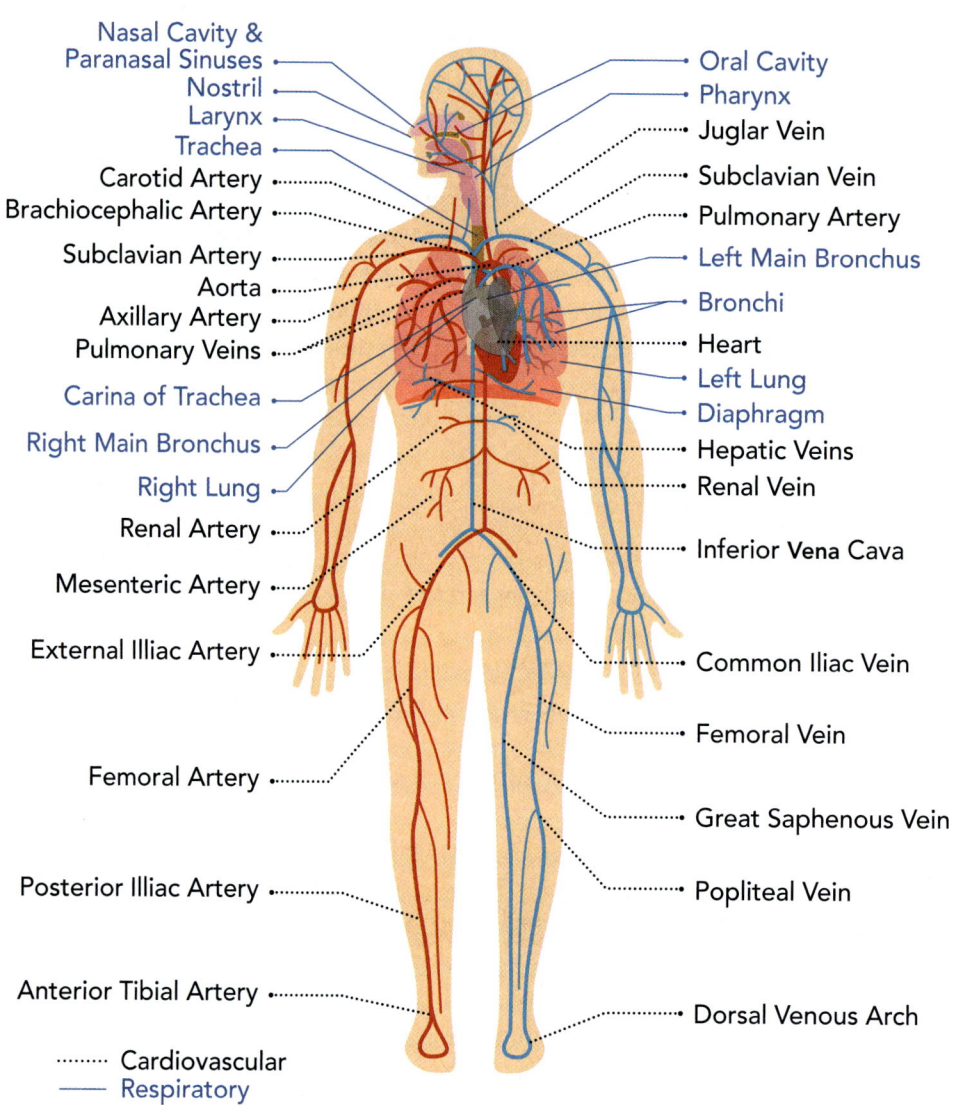

Nasal Cavity & Paranasal Sinuses
Nostril
Larynx
Trachea
Carotid Artery
Brachiocephalic Artery
Subclavian Artery
Aorta
Axillary Artery
Pulmonary Veins
Carina of Trachea
Right Main Bronchus
Right Lung
Renal Artery
Mesenteric Artery
External Illiac Artery
Femoral Artery
Posterior Illiac Artery
Anterior Tibial Artery

Oral Cavity
Pharynx
Juglar Vein
Subclavian Vein
Pulmonary Artery
Left Main Bronchus
Bronchi
Heart
Left Lung
Diaphragm
Hepatic Veins
Renal Vein
Inferior **Vena** Cava
Common Iliac Vein
Femoral Vein
Great Saphenous Vein
Popliteal Vein
Dorsal Venous Arch

.... Cardiovascular
—— Respiratory

FIGURE 5.11 The Cardiorespiratory System

In group fitness classes, you can assist your participants in determining the appropriate intensity that will help them improve their health and fitness. Heart rate is one method you can use. These specific variables will be covered in more detail in subsequent content. As a fitness professional, it is important to know that an improvement in stroke volume is just one of the many positive physiological adaptations your participants will experience.

Lesson 3: Metabolism and Bioenergetics

Exercise Metabolism/ Bioenergetics

Everything that we do requires our body to convert the food we eat into a form of energy that our cells can use. **METABOLISM** is the series of chemical reactions that take place in the body to provide this energy to the cells to keep us alive and allow vital functioning. Proteins in the body known as enzymes are the keys that allow this metabolic process to take place by catalyzing, or accelerating, the rate of metabolic reactions.

This may seem like an overwhelming concept at first, but it is essentially how the body fuels activity. Instructors who take the time to learn, understand, and apply the science will find that it not only makes classes easier to create, but it also makes them significantly more effective. Knowledge of energy systems will help you plan intelligent interval sets, understand and explain the importance of building endurance, and give context to provide specific cues about the way participants should feel during varying levels of intensity. In short, this knowledge removes some of the guesswork and replaces it with the science of achieving results.

Although it is not necessary to fully comprehend the specific complexities of the chemical processes involved, it is helpful to understand the fundamentals as they directly relate to such things as the appropriate length of recovery from certain types of efforts and why muscles have a burning sensation at higher levels of intensity. Equipped with the basic knowledge of these principles, you can deliver classes that are both challenging *and* effective.

AEROBIC VERSUS ANAEROBIC ENERGY PATHWAYS

Although the terms *aerobic* and *anaerobic* may be familiar to most instructors, it is important to understand what they really mean when it comes to creating intensity and designing classes. To deliver well-rounded, results-oriented classes, in addition to being familiar with the terms, it is important that you know why and when each metabolic pathway (how the body utilizes fuel for energy) is used.

The term **AEROBIC** means "with oxygen," and refers to those metabolic processes that require oxygen in order to produce energy. Conversely, the term **ANAEROBIC** refers to those metabolic processes that do not require oxygen to produce energy (Allen & Cheung, 2012). This does not mean that there is no oxygen in the body; rather, it means that a particular metabolic process does not require oxygen to produce energy. Typically, aerobic exercise is associated with long, slow, steady efforts, and anaerobic exercise is associated with short, fast, intense efforts (Comana, 2019). This is not always the case, however. Consider the popular method of **INTERVAL TRAINING**. Although it is common to associate this training method almost exclusively with shorter, high-intensity efforts, in truth, the intervals can be performed aerobically or anaerobically depending on duration and level of effort. Aerobic and anaerobic exercise are both beneficial, but in different ways. The well-informed instructor should understand how and why.

The anaerobic and aerobic energy pathways that the body uses to create energy are comprised of two anaerobic energy systems and one aerobic energy system. These systems work interdependently to meet the energy demands of exercise.

Energy Systems

A general understanding of the body's energy systems (and why it matters in class design) begins with **ADENOSINE TRIPHOSPHATE (ATP)**. ATP is the chemical currency that fuels all functions of the body and all forms of movement including the varying intensities of exercise (Allen & Cheung, 2012). For every activity, from a low-intensity stretching class to a heavy set of squats, the body uses ATP to fuel it. However, depending on how much it needs and how quickly it needs it, the body produces ATP differently using three distinct but interrelated energy systems used to create energy based on physiological demand: the **ATP-PC SYSTEM** (also referred to as the phosphagen system or ATP-CP), the **GLYCOLYTIC (ANAEROBIC) SYSTEM**, and

ADENOSINE TRIPHOSPHATE (ATP)

The unit of energy created, stored, and used by the body to support all functions of living, including exercise and physical activity.

ATP-PC SYSTEM

One of the body's three energy systems. This anaerobic system produces energy very rapidly but in extremely limited amounts. It is fueled by adenosine triphosphate (ATP) and phosphocreatine. Also known as the ATP-CP and phosphagen systems.

GLYCOLYTIC (ANAEROBIC) SYSTEM

One of the body's three energy systems. This anaerobic system produces energy rapidly through anaerobic glycolysis, which uses carbohydrate as fuel to produce energy.

AEROBIC (OXIDATIVE) SYSTEM

One of the body's three energy systems. This energy system is fueled by fats, carbohydrates, and proteins and requires oxygen. It can produce a seemingly limitless supply of energy but it does so at a slower rate than the other two systems.

MACRO-NUTRIENTS

Nutrients required in large amounts in the diet; include carbohydrate, fat, and protein.

GLUCOSE

A simple sugar that is the main fuel for the body's cells. It is produced by the breakdown of complex carbohydrates.

GLYCOGEN

A complex carbohydrate stored in the muscles and liver that is used in energy production.

the **AEROBIC (OXIDATIVE) SYSTEM**. These systems take various fuel sources and convert them to ATP. **Figure 5.12** provides a high-level overview of the energy pathways and the three systems within them (one aerobic system and two anaerobic systems).

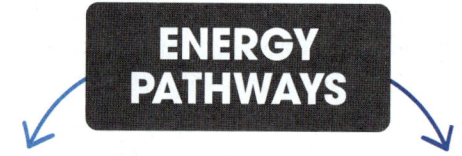

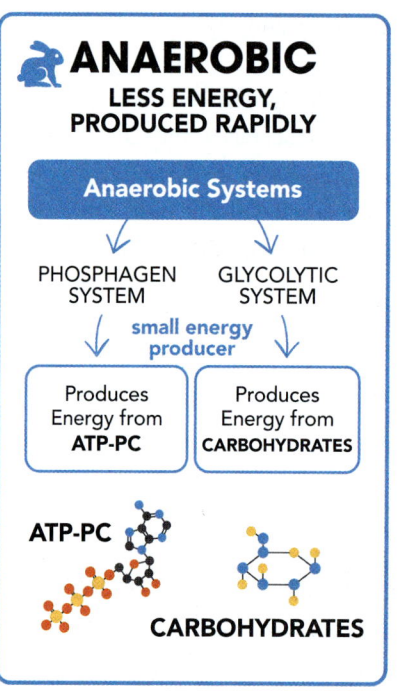

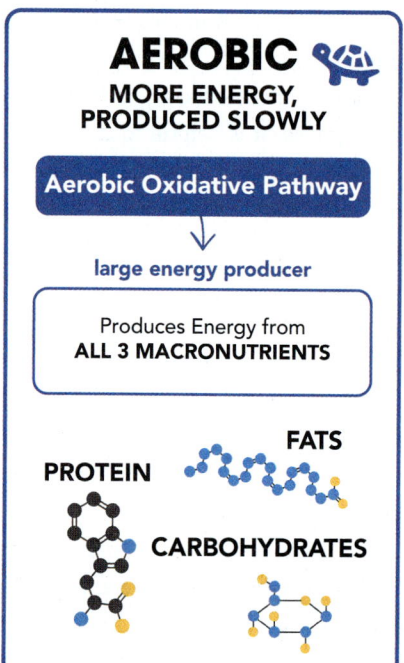

FIGURE 5.12 Energy Systems Overview

✓ CHECK IT OUT

All movement starts out as an anaerobic activity. When you first begin an exercise (no matter how easily), the anaerobic system is the first to respond to produce the initial change in energy demand. However, as the movement continues for several minutes, provided there are no major changes in intensity, the aerobic system will catch up and take over energy production until the demand changes again, such as increasing weight or intensity (Comana, 2019).

Note that the aerobic pathway produces significantly more energy than the anaerobic pathway and can use all three **MACRONUTRIENTS** (i.e., carbohydrate, fat, and protein) for fuel. It can produce an almost endless supply of energy, but it does so at a much slower rate than the anaerobic pathway. Conversely, although the anaerobic pathway produces energy very quickly, it produces limited amounts, and the only macronutrient this system uses is carbohydrates (sugars in the form of **GLUCOSE** or **GLYCOGEN**).

Moreover, the anaerobic glycolytic system comes with a metabolic byproduct (**LACTATE**) that is related to, but not responsible for, the burning sensation in the muscles that forces exercisers to stop or slow down when they go too hard for too long. These features make prolonged anaerobic energy production not only unsustainable but uncomfortable. This is important when prescribing realistic intensity levels for participants in classes. While it is not necessary to understand the scientific concepts related to the body's metabolic response (reaction to a stimulus or influence) to exercise such as **LACTATE THRESHOLD** or **ANAEROBIC THRESHOLD** in most group fitness settings, it can be useful when speaking with other professionals.

🤖 GETTING TECHNICAL

Although the lactate threshold occurs earlier in exercise than the anaerobic threshold, many fitness and coaching professionals refer to these thresholds interchangeably. For the purposes of this content, they will be referred to as the same point in the body's metabolic response to exercise demand. This threshold marks the point where the amount of lactate in the blood overwhelms the body's ability to neutralize it. Activity at this level of intensity is not sustainable for long (generally less than 2 minutes). The body's maximal *sustainable* effort will occur just below this threshold.

The lactate threshold is often used as a trainable fitness adaptation; that is, a person's fitness level can be improved by reducing how quickly the body produces lactate and/or by increasing how quickly it is neutralized in the blood. This allows the exerciser to accomplish more work at a higher intensity. In other words, the lactate threshold is the point when the dominant energy system fueling exercise becomes anaerobic glycolysis, or the activity level shifts from being sustainable to unsustainable. From a practical standpoint, participants will be breathing rapidly and have trouble catching their breath. A participant's appearance is the quickest and easiest indicator of which energy system is dominant for them. Intervals created at an anaerobic threshold are of short duration and high intensity.

Because the pathway used by the body is related to the demand and the duration of the activity, it is important to begin with the body's most immediately available energy source: the ATP already stored in the cells of the body (particularly the muscles). When the energy demands of the body change rapidly, those needs are met by the first anaerobic pathway, the ATP-PC system. For example, if you have your class do a set of high-intensity burpees, those energy needs will be met by the ATP-PC system. However, because the amount of stored ATP is depleted within seconds, the body needs another system to quickly replenish it. Using the same example, if the participant continued at that increased intensity for longer than 15–20 seconds, the body would shift into the second anaerobic pathway, the glycolytic system, to continue fueling the higher intensity (Allen & Cheung, 2012). If they attempted to continue at that high intensity for more than a minute or two, they would either be forced to stop or slow down to recover. As they recovered, the aerobic system would again become dominant until they initiated the next major intensity change. As detailed in **Figure 5.13**, energy and the primary metabolic pathways that produce it ultimately become a function of time and intensity (Comana, 2019).

LACTATE

A by-product of anaerobic energy production. Also known as lactic acid.

LACTATE THRESHOLD

The point during high-intensity activity when the body can no longer meet its demand for oxygen and anaerobic metabolism predominates.

ANAEROBIC THRESHOLD

The exercise intensity at which glycogen via the anerobic glycolysis energy system becomes an exerciser's dominant fuel source.

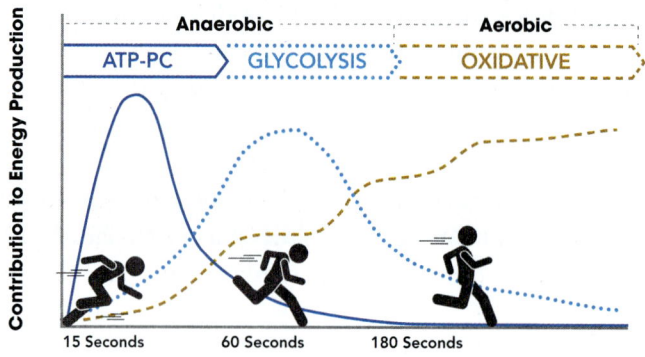

Duration of Maximal Sustainable Performance

FIGURE 5.13 Energy System Usage by Duration

⚠ CRITICAL

The activity's duration and intensity are the main determinants of which energy system is dominant. Although it is tempting to envision the energy pathways as working in a linear fashion and one at time—with one switching *off* as the other is turning *on*—this is not the case. For example, the body does not completely switch off the anaerobic system after 3 minutes. Energy pathways do not work in isolation, but rather simultaneously, with one becoming dominant but not exclusive. As energy demands shift, the dominant pathway changes in response (Allen & Cheung, 2012).

☰ INSTRUCTOR TIP

To gain a better understanding of the energy pathways at work, start by observing yourself. Although you may not have known why, you experience the effects of these systems all the time. Perhaps you feel winded walking up the stairs after being at rest, even though you know that you are fit enough. Maybe you have participated in a sport such as soccer or basketball where you had lots of rapid stops and starts. Or maybe you have trained for a longer endurance event such as a half-marathon or marathon. Did you ever participate in a class that did not provide an adequate warm-up, where you felt breathless (and miserable) instantly at an intensity that would normally feel fine? All these experiences can help you to better understand the interplay of these systems—most notably with regard to intensity and duration. They will also help you to better explain how each system feels to participants.

Remember that as a duration demand increases, intensity must concurrently decrease, and an increase in intensity shortens duration. When cueing every level of intensity, *how long* really does matter (**Table 5.6**).

TABLE 5.6 General Time Limits for Each Energy Pathway

Effort Duration	Effort Intensity	Dominant Energy System
0–6 seconds	Extremely high	ATP-PC
6–30 seconds	Very high	ATP-PC first and glycolytic (anaerobic) second
30–120 seconds	High	Glycolytic (anaerobic)
2–3 minutes	Moderate	Glycolytic (anaerobic) first and oxidative second
> 3 minutes	Low	Oxidative (aerobic)

Comana, F. (2019). *National Academy of Sports Medicine cardio programming.* [Unpublished Manuscript]. National Academy of Sports Medicine.

To summarize this information and apply it to group fitness, you simply need to remember that varying levels of intensity and duration require the body to produce energy in different ways. Each energy system has its own unique features, limitations, and benefits. When designing and coaching classes, you should strive to keep varied energy production in mind and allow it to appropriately inform the choices you make regarding class design and intensity and recovery cues.

PRACTICE THIS

To experience the energy systems in action, use a piece of cardio equipment. Start at a very light intensity and progress slightly every 2 minutes until you achieve your hardest sustainable effort. You will recognize the energy system's work by the need for intense focus to maintain the pace. At that point, begin to increase speed and or incline/resistance every 2 minutes until you find an effort that feels very intense, with heavy breathing and even more focus and noticeable burning sensations in your working muscles. Then, to complete the process, try pushing your intensity to a maximal effort that you can only hold for 10–15 seconds until you are forced by the burning of the muscles to slow down or stop—regardless of desire. Throughout the process, make note of how you feel at each stage, in your muscles, your breathing rate, and your mental focus. If you have a heart rate monitor and/or power meter, you can get even more information by watching the numbers and noting what you see at each level.

AEROBIC VERSUS ANAEROBIC PATHWAYS IN CLASS

Instructors should be aware of the goals of the format they are teaching and design classes around the desired outcome. An aerobic-focused class will have a different intensity and feel compared to an anaerobic-based class. Often, aerobic-based classes will keep a moderate intensity for the duration of the class, and the tone and cueing for this format should match that intensity. Consider the following example cues: "You should feel like the intensity is challenging, but sustainable," "You might notice a slight burning in your legs, but nothing you can't get through," or "If you are already breathless, you are going too hard and you will burn out before this interval is over."

In another example, if the class is a high-intensity interval training (HIIT) class, you want to make sure that there are portions of high-intensity bursts to train the anaerobic energy system, followed by recovery intervals to allow the participants to reset and prepare for the next effort. The cues and coaching for this type of class will also be very different from an aerobic-based class. Often at this intensity, time is very important, and you will want to inform your participants how many repetitions they will be performing or how long they will be working at that intensity. This will allow the participants to put an appropriate amount of effort into the work intervals.

Training with multiple intensities has great benefits, and having knowledge of these principles will help you create—and cue—more interesting and effective classes.

SUMMARY

Several benefits can be obtained from a single group fitness class or with continued and consistent participation. After only one workout, exercise participants will experience an improvement in mood, stress management, sleep quality, and energy. With continued participation, exercise participants will witness an improved mind–body connection, decreased risk for chronic disease, and improvement in body composition. You should understand and communicate these benefits to your participants in meaningful ways to help improve adherence.

Group Fitness Instructors and other fitness professionals must be familiar with the basic principles of kinesiology and be able to apply them to class design as well as help to answer any participant questions. This includes understanding the human movement system and how you can ensure that your classes are safe and effective for all participants. Once you understand how the body responds during exercise, you will be better able to provide effective classes that use science and not guesswork. The science of kinesiology affects every aspect of group fitness classes, from the planning stages of class design to the delivery stages with coaching and cueing. A basic understanding of how the body meets the increased physiological needs brought on by exercise helps you relate to your participants' experiences and create classes that are scientifically sound, are safe, and have clear objectives.

REFERENCES

Allen, H., & Cheung, S. S. (2012). *Cutting-edge cycling: Advanced training for advanced cyclists.* Human Kinetics.

Besedovsky, L., Lange, T., & Born, J. (2012). Sleep and immune function. *Pflügers Archive: European Journal of Physiology, 463*(1), 121–137. https://doi.org/10.1007/s00424-011-1044-0

Booth, F. W., Roberts, C. K., & Laye, M. J. (2012). Lack of exercise is a major cause of chronic diseases. *Comprehensive Physiology, 2*(2), 1143–1211. https://doi.org/10.1002/cphy.c110025

Breus, M. J., & O'Connor, P. J. (1998). Exercise-induced anxiolysis: A test of the "time out" hypothesis in high anxious females. *Medicine & Science in Sports & Exercise, 30*(7), 1107–1112. https://doi.org/10.1097/00005768-199807000-00013

Brooks, G. A., Fahey, T. D., & Baldwin, K. M. (2004). *Exercise physiology: Human bioenergetics and its applications* (4th ed.). McGraw-Hill Education.

Bryant, P. A., Trinder, J., & Curtis, N. (2004). Sick and tired: Does sleep have a vital role in the immune system? *Nature Reviews. Immunology, 4*(6), 457–467. https://doi.org/10.1038/nri1369

Centers for Disease Control and Prevention. (2022, January). *National Center for Health Statistics: Leading causes of death.* https://www.cdc.gov/nchs/fastats/leading-causes-of-death.htm

Chekroud, S. R., Gueorguieva, R., Zheutlin, A. B., Paulus, M., Krumholz, H. M., Krystal, J. H., & Chekroud, A. M. (2018). Association between physical exercise and mental health in 1·2 million individuals in the USA between 2011 and 2015: A cross-sectional study. *The Lancet. Psychiatry, 5*(9), 739–746. https://doi.org/10.1016/S2215-0366(18)30227-X

Childs, E., & de Wit, H. (2014). Regular exercise is associated with emotional resilience to acute stress in healthy adults. *Frontiers in Physiology, 5*, 161. https://doi.org/10.3389/fphys.2014.00161

Cochrane, A., Robertson, I. H., & Coogan, A. N. (2012). Association between circadian rhythms, sleep and cognitive impairment in healthy older adults: An actigraphic study. *Journal of Neural Transmission, 119*(10), 1233–1239. https://doi.org/10.1007/s00702-012-0802-2

Comana, F. (2019). *National Academy of Sports Medicine cardio programming.* [Unpublished Manuscript]. National Academy of Sports Medicine.

Costill, D. L., Daniels, J., Evans, W., Fink, W., Krahenbuhl, G., & Saltin, B. (1976). Skeletal muscle enzymes and fiber composition in male and female track athletes. *Journal of Applied Physiology, 40*(2), 149–154. https://doi.org/10.1152/jappl.1976.40.2.149

Elsenberger, N. I., Taylor, S. E., Gable, S. L., Hilmert, C. J., & Lieberman, M. D. (2007). Neural pathways link social support to attenuated neuroendocrine stress responses. *NeuroImage, 35*(4), 1601–1612. https://doi.org/10.1016/j.neuroimage.2007.01.038

Esch, T., & Stefano, G. B. (2010a). Endogenous reward mechanisms and their importance in stress reduction, exercise and the brain. *Archives of Medical Science, 6*(3), 447–455. https://doi.org/10.5114/aoms.2010.14269

Esch, T., & Stefano, G. B. (2010b). The neurobiology of stress management. *Neuro-Endocrinology Letters, 31*(1), 19–39.

Eugene, A. R., & Masiak, J. (2015). The neuroprotective aspects of sleep. *MEDtube Science, 3*(1), 35–40.

Firth, J., Solmi, M., Wootton, R. E., Vancampfort, D., Schuch, F. B., Hoare, E., Gilbody, S., Torous, J., Teasdale, S. B., Jackson, S. E., Smith, L., Eaton, M., Jacka, F. N., Veronese, N., Marx, W., Ashdown-Franks, G., Siskind, D., Sarris, J., Rosenbaum, S., Carvalho, A. F., & Stubbs, B. (2020). A meta-review of "lifestyle psychiatry": The role of exercise, smoking, diet and sleep in the prevention and treatment of mental disorders. *World Psychiatry, 19*(3), 360–380. https://doi.org/10.1002/wps.20773

Harris, M. L., Oldmeadow, C., Hure, A., Luu, J., Loxton, D., & Attia, J. (2017). Stress increases the risk of type 2 diabetes onset in women: A 12-year longitudinal study using causal modelling. *PLoS ONE, 12*(2), e0172126. https://doi.org/10.1371/journal.pone.0172126

Hirshkowitz, M., Whiton, K., Albert, S. M., Alessi, C., Bruni, O., DonCarlos, L., Hazen, N., Herman, J., Katz, E. S., Kheirandish-Gozal, L., Neubauer, D. N., O'Donnell, A. E., Ohayon, M., Peever, J., Rawding, R., Sachdeva, R. C., Setters, B., Vitiello, M. V., Catesby Ware, J., & Adams Hillard, P. J. (2015). National Sleep Foundation's sleep time duration recommendations: Methodology and results summary. *Sleep Health, 1*(1), 40–43. https://doi.org/10.1016/j.sleh.2014.12.010

Holt-Lunstad, J., Smith, T. B., Baker, M., Harris, T., & Stephenson, D. (2015). Loneliness and social isolation as risk factors for mortality: A meta-analytic review. *Perspectives on Psychological Science, 10*(2), 227–237. https://doi.org/10.1177/1745691614568352

Kim, J. Y., Han, S.-H., & Yang, B.-M. (2013, Aug.). Implication of high-body-fat percentage on cardiometabolic risk in middle-aged, healthy, normal-weight adults. *Obesity, 21*(8), 1571–1577. https://doi.org/10.1002/oby.20020

Kline, C. E. (2014). The bidirectional relationship between exercise and sleep: Implications for exercise adherence and sleep improvement. *American Journal of Lifestyle Medicine, 8*(6), 375–379. https://doi.org/10.1177/1559827614544437

Kredlow, M. A., Capozzoli, M. C., Hearon, B. A., Calkins, A. W., & Otto, M. W. (2015). The effects of physical activity on sleep: A meta-analytic review. *Journal of Behavioral Medicine, 38*(3), 427–449. https://doi.org/10.1007/s10865-015-9617-6

Laksono, S., Yanni, M., Iqbal, M., & Prawara, A. S. (2022). Abnormal sleep duration as predictor for cardiovascular diseases: A systematic review of prospective studies. *Sleep Disorders, 2022*, Article 9969107. https://doi.org/10.1155/2022/9969107

Li, A. W., & Goldsmith, C.-A. W. (2012). The effects of yoga on anxiety and stress. *Alternative Medicine Review, 17*(1), 21–35.

Li, C.-I., Lin, C.-C., Liu, C.-S., Lin, C.-H., Yang, S.-Y., & Li, T.-C. (2022). Sleep duration predicts subsequent long-term mortality in patients with type 2 diabetes: A large single-center cohort study. *Cardiovascular Diabetology, 21*(1), 60. https://doi.org/10.1186/s12933-022-01500-0

Luyster, F. S., Strollo, P. J., Jr., Zee, P. C., & Walsh, J. K. (2012). Sleep: A health imperative. *Sleep, 35*(6), 727–734. https://doi.org/10.5665/sleep.1846

Miller, K. R., McClave, S. A., Jampolis, M. B., Hurt, R. T., Krueger, K., Landes, S., & Collier, B. (2016). The health benefits of exercise and physical activity. *Current Nutrition Reports, 5*, 204–212. https://doi.org/10.1007/s13668-016-0175-5

Moore, M. (2007). Golgi tendon organs neuroscience update with relevance to stretching and proprioception in dancers. *Journal of Dance Medicine & Science, 11*(3), 85–92.

O'Connor, P. J., & Puetz, T. W. (2005). Chronic physical activity and feelings of energy and fatigue. *Medicine & Science in Sports & Exercise, 37*(2), 299–305. https://doi.org/10.1249/01.mss.0000152802.89770.cf

Padwal, R., Leslie, W. D., Lix, L. M., & Majumdar, S. R. (2016, April). Relationship among body fat percentage, body mass index, and all-cause mortality: A cohort study. *Annals of Internal Medicine, 164*(8), 532–541. https://doi.org/10.7326/M15-1181

Paillard, T., Rolland, Y., & de Souto Barreto, P. (2015). Protective effects of physical exercise in Alzheimer's disease and Parkinson's disease: A narrative review. *Journal of Clinical Neurology, 11*(3), 212–219. https://doi.org/10.3988/jcn.2015.11.3.212

Piscean. (2012, October 6). Organization of the autonomic nervous system. *Pharmacology.* https://pharmacology-notes-free.blogspot.com/2012/10/organization-of-autonomic-nervous-system.html

Puetz, T. W., O'Connor, P. J., & Dishman, R. K. (2006). Effects of chronic exercise on feelings of energy and fatigue: A quantitative synthesis. *Psychological Bulletin, 132*(6), 866–876. https://doi.org/10.1037/0033-2909.132.6.866

Schmid, S. M., Hallschmid, M., Jauch-Chara, K., Born, J., & Schultes, B. (2008). A single night of sleep deprivation increases ghrelin levels and feelings of hunger in normal-weight healthy men. *Journal of Sleep Research, 17*(3), 331–334. https://doi.org/10.1111/j.1365-2869.2008.00662.x

Spalding, T. W., Lyon, L. A., Steel, D. H., & Hatfield, B. D. (2004. July). Aerobic exercise training and cardiovascular reactivity to psychological stress in sedentary young normotensive men and women. *Psychophysiology, 41*(4), 552–562. https://doi.org/10.1111/j.1469-8986.2004.00184.x

Spiegel, K., Knutson, K., Leproult, R., Tasali, E., & Van Cauter, E. (2005, Nov.). Sleep loss: A novel risk factor for insulin resistance and Type 2 diabetes. *Journal of Applied Physiology, 99*(5), 2008–2019. https://doi.org/10.1152/japplphysiol.00660.2005

Stehr, M. D., & von Lengerke, T. (2012, May). Preventing weight gain through exercise and physical activity in the elderly: A systematic review. *Maturitas, 72*(1), 13–22. https://doi.org/10.1016/j.maturitas.2012.01.022

U.S. Department of Health and Human Services. (2018). *Physical activity guidelines for Americans,* 2nd ed. https://health.gov/sites/default/files/2019-09/Physical_Activity_Guidelines_2nd_edition.pdf

U.S. Department of Health and Human Services. (2019). *Move your way: What's your move?* https://health.gov/sites/default/files/2019-11/PAG_MYW_Adult_FS.pdf

Wang, F., Lee, E.-K. O., Wu, T., Benson, H., Fricchione, G., Wang, W., & Yeung, A. S. (2014). The effects of tai chi on depression, anxiety, and psychological well-being: A systematic review and meta-analysis. *International Journal of Behavioral Medicine, 21*(4), 605–617. https://doi.org/10.1007/s12529-013-9351-9

Wang, H., Sun, J., Sun, M., Liu, N., & Wang, M. (2021). Relationship of sleep duration with the risk of stroke incidence and stroke mortality: An updated systematic review and dose–response meta-analysis of prospective cohort studies. *Sleep Medicine, 90,* 267–278. https://doi.org/10.1016/j.sleep.2021.11.001

Williamson, A. M., & Feyer, A. M. (2000, Oct.). Moderate sleep deprivation produces impairments in cognitive and motor performance equivalent to legally prescribed levels of alcohol intoxication. *Occupational and Environmental Medicine, 57*(10), 649–655. https://doi.org/10.1136/oem.57.10.649

Yang, H.-J., Koh, E., & Kang, Y. (2021). Susceptibility of women to cardiovascular disease and the prevention potential of mind–body intervention by changes in neural circuits and cardiovascular physiology. *Biomolecules, 11*(5), 708. https://doi.org/10.3390/biom11050708

Yang, P.-Y., Ho, K.-H., Chen, H.-C., & Chien, M.-Y. (2012). Exercise training improves sleep quality in middle-aged and older adults with sleep problems: A systematic review. *Journal of Physiotherapy, 58*(3), 157–163. https://doi.org/10.1016/S1836-9553(12)70106-6

Yaribeygi, H., Panahi, Y., Sahraei, H., Johnston, T. P., & Sahebkar, A. (2017). The impact of stress on body function: A review. *EXCLI Journal, 16,* 1057–1072. https://doi.org/10.17179/excli2017-480

Zadra, J. R., & Clore, G. L. (2011). Emotion and perception: The role of affective information. *Wiley Interdisciplinary Reviews. Cognitive Science, 2*(6), 676–685. https://doi.org/10.1002/wcs.147

Zhang, X., Zong, B., Zhao, W., & Li, L. (2021, Feb.). Effects of mind–body exercise on brain structure and function: A systematic review on MRI studies. *Brain Sciences, 11*(2), 205. https://doi.org/10.3390/brainsci11020205

Zhao, E., Tranovich, M. J., & Wright, V. J. (2014). The role of mobility as a protective factor of cognitive functioning in aging adults: A review. *Sports Health, 6*(1), 63–69. https://doi.org/10.1177/1941738113477832

CHAPTER 6

TRAINING SCIENCE

LEARNING OBJECTIVES

The intent of this chapter is to provide basic training principles and how they influence participant outcomes. This chapter will also go over acute variables, integrated fitness, and how to accommodate all participant levels through modification.

After reading this content, students should be able to demonstrate the following objectives:

- **Describe** training principles and their relationship to group fitness.

- **Explain** the relationship between training principles and group fitness outcomes.

- **Identify** the various components of integrated fitness.

Lesson 1: Training Principles and Fitness Outcomes

Introduction

As a Group Fitness Instructor, you will have a variety of individuals who will look to you for guidance and motivation. Group fitness classes can be designed to support a myriad of health and fitness goals for a wide range of individuals. This opportunity—to positively influence the lives of others—is truly special. Scientific training concepts influence major aspects of class design and delivery, including exercise selection, challenge level, variety, long- and short-term planning, and more.

Classes can be developed with varying goals, ranging from enhancing athletic performance, improving general conditioning, enhancing daily function, to even maintaining independence later in life. However, these goals are all similar in that each requires change or improvement in the human movement system. By keeping these different goals in mind, you can apply scientific principles when designing long-term class objectives as well as objectives for each individual class. Training principles will also allow you to add

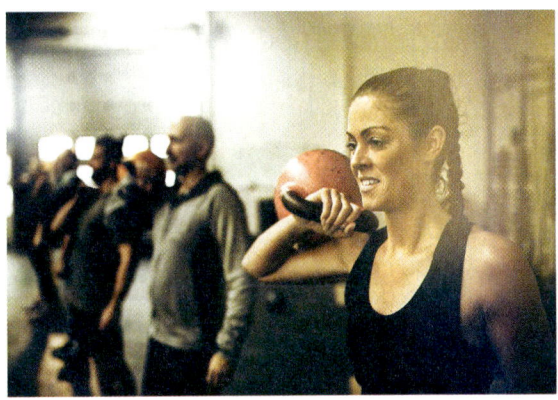

© Ground Picture/Shutterstock

variety and appropriate challenges for more advanced participants and those who attend your classes regularly.

Training Principles

No matter what format of group fitness is being taught, training outcomes can be maximized by using sound training principles when designing classes. These basic training principles will help you plan and structure a more deliberate workout.

As a starting point, you must understand that a degree of overload is required to create change. Recall that exercise is a form of eustress on the body, and fitness professionals are, essentially, "stress and recovery designers." The merging of training science, workout design, and instructor engagement benefits participants. Without science, fitness professionals would have to randomly apply stress to find proper fitness adaptations and progressions. Additionally, for specific adaptations to take place, there must be specific stimuli. In other words, to improve aerobic endurance, the training must be of appropriate intensity and duration to stimulate that adaptation.

If the primary goal is improved muscular strength, then that skill must be emphasized with appropriate resistance, rest, and repetitions. Both are excellent goals that contribute to well-rounded fitness, but it is helpful to understand that to best achieve them they must be targeted with specificity and repetition. Again, although teaching a group fitness class to the general population should not be confused with training competitive athletes, the principles of training outlined in this chapter can be applied to support variety, balance, and better results (**Table 6.1**).

TABLE 6.1 Principles of Training

- Adaptation
- Overload
- Progression
- Specificity

Adaptation

A well-planned, structured, and repeated training program will lead to long-term changes in physiology and structure. Each component of the human movement system will adapt and change in ways that are specific to the type of demands (e.g., exercise) performed. The **PRINCIPLE OF ADAPTATION** indicates that the body responds to various forms of eustress with improvements in function and performance (Fahey, 1998).

With every bout of exercise, the human movement system will have a number of short-term responses. Each system in the body will respond in unique ways to meet the demands of the exercise being done. These acute responses vary depending on the type of workout but can include the production of hormones, an increase in heart rate, damage to the cell membrane of the muscle cells, a change in muscle tension, and many others. When the body is exposed to these responses consistently, it will begin to change to be better able to cope with the demands of exercise. Over time, these changes will result in adaptation (Hawley, 2002).

The idea of adaptation comes from research on the body's immune system performed in the early 20th century by Dr. Hans Selye (1950). His research suggested that as the body is exposed to a stressor, such as the eustress of exercise, it will go through three distinct stages that allow for adaptation to occur. The stages of the **GENERAL ADAPTATION SYNDROME** are summarized in **Figure 6.1** and **Table 6.2**.

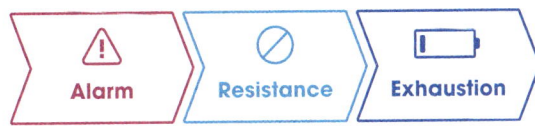

FIGURE 6.1 General Adaptation Syndrome Stages

TABLE 6.2 General Adaptation Syndrome and Exercise

Stage	Body's Response to Exercise
Alarm	Exercise performed upsets the body's cellular balance and homeostasis.
Resistance	The body adjusts to overcome or accommodate the stress (muscles become stronger, the cardiorespiratory system becomes more efficient, etc.).
Exhaustion	Adequate rest between workouts is required to allow for recovery and proper adaptation. Without this, eustress can turn into distress, and chronic distress may lead to issues such as overtraining or injury.

Long-term exercise results in adaptations that change both the structure and the function of the human movement and cardiorespiratory systems.

NERVOUS SYSTEM ADAPTATIONS

The nervous system works along with the muscular system to create movement. The long-term adaptations of the nervous system make movements more efficient. The nervous system becomes better able to stimulate force production by increasing **NEURAL DRIVE**, motor unit synchronization, and recruitment, and it works with the muscular system to refine movements so that they become more coordinated (Del Vecchio et al., 2019). This improvement in neuromuscular control makes movement more automatic and fluid. Think about a toddler trying to learn how to walk. With early attempts, the child has to work very hard to figure out how they can pick their feet up and move forward with a changing base of support. Over time, this movement becomes so natural that the child does not even think about it. This is a great example of adaptations in neuromuscular control.

The increases in strength that are evident in the early stages of exercise are largely from neural changes (Gabriel et al., 2006). Before significant increases in muscle mass occur, force production increases due to the nervous system's ability to activate the agonist muscles.

CARDIORESPIRATORY SYSTEM ADAPTATIONS

A properly designed training program results in positive adaptation and improvement in the cardiovascular and respiratory systems. The type and degree of improvement varies greatly based on the particular program's demands, but the heart and lungs generally become more efficient, resulting in an increase in aerobic endurance and power (Hellsten & Nyberg, 2015). As a result of these improvements, group fitness participants can see enhanced daily function and the capacity to perform activities of daily living (ADLs) without undue fatigue.

How the body responds to imposed demands to accommodate future application of similar stressors. Characterized by the three stages of alarm, resistance, and exhaustion.

NEURAL DRIVE

The signals from the nervous system that activate the muscle fibers.

The muscular system can adapt in several ways, depending on the type of exercise performed. Changes can include an increase in the cross-sectional area of the muscles, known as **HYPERTROPHY**; an increase in force production; or an increase in muscular endurance (Hawley, 2002; Holtermann et al., 2007; Kraemer et al., 2004). Muscle fiber types (slow twitch or fast twitch) may change to better prepare the muscle for the type of training being performed. Tendons and ligaments also increase in strength to better withstand the amount of force being transferred from the muscle to the bones (Kongsgaard et al., 2005). This all results in better muscular performance and improved physique.

HYPERTROPHY

Skeletal muscle fiber enlargement.

PRINCIPLE OF OVERLOAD

To create physiological changes, an exercise stimulus must be applied at an intensity greater than the body is accustomed to receiving.

REPETITION

One complete movement of a single exercise.

SET

A group of consecutive repetitions.

🤖 GETTING TECHNICAL

Researchers generally accept that training can change the properties of muscle fiber types within classifications, but not across classifications (Wilson et al., 2012). For example, training can influence the conversion of Type IIa to IIx and vice versa. However, it has not been confirmed that training can convert between Type I and II muscle fibers.

Overload

The **PRINCIPLE OF OVERLOAD** has been recognized for many years as a necessary component to induce change and adaptation. For the body to recognize a need for improvement, the training stimulus must be adequate and the available recovery resources must support the necessary changes. This means that the body needs to be challenged to do more than it is accustomed to by assigning a workout that is greater in intensity and/or duration than usual. The level or threshold for change will depend on several individual factors, such as the individual's current fitness level, age, health status, and genetics, as well as several social and psychological factors.

Overload can be applied by manipulating the various training variables, such as increasing the number of **REPETITIONS** (or *reps*) and **SETS** of an exercise, increasing resistance load, decreasing rest periods between efforts, increasing the frequency of training, and changing the type of exercise. In a group fitness class, this can be challenging because many of the participants will be at different levels. However, cueing, coaching, and exercise selections can be used in the group fitness class to help the participants understand how the right amount of challenge should feel.

Overload and recovery are important principles to understand as an instructor. The human body is very good at adapting if it is given sufficient reason. When the system is stressed with exercise (overloaded), it responds by becoming better able to handle that stress, which is how results are created. To get these results, however, it must also recover (Carmichael & Rutberg, 2012). Instructors should keep this in mind and coach participants to avoid going to their limit in every class, particularly over consecutive classes within a week. Eventually, there will be diminishing returns if their intensity is always high. Wise coaches will know which participants work too hard too often and will provide coaching that speaks to that. For example, if on the day following a very high-intensity workout an instructor sees one or more of the same participants in their scheduled class and has

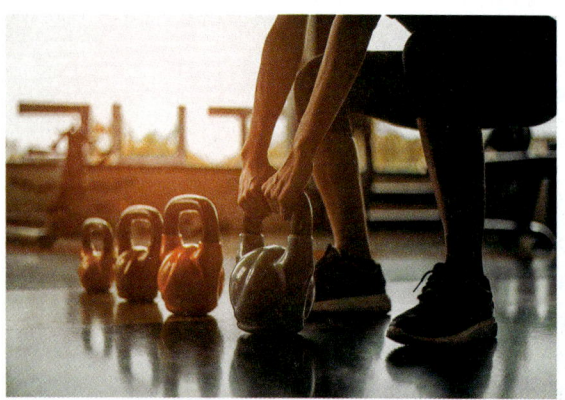

© Day Of Victory Studio/Shutterstock

another intense workout planned, their class welcome might include a statement such as, "if you were in class last night and really pushed yourself, take it a little easier today. When we perform the hard sets, avoid maxing out. You will be stronger for it next week!"

Progression

The **PRINCIPLE OF PROGRESSION** takes the concept of overload a step further and states that as the body adapts and changes in response to stress, the current level will no longer produce overload. At this point, the adaptations will decline or stop because the imposed demands no longer produce a sufficient stimulus to require change. To ensure continuous improvements, there must be an increase in the difficulty or demands of the activity (Rhea et al., 2003). Although most people think first of load or intensity to increase the challenge, progression can come from adjusting any of the acute program variables, such as altering the frequency of training, rest between bouts, the complexity of the movement, or the volume of training (Kraemer & Ratamess, 2004). Progression is a form of systematic overload that is gradual, evidence based, and encourages the body to make incremental performance improvements over time. Using proper progression will ensure that your participants do not plateau or become bored with the workout, and it will reduce the likelihood of overtraining and the incidence of injury.

Although instructors in most class settings will not have the ability to truly progress all individuals at the same rate, they should coach participants to observe and apply these principles for themselves. Your goal is to help each participant understand how to progress and regress an exercise to find the right challenge level. Offering progression options throughout class is one way to do this, along with coaching participants on how they should be feeling throughout an exercise. Progression for a group fitness participant might mean starting with attending class two times per week and working their way up to four times per week over the course of a few months. It might also mean cueing new participants to take longer recovery periods between exercise sets or intervals. A systematic approach for a new participant might be to stay for 30 minutes of a 60-minute class and add 5 minutes a week until they can do the whole class. It might also mean telling the class that each week for a month the workout will feature progressively longer intervals at the same intensity. By applying the science of progression, even at its most basic level, instructors can help guide participants to the outcomes they are seeking.

> ⚠️ **CRITICAL**
>
> Increasing load or intensity is not the only way to progress the challenge level of an exercise.

PRINCIPLE OF PROGRESSION

An option that allows the fitness class participant to increase complexity, impact, or intensity of a movement or movement patterns.

Specificity

The principle of specificity states that the type of exercise stimulus will determine the expected physiological and structural outcomes. This is also referred to as the SAID (specific adaptation to imposed demands) principle. Although there is a training effect when considering general fitness and overall health, to improve the performance of a specific activity, the more similar the training is to the activity, the more beneficial the exercise will be (McCafferty & Horvath, 1977). For example, a participant who plays tennis would benefit from exercises that use rapid changes in direction or speed.

The principle of specificity means that if an individual is seeking a specific result, then they must train for it. In the case of group fitness, this means that if a person wants to improve one component of fitness, then they should focus on doing exercises that challenge those systems of the body. An instructor can support that process by sharing the benefits of each type of exercise or class and reminding participants that if they want to get better at it, then they will have to focus on it, even if it is not easy for them. In practice, it might sound something like this: "This next exercise is going to help improve your core muscular endurance. If you want to improve your endurance, then you want to make sure to really challenge yourself and hold as long as you can. When we push ourselves with this exercise, we will improve our core stability and keep our posture muscles strong!"

An important consideration of this training principle is that only the muscles that are trained will adapt, emphasizing the need to train all the muscles in the body and use multiple planes of motion (Kraemer et al., 2004). Each component of the human movement system will adapt to the demands in unique ways. Adaptations will include both structural (physical) changes and physiological (functional) changes. The body will adapt and respond to the specific biomechanics, neuromuscular recruitment, and metabolic pathway required by the activity (Coyle et al., 1981; Cronin et al., 2002; Hawley, 2002; Tesch et al., 1989) (**Table 6.3**).

You can use the principle of specificity to plan effective classes that enable the participants to reach the goals set forth in the class title or description. Your participants will better know what to expect when they come to your class, and they will keep coming back when they achieve the results that they are looking for.

TABLE 6.3 Specific Adaptations to Exercise

Type of Adaptation	Description
Biomechanics	Refers to the joint actions performed and plane of motion. For example, to improve an older adult's ability to climb stairs, they should improve single-leg hip and knee extension in the sagittal plane.
Neuromuscular	Refers to specific movement patterns performed and the speed of movement as they are completed. For example, to improve jump height, it is important to train the muscles of the lower body to work together to produce force quickly.
Metabolic	Refers to the energy demand placed on the body. For example, to improve aerobic endurance, long-duration activities of low to moderate intensity should be performed.

Planning for Fitness Training Outcomes

With the principles of training in mind, the fitness professional can look toward understanding the various goals and adaptations that are expected from group fitness classes. Regardless of class format type, understanding how to apply these fundamental principles will help you design more effective and engaging classes that will yield real results for participants.

With proper programming and consistent participation, the body will improve in multiple dimensions. The outcomes that participants seek can be classified as one or more fitness training outcomes. Whether the individual's goal is improved general fitness, body composition change, or sport-specific performance, the human movement and cardiorespiratory systems will become **CONDITIONED** based on the physical activity performed. This means they will be better able to perform activities that are related to that fitness component.

You can design workouts, tailor your class recommendations, and be more effective with coaching and motivating participants if you know their goals. You should be familiar with the differences between endurance and strength, and consider how you can modify your class design to focus on developing one over the other or both in combination. With a thorough understanding of the fitness outcomes that can be gained through group fitness, you will be both effective and confident.

Endurance

ENDURANCE refers to the ability to sustain a given effort for an extended period or to resist fatigue. By improving endurance, the body is better able to withstand submaximal effort for a longer duration (Hughes et al., 2018). Metabolically speaking, this taps into aerobic energy production and relies on the body's ability to provide a constant stream of adenosine triphosphate (ATP) that is being produced as needed. The adaptations seen with endurance training enhance the cardiorespiratory system by increasing capillary density, the number and size of mitochondria, and the efficiency of the heart and lungs, and improving circulatory function (Joyner & Coyle, 2008). Endurance is needed for everyday function because most of us are moving at a submaximal level for the majority of the day. As endurance improves, we become better able to complete the things that we *need* to do every day and still have adequate energy left over to pursue the things that we *want* to do. Improved endurance can make a huge functional difference in your participants' overall wellness.

Endurance-based group fitness classes combine low- to moderate-intensity effort for an extended duration. The combination of the level of effort (intensity) and length of the work (duration) is used to provide sufficient overload to the cardiorespiratory and human movement systems. Beginners should start with a lower level of intensity and can be coached to maintain a challenging but doable effort for the class. As participants progress, you can coach them to increase either intensity or duration. This can look like, "If you've been coming for a while and you're ready for an extra challenge today, let's try to push our pace a little faster for this section."

Endurance-based classes can be either cardio or muscular endurance based. With cardio-based endurance, the effort will be relatively similar throughout the class, and you will keep participants at a level that they can maintain. With muscular endurance–based classes, the weights lifted will allow for a high number of repetitions and give a small amount of recovery between sets. Resistance can come from equipment or even body weight with these classes. Keep in mind that endurance training is only one aspect of class design; strength and/or other goals can be interspersed in the workout at different points should that align with the class's purpose. This can meet participants' functional needs because both endurance and strength are needed in daily activities.

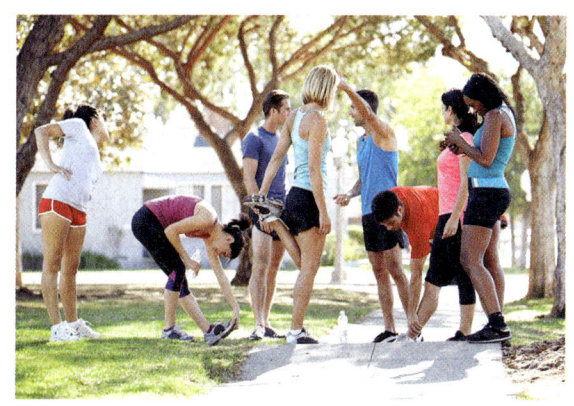

© Monkey Business Images/Shutterstock

CONDITIONED

A state in which the body has proportionately adapted to imposed demands through practice and repeated exposure.

ENDURANCE

The ability to sustain a given effort for an extended period of time or to resist fatigue.

Strength

Unlike endurance, strength improvements require effort, usually of higher intensity, in overcoming an external force over a short duration of time. Strength is a paramount health-related component of fitness because it is what allows us to carry out everyday tasks, maintain work capacity, and improve our durability (National Institute on Aging, 2020; Pimenta et al., 2019). **STRENGTH** is defined as the ability of the neuromuscular system to produce force or the maximal amount of force that can be generated. Every time we pick up and move an object, we must have adequate strength to overcome the force of gravity. With aging, there is a selective loss of Type II muscle fibers, which contribute to strength and high force production. This highlights the importance of strength training later in life to help maintain independence, reduce the chance of falling, and maintain quality of life (Sherrington et al., 2019; Spirduso, 2001).

Adaptations that improve strength involve both the nervous system and the muscular system. When an individual begins a training program, strength increases rapidly as the nervous system learns the needed movement pattern and coordinates muscular recruitment to produce force (Folland & Williams, 2007). Strength can continue to increase as the muscles become larger (hypertrophy) if there is progressive overload, adequate recovery, and nutrition to support it. This overload can be accomplished using low-to-moderate repetition ranges and moderate-to-heavy loads *for that individual* and that muscle group (Kraemer & Ratamess, 2004). The appropriate load and repetition ranges for each individual will change over time, emphasizing the importance of progression and continual challenge by manipulating exercise variables such as volume, complexity, and exercise selection.

Group fitness formats that improve strength will often use resistance training that includes body weight or equipment such as barbells, dumbbells, kettlebells, and other tools. However, several other class formats can include strength as a component, such as a yoga class that includes strength-building poses or cycle classes that have drills with heavy resistance and a slow cadence.

Neuromuscular Efficiency

The nervous system and muscular system work together to control movement. When an individual is first learning a new movement, they might make a lot of errors, and the movement may feel very difficult and shaky and require their attention. Luckily, the body can adapt to demand by improving the communication and cooperation between these two systems. With each repetition, the nervous system will refine and improve its control of the muscular system, and the muscles used will improve in work capacity and coordination. **NEUROMUSCULAR EFFICIENCY** is the ability of the neuromuscular system to enable muscles to efficiently work together in all planes of motion. This adaptation allows the muscles to produce the appropriate amount of force in the desired direction, smoothing out the movement, and making it feel effortless. This adaptation takes place earlier than morphological changes, such as an increase in muscle mass, and these account for the early improvements in strength and performance when an exercise program is established. Many of those new to exercise often feel that their strength takes a big jump in the first weeks of starting class.

In group fitness, new participants will often be working hard to not only keep up with the fitness components of class, but also to learn the movements being performed. You can help new participants by keeping an eye on them (often those in the back of the class), modeling the new exercises with proper form, and using cues that will help them to learn the new movement. These cues should describe how the exercise should look and feel and help to prevent common errors (**Table 6.4**) that might occur when learning a new exercise. A new participant can then use this feedback to help refine the exercise and become more efficient.

STRENGTH

The ability of the neuromuscular system to produce force; the maximal amount of force that can be produced.

NEUROMUSCULAR EFFICIENCY

The ability of the neuromuscular system to enable all muscles to work in a coordinated manner in all planes of motion.

TABLE 6.4 Common Movement Errors in Group Fitness Classes

Movement Type	Common Errors	Helpful Cues
Upper body pushing and pulling	Shoulders elevate (move toward ears) Shoulders round forward Head juts forward	"Keep your shoulders away from your ears as you push." "Keep the shoulders down and back as your elbows come back toward your body" "Try to put your shoulder blades in your back pocket as you pull." "Keep your chin back."
Lower body squatting and lunging	Knee valgus (caves in) Heel rises off the floor Feet turn out (often seen with knee valgus)	"Keep your knees in line with your toes." "Push with your whole foot." "Keep your feet pointing forward."

Power

When it comes to improving performance, power is an important training outcome that cannot be overlooked. **POWER** is the amount of force produced in a specific amount of time and is dictated by how quickly the muscles can develop force. Power can be increased by lifting the same amount of weight in less time or by lifting more weight in the same amount of time. Strength has a direct effect on power and should be considered a prerequisite to power training.

Power is important for athletes performing sports skills because, quite often, how quickly a move can be done effectively will determine how successful an athlete is in the sport. However, power is also important in everyday life when thinking about quickly reacting to our environment. A good example is a reaction to a loss of balance. It is not only important to have the strength to catch your body weight but also to be able to respond quickly enough with enough opposing force and do so before falling to the ground.

Power can be improved by training with a low-to-moderate amount of resistance and fast velocity. The method used to improve power must include a speed-based or reduced-time component in order for the nervous and muscular systems to make the appropriate adaptations. Typical exercises that increase power are plyometrics and other forms of jump training. However, no special exercises are required, because performing multiple strength or endurance-based exercises can improve power if they are done with the right velocity and technique.

Group exercise classes that have power as a component include kickboxing, cycling, high-intensity interval training (HIIT), and many strength-based classes. Beginners should focus on building a base of strength and learning proper form before increasing intensity via velocity. Those who wish to improve their power should be encouraged to move with explosive but controlled efforts within a safe range of motion, which will depend on the exercise and format.

Flexibility

Flexibility is a health-related component of fitness, which means that it affects wellness, function, and overall quality of life. The terms *flexibility* and *stretching* are often confused. **FLEXIBILITY** has been defined in scientific literature as the physical feature responsible for

> **POWER**
>
> The amount of force produced in a given amount of time.

> **FLEXIBILITY**
>
> The present state or ability of a joint to move through a range of motion.

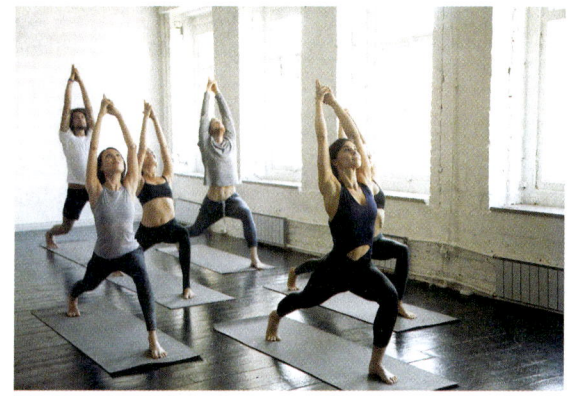
© Fizkes/Shutterstock

voluntary movement through a person's available joint range of motion without injury and within a person's normal structural limits (Dantas et al., 2011). Thus, the term *flexibility* generally refers to the present state or ability of a joint to move through a range of motion. **STRETCHING**, in contrast, is an active or passive process to elongate muscles and connective tissues to increase that present state of flexibility. Stretching is a form of training that improves flexibility.

⚠ CRITICAL

It is essential to keep the following training principles in mind when developing stretching programs to enhance flexibility:

- **Adaptation:** Each stretching session will result in short-term improvement in the extensibility of the muscles. Although this improvement does not last long, a properly structured long-term flexibility program will induce chronic increases in flexibility of the targeted muscle (Depino et al., 2000; Meideiros et al., 2016; Sainz de Baranda & Ayala, 2010).
- **Specificity:** Only the muscle groups that are stretched will improve in flexibility; thus, it is recommended to stretch all the major muscle groups at least two times per week. As an instructor, it is important to plan stretches that affect the muscle groups that are trained during that group fitness class.
- **Overload:** Use a proper intensity when stretching to ensure that benefits are received. This includes stretching to the point of tension but not pain. You want to cue this properly with your classes to ensure that your participants reap the benefits without increased injury risk.
- **Progression:** Flexibility, like the other components of fitness, will result in adaptation to the exercises completed. If continued flexibility work is desired (within safe limits), flexibility may be progressed by using a different tool for self-myofascial techniques, increasing the time spent performing the exercises, or progressing to a group fitness class that is designed specifically to improve flexibility.

Lesson 2: Acute Training Variables

Acute Program Variables

You will use the training principles just described to plan and design workouts and group fitness programs. Each individual workout should be structured in a manner that will produce short-term responses during and after the workout that, over time, will lead to adaptation. It is the short-term (or acute) program variables that will ultimately drive this adaptation. Fitness professionals make strategic adjustments and progressions to acute program variables to provide overload, specificity, and progression.

ACUTE PROGRAM VARIABLES are the aspects of each individual workout that fitness professionals can plan, adjust, and manipulate to get the responses they are looking for.

Put simply, program variables are the levers you pull to encourage the body's adaptation to the workouts. For example, to improve endurance, you would select variables that would stress the oxidative metabolic pathway, choosing a low-to-moderate intensity and an extended duration for the workout. To improve strength, you would select heavier weights, fewer repetitions, and longer rest intervals between sets. These short-term decisions in program design will ultimately determine how the body will adapt and change.

Exercise Selection

EXERCISE SELECTION is typically the first decision that is made when developing programming. Fitness professionals choose exercises based on the goals that they are looking to achieve and the class environment. Several factors will help determine what exercises are best for the class you are teaching, such as what muscle groups are targeted, what the goal is for the class format, and the population in attendance. For example, for a beginner strength class, consider simple, single-joint exercises that are easy to learn and low-to-moderate intensity. For a more advanced class, more technical exercises that target several major muscle groups and involve complex movement patterns that rely heavily on solid technique would be effective. In many group exercise settings, it is appropriate to have multiple options and progressions to offer to participants so that they can tailor the workout to their unique needs and abilities (with your guidance, of course!). Exercise selection is an important part of class planning.

Frequency of Training

To offer the body enough time to adapt to the selected workouts, consistency is key. This is where the frequency of training plays a role (**Table 6.5**). Quite often, this can be a variable that new participants can focus on first, because it will help set them up for success moving forward. Focusing on the frequency of training can help with setting a workout habit. As with all other variables, frequency of training should be progressed as the individual adapts and can be adjusted based on the intensity and duration of the workouts being completed. Newer exercisers do not need as much frequency as those who are experienced, and they should be encouraged to work up to a higher frequency of training as their body adapts.

TABLE 6.5 Frequency of Training: Goals to Work Up To

Fitness Component	Frequency	Notes
Cardiorespiratory	3–5 days per week	Depending on the duration and intensity
Muscular	2–3 days per muscle group per week	Can be completed as full-body training days or split between days
Flexibility	2–7 days per week	Muscle groups stretched should reflect those that are trained.

Intensity of Training

The intensity of training is arguably one of the most important acute program variables because it will determine if overload is achieved. Recall that overload is necessary to lead to adaptation, and the body will remain stagnant if this training principle is not considered. Intensity can be measured using several methods, depending on the fitness component, and should be coached appropriately, depending on the class format and goal.

CARDIORESPIRATORY TRAINING

To achieve the desired physical and physiological adaptations of cardiorespiratory overload, intensity must be adequate. The appropriate intensity depends heavily on the individual's training status, as well as the intent of the class being taught (Blair & Connelly, 1996). For a steady-state or continuous-intensity class, plan for light-to-moderate intensity. For an interval training class, you might alternate between light-to-moderate and moderate-to-vigorous intensity. All of these training modalities are relative to the individual and can be measured and coached using multiple methods that often incorporate some version of training zones. Training zones can be based on heart rate (HR), **RATING OF PERCEIVED EXERTION (RPE)**, or a talk test. Time spent in specific zones creates specific adaptations in the cardiorespiratory system and overall conditioning of participants. Training zones vary based on the population (e.g., recreational exerciser vs. competitive bicyclist) and the training objectives. Given the variability in conditioning scenarios and individual differences in cardiorespiratory response, some methods of measuring intensity and coaching training zones work better than others in group settings. Regardless of the participant's long-term goal, it is a good idea to first build an aerobic base, or initial aerobic work capacity, as a foundation for higher-intensity work (Swain & Franklin, 2002). Refer to **Table 6.6** for basic cardiorespiratory training zone categories.

RATING OF PERCEIVED EXERTION (RPE)
A subjective measurement of physical activity intensity that uses a numeric scale to rate exercise intensity.

TABLE 6.6 Cardiorespiratory Training Zones

Training Zone	Cardiorespiratory Intensity	Notes
Zone 1	Aerobic base, active recovery, and warm-up	New participants can be encouraged to work at an intensity that is challenging but doable because there are benefits from light intensity at the onset of training (Swain & Franklin, 2002).
Zone 2	Moderate-to-hard effort	
Zone 3	Hard-to-very hard effort	
Zone 4	Very hard-to-maximal effort	

MUSCULAR FITNESS TRAINING

When building muscular fitness in group settings, intensity is often expressed as the number of repetitions that can be completed for a given load with proper form and before failure. If someone is lifting for a repetition count of 10 for example, that means they are able to complete roughly 10 repetitions with that given weight with good technique and they should be fatigued, but not failing, by the end of that set. Depending on the goal of the class (e.g., strength, hypertrophy, endurance, or power), the intensity will change (Campos et al., 2002; Cormie et al., 2007; Peterson et al., 2005; Wernbom et al., 2007). Refer to **Table 6.7** for ranges related to different training goals. Note that the recommended repetition ranges represent a spectrum of fitness adaptations. For example, hypertrophy does not stop as soon as 15 repetitions are used for a set. The ranges reflect the *primary* fitness adaptation seen at those repetition counts, not the *only* ones.

TABLE 6.7 Resistance Training Goal and Recommended Ranges

Goal	Repetition Range	Notes
Endurance	15–25	The goal of training determines the repetition range used.
Strength	8–12 (lower for advanced lifters)	The correct intensity is achieved when the participant reaches the point of fatigue or loss of technique that is just short of failure at the desired repetition range.
Hypertrophy	8–12	
Power	3–6	

 INSTRUCTOR TIP

Group Fitness Instructors occasionally hear that participants do not want to appear *bulky*, so they avoid moderate-to-heavy weight selections. Remember that building strength offers a multitude of benefits for longevity and overall health. Additionally, strength training is not the only factor that goes into building "too much muscle." Factors such as genetics, nutrition habits, workout volume, hormone levels, and more all play a role in building muscle. Most participants will not bulk up and will reap tremendous benefits from improving their muscular endurance and strength. These factors vary from person to person, so participants who are concerned about gaining too much bulk may benefit from consulting with their primary care physician for individualized exercise guidelines.

FLEXIBILITY TRAINING

Flexibility can be improved by performing stretches or other flexibility techniques (e.g., foam rolling) for the desired muscle group. Stretches should be done with proper alignment, posture, and breathing, and the muscle should be lengthened to the first point of feeling tension or tightness but not to the point of pain.

Time

The amount of time, or duration of training, affects the overall volume of stress placed on the system being trained. At the beginning of an exercise program, exercisers will not need long durations because any activity above what they are accustomed to will provide overload. However, as adaptation takes place, duration volume will be an important variable in programming for continual improvements. Time is also inversely related to the intensity of a particular exercise or workout. As physical demands increase, the body's ability to sustain those higher levels of effort decreases. This is also why interval training requires both work and recovery segments to give the body's ATP-producing pathways the opportunity to catch up and prepare for the next bout of effort.

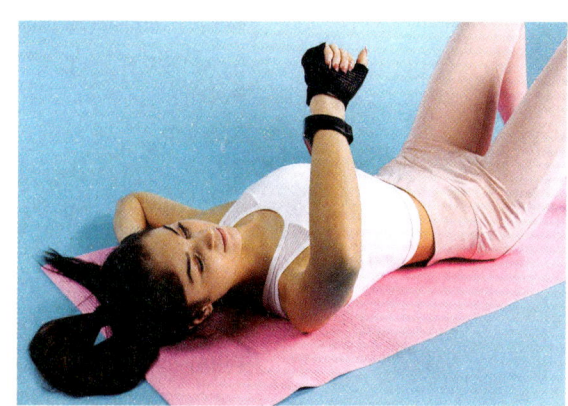

© PixelsMD Production/Shutterstock

EFFECTIVE REPETITION RANGES FOR RESISTANCE TRAINING

The number of repetitions performed during a resistance training workout will determine the metabolic and structural changes that will take place with adaptation. With higher repetitions, muscles preferentially develop endurance and will be able to delay fatigue for longer durations. With moderate-to-high loads and lower repetitions, muscles improve in strength and size. An inverse relationship exists between the amount of weight lifted and the number of repetitions that will be possible. To program effectively, you want to encourage your class to use a weight that is challenging for the desired number of repetitions to fatigue but not exhaustion. The guidelines provided in Table 6.7 can help you plan for the desired adaptations.

EFFECTIVE DURATION FOR CARDIORESPIRATORY EXERCISE

Overload and energy pathway selection are dependent on intensity and duration. Higher intensities will require less duration, and lower intensities will require more time. The two primary arrangements for cardiorespiratory exercise duration in group fitness are interval training and steady-state (continuous) training. Both have benefits for health and fitness, and, ultimately, the style of training will depend on the class format and goal.

Steady-state cardio is done at a low-to-moderate intensity that is maintainable for a long duration. At this intensity, the body will be able to produce adequate energy through aerobic pathways, and the body can clear byproducts of energy metabolism faster than, or at the same rate as, energy is produced (i.e., below the lactate threshold). A recent meta-analysis found that this style of training is superior to interval training when it comes to long-term glucose metabolism, which is a health marker for preventing or managing diabetes (Maturana et al., 2021). This style of training may be more enjoyable for some and benefit mental health and stress levels.

Interval training, in contrast, uses higher bouts of intensity interspersed with periods of the lower-intensity recovery effort. This style of training has been found to be better for improving cardiorespiratory fitness (VO_{2max}), especially in older populations (Maturana et al., 2021). It is also time efficient because significant improvements in fitness can be attained in a shorter amount of time. However, the higher intensity will create more fatigue and require longer recovery time between sessions.

Adherence is a significant factor with either form of cardiorespiratory programming. Cardio-based classes will only be effective if the participant is consistent enough to allow for adaptations. Some research has found that although interval training was more uncomfortable than continuous training, those who participated in interval training reported being more likely to continue training, which suggests that those individuals may have a higher chance of adherence to the exercise (Heinrich et al., 2014). However, for newer exercisers, steady-state cardio can be more comfortable, which may increase exercise adherence (De Feo, 2013). This highlights the fact that there is a level of participant preference that should be taken into consideration. Fitness instructors can educate participants about the benefits of both methods as well as encourage them to find an enjoyable activity they are likely to stick to.

Also note that research has found no significant difference in body composition changes between interval and continuous training (Maturana et al., 2021). Those who wish to use cardio as a method of changing body composition should choose the style that they are most likely to be consistent with and enjoy. Participant enjoyment, preferences, goals, and energy level will ultimately determine which training duration they gravitate toward. It is also a great idea to encourage participants to try both interval and continuous training because both have benefits, and using a combination can prevent boredom by providing variation in training times.

EFFECTIVE TIME FOR FLEXIBILITY TRAINING

To properly perform static stretching, the stretch is held at the first point of tension, or resistance barrier, for a specific amount of time (e.g., 30 seconds). It is theorized that this form of training improves flexibility via several mechanisms, including neural, mechanical, and psycho-physiological, but each method highlights the importance of using an adequate amount of time during the stretch.

Neurologically, static stretching of muscle and myofascial tissues to the end range of motion appears to decrease motor neuron excitability. With passive static stretching, the muscle is typically extended at a slow-to-moderate rate into an elongated position and held for an extended period (Alter, 2004; Behm, 2018; Behm et al., 2016). When the static stretch is held for a prolonged period (e.g., 30–60 seconds), the muscle spindle reflexes are less active. This allows the muscle to relax more, providing less resistance to lengthening or stretching.

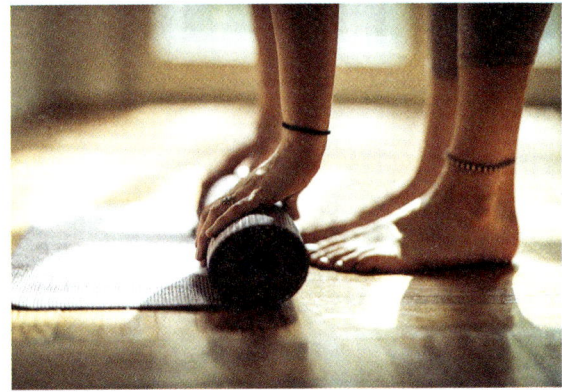

© MilanMarkovic78/Shutterstock

In addition to mechanical and neural responses to stretching, psycho-physiological mechanisms can lead to increases in stretch tolerance. Some researchers believe that stretch tolerance is the greatest contributor to increased range of motion (Magnusson, Simonsen, Aagaard, & Kjaer, 1996; Magnusson, Simonsen, Aagaard, Sorensen, et al., 1996; Magnusson, Simonsen, Aagaard, Dyhre-Poulsen, et al., 1996). The term **STRETCH TOLERANCE** means that the client or athlete can tolerate greater discomfort and then push themselves through a greater range of motion.

This effect can be psychological as the person becomes more accustomed to the discomfort as they hold a static stretch for a longer period of time (e.g., 30–60 seconds). It can also be physiological because prolonged activation of the pain receptors can decrease their firing frequency or discharge as well as signal the release of endorphins and enkephalins (opioids made by the body) that reduce pain and discomfort throughout the body (Melzack & Wall, 1965). Thus, increased stretch tolerance is considered psycho-physiological because both psychological and physiological factors may contribute.

> **STRETCH TOLERANCE**
>
> A person's ability to experience the physical sensations associated with stretching and increase their comfort at end-range.

Exercise Tempo

Exercise tempo refers to the speed at which each repetition is performed (**Table 6.8**). This is an important variable for achieving training goals such as endurance, muscle growth, strength, and power. The movement occurs at different speeds in order to get the appropriate results from the training.

TABLE 6.8 Exercise Tempos for Adaptations of Integrated Fitness

Speed	Exercise Tempo (E/I/C)	Exercise Tempo with Music (E/C)	Adaptation
Slow	4/2/1	3/1	Endurance
Moderate	2/0/2	2/2	Strength
Fast	x/x/x	1/1 or 1/2/1/2	Maximal strength, power

Slower training tempos are better for increasing endurance and initially developing motor control. A slower tempo, especially during eccentric contractions, is recommended for stabilization endurance training and when working with untrained individuals.

Tempo is specified by three numbers representing the eccentric/isometric/concentric (E/I/C) phases of an exercise (e.g., 2/1/1, 2/0/2, and so on). The first number represents the seconds for the eccentric (E) portion of the exercise. The middle number represents an isometric (I) hold at the transition point of the exercise. The last number represents the number of seconds spent on the concentric (C) portion of the exercise. The tempo x/x/x indicates the exercise should be performed as fast as can be controlled.

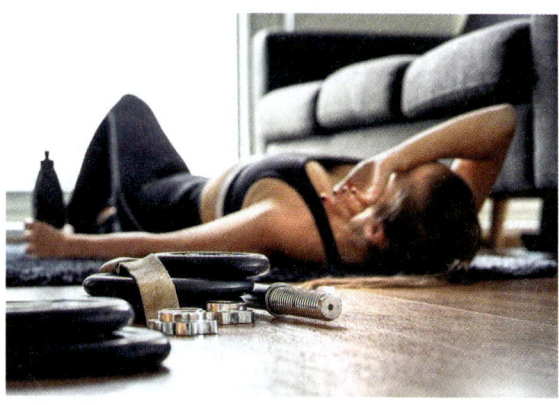

© Tero Vesalainen/Shutterstock

Rest/Recovery

A rest period is a short amount of time taken between sets or exercises to rest or recover. The length of the rest period can influence the adaptations and response to exercise. Rest periods are directly related to bioenergetic pathways and energy production and are indirectly related to load and **TRAINING INTENSITY**. Exercises at a lower intensity can be performed for longer periods of time because the body is able to use aerobic energy pathways and, therefore, does not require as much rest to recover. When exercises are performed at a much higher intensity for shorter periods of time, anaerobic energy production may not meet the demand, stores are quickly depleted, and the body will require longer rest periods.

 INSTRUCTOR TIP

Because rest and intensity are inversely related, an easy way to plan for rest is to think about how hard you want your participants to work during the next bout of exercise. If a higher intensity is demanded in the next bout of exercise, such as a sprint or the use of heavier weights, it makes sense to plan for a longer active recovery set (or rest) to allow preparation (physically and mentally) for the push ahead. Offering participants a time frame for the work ahead or the rest also will help them place adequate focus on both rest and the subsequent effort.

Lesson 3: Integrated Training Concepts

Integrated Training Concepts

Integrated fitness is a comprehensive approach that combines multiple types of exercise to help a participant achieve higher levels of function, conditioning, and resistance to injury (**Infographic 6.1**) (Sutton, 2022). Some class formats will emphasize one or two specific

1   MOVEMENT PREPARATION

Movement preparation is often used interchangeably with warm-up, but it carries a more specific purpose for the upcoming workout. A general warm-up can be a few minutes of walking or jogging to increase heart rate, body temperature, and breathing rate to prepare for increased work. Movement prep incorporates elements of a warm-up with targeted exercises to get you ready for how you'll be moving. Movement prep includes exercises targeting flexibility, core activation, balance, and plyometric training related to the movement demands and patterns of the workout and format.

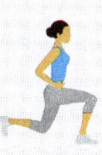

2   CORE TRAINING

All movement begins with the core and trunk. Adequate core activation harnesses the full strength of our prime movers. Core training can occur anywhere in the workout, but it can be especially helpful early on to "wake up" (but not fatigue) core muscles in preparation for more intense movement demands.

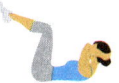

3   BALANCE TRAINING

Balance training uses slightly unstable (and controllable) stances to improve how well the body reflexively maintains its equilibrium. Balance training reinforces the communication between the nervous and muscular systems to recruit the right muscles, at the right time, with the right amount of force. Balance training can be easily incorporated by using narrow or single-leg stances while performing exercises.

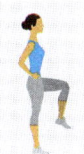

4   PLYOMETRIC TRAINING

Plyometric training enhances the speed at which motor units are recruited. It teaches the body to quickly respond to the changes in the environment that we encounter during functional activities at realistic speeds. Plyometric training can be used as part of movement prep or in the body of the workout depending on the format and demands of the class.

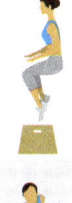

5   SAQ TRAINING

Speed, Agility, and Quickness (SAQ) training teaches the body to quickly change direction, produce speed in multiple directions, and quickly accelerate and decelerate. Drills that use cones, low hurdles, or ladders are common in SAQ training. These can be used to improve conditioning and inject a little fun into classes and as part of movement prep or body of the workout.

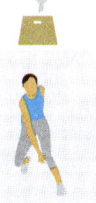

6   CARDIORESPIRATORY TRAINING

Cardiorespiratory training creates foundational aerobic work capacity along with conditioning for higher-demand activities and energy systems. The benefits are numerous and are not limited to weight management, reduction of cardiovascular risk factors, stress management, and overall performance.

7   RESISTANCE TRAINING

Resistance training is an integral part of maintaining health and overall physical capacity, injury risk reduction, self-efficacy, and self-confidence. Resistance training programs should be carefully planned and progressed to match your participants' current capabilities to your class format's objectives. Numerous training systems can be used to create a workout and multiple human movement system adaptations can be yielded including stabilization, endurance, strength, muscle growth (hypertrophy), and power.

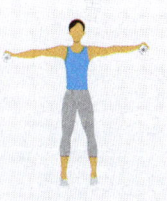

INFOGRAPHIC 6.1 Components of Integrated Fitness

components, whereas others may balance multiple integrated fitness components. Training components include the following:

- Cardiorespiratory
- Flexibility
- Core
- Balance
- Plyometric
- Resistance
- Speed, agility, and quickness (in some instances)

FUNCTION is an important component of an individual's everyday performance. Integrated fitness addresses function with a well-rounded approach that meets everyday movement needs. Integrated training sets the stage for multiple fitness adaptations that benefit our longevity, work capacity, movement quality, and resilience. Group fitness classes do not leave a lot of room for instructors to offer as much individualized attention as they might like while teaching. Due to this, it is important to be mindful of the various levels of fitness that may be in attendance. As an instructor, it is essential to offer options (i.e., progressions) for difficult exercises while also using language that withholds judgment. Group fitness instruction requires knowledge of how to make exercises less (regress) or more (progress) challenging to accommodate a variety of class participants. Some exercisers will not want to take a regression or modification, but they may be encouraged to take an *option* to decrease impact or to help them maintain proper form. Demonstrating options during class can be an effective way to allow everyone to pick the level that is right for them. Choosing the right progression is not the same thing as making an exercise easier or harder. In fact, it often makes an exercise more effective, and feel more challenging, because it allows for proper form and execution, thereby maximizing its benefit to the participant.

Cardiorespiratory Training

Cardiorespiratory fitness is a health-related component of fitness because it has a direct correlation with overall health and well-being. Many participants will have goals that can be achieved with cardiorespiratory training. Instructors should be familiar with the various training methods and understand how the training principles apply to programming for these types of classes. *Cardiorespiratory fitness* is the ability to perform large muscle, dynamic, rhythmic, and continuous moderate-to-vigorous intensity exercise for an extended period. Cardio classes will challenge the cardiovascular and respiratory systems with increases in heart rate, respiration, and the ability to deliver and use oxygen in the exercising muscle groups.

Benefits from cardiorespiratory training include the following (Anderson et al., 2016; Thorogood et al., 2011; Warburton et al., 2006):

- Decreased cardiovascular risk factors (high blood pressure, poor blood lipid profile, or unhealthy body composition)
- Decreased risk for overall morbidity and mortality
- Improved mood and mental health
- Improvement in performance in work, life, and sports

© Satyrenko/Shutterstock

TYPES OF CARDIORESPIRATORY TRAINING

To help participants attain these benefits and reach their goals, instructors for these formats should understand how to implement both steady-state and interval training and be comfortable programming for both methods.

AEROBIC ENDURANCE TRAINING

To improve aerobic endurance, instructors should plan classes with moderate resistance and long duration. By nature, aerobic efforts are performed below the anaerobic or lactate threshold. However, at higher endurance ranges, the effort should feel challenging, and participants should still perceive the effort as sustainable, even if moderately uncomfortable.

Aerobic endurance is the foundation of cardiovascular exercise and, typically, should make up a significant proportion of an individual's workout program (Allen & Coggan, 2010), particularly in the beginning. Classes can be designed to sustain this submaximal effort for the duration of the class, or they can have portions that are performed at this intensity with options to include intervals within the same class.

AEROBIC INTERVAL TRAINING

Interval training is a popular and effective form of exercise that can be used to improve both health and fitness levels. Unfortunately, with the immense enthusiasm for interval training, many instructors apply this training method without understanding the principles behind it (Comana, 2019). Although the benefits of steady-state training continue to be notable and embraced by many, some group fitness classes focus heavily on HIIT. HIIT certainly has many benefits, most notably time efficiency. However, when overdone or used in the wrong way, it can simultaneously increase the risk of injury for some participants, diminish the exercise experience for other participants, and detract from the opportunity to attain specific goals for others (Comana, 2019). With an improved understanding of appropriate interval intensity, recovery ratios, and proper training load, instructors can design classes that use (but do not abuse) this popular training method.

To ensure that proper recovery time is provided, instructors should keep in mind the general principle that the more intense the effort, the longer the amount of recovery time needed. See **Table 6.9** for sample recommendations (Comana, 2019).

TABLE 6.9 Example Ratios of Work to Recovery

Interval Intensity	Work-to-Recovery Ratio	Example Intervals
Moderate aerobic intervals	2:1 to 4:1	4-minute work, 2-minute recovery 8-minute work, 2-minute recovery
Anaerobic intervals (above threshold)	1:1 to 1:2	1-minute work, 1-minute recovery 45-second work, 90-second recovery
Extremely high-intensity anaerobic intervals	1:4 to 1:8	15-second work, 60-second recovery 10-second work, 80-second recovery

EXAMPLES OF CARDIORESPIRATORY TRAINING FORMATS

Cardiorespiratory training classes are popular in group fitness and include dance-based classes, indoor cycling, step-based classes, kickboxing, and many more. Each class provides large muscle, dynamic, and continuous bouts of effort that place overload on the cardiovascular and respiratory systems at various intensities.

PROGRESSION, REGRESSION, AND MODIFICATION IN CARDIORESPIRATORY TRAINING

To provide options for participants, instructors must be clear on the intensity level during each exercise and use coaching methods that drive the proper intensity for the class format. For example, in a cycle class, the instructor can explain the drill coming up and offer instruction for how hard the participants should push during each work interval, whether it is a steady-state portion of the class or an interval. This can be combined with information about how long the work and rest intervals will be so everyone can prepare for the effort ahead. To give various levels of challenge, guidance as to how to make the exercise more challenging or to pull back the intensity is also essential. Although each format has a unique method for increasing intensity, overall, the workload and duration of the work will determine the difficulty.

 INSTRUCTOR TIP

Depending on the format, it can be more effective to speak to how participants are feeling during an effort, rather than targeting a metric (e.g., specific heart rate). For example, an instructor might say, "Okay team, we have 1 minute of hard work coming up! You should be breathing hard, but not breathless. Choose the pace that gets you there. Let's go!"

STATIC STRETCHING

The process of passively taking a muscle to the point of tension and holding the stretch for a minimum of 30 seconds.

DYNAMIC STRETCHING

The active extension of a muscle, using a muscle's force production and the body's momentum, to take a joint through the full available range of motion.

SELF-MYOFASCIAL ROLLING (SMR)

A self-induced rolling technique to inhibit overactive muscles and improve flexibility.

Flexibility Training

To improve the range of motion throughout a joint or a series of joints, it is important to include flexibility techniques in group fitness classes. Several techniques can be used in group fitness to help improve flexibility, depending on the class format. Although each technique generates specific adaptations, they share similar benefits (Behm et al., 2016; Cheatham et al., 2015; Opplert & Babault, 2018):

- Correct and prevent muscle imbalances
- Increase joint range of motion
- Decrease muscle soreness
- Relieve joint stress
- Improve muscle extensibility
- Maintain the functional length of all muscles

Inadequate flexibility will compromise musculoskeletal function and, therefore, movement quality, making everyday activities, exercise, or sports performance more difficult and less efficient.

TYPES OF STRETCHING

Several techniques are used in fitness programming to enhance flexibility (**Table 6.10**). The most common flexibility techniques in group fitness include **STATIC STRETCHING**, **DYNAMIC STRETCHING**, and **SELF-MYOFASCIAL ROLLING (SMR)**. Although the goal of each technique is ultimately the same (improving available range of motion at a joint, increasing tissue extensibility, decreasing muscle and tendon injury risk, and enhancing neuromuscular efficiency), each method can be used separately or integrated with other techniques to achieve individualized program goals.

The movement preparation section of the class is a great time to include dynamic stretching because it will help to prepare the body for more intense exercise and ranges of motion. SMR can be used, when available, to assist with increased mobility at the start or end of class. Static stretching is the most common form of stretching and should primarily be done at the end of the workout session or at least when the muscles are warm. The technique(s) to be used will be determined by the Group Fitness Instructor based on the area being emphasized, effectiveness, client goals, and the level of client adherence to the program.

TABLE 6.10 Description of Flexibility Techniques

Technique	Description
Static stretching	Static stretching combines low-to-moderate forces with long duration using a variety of neural, mechanical, and psycho-physiological mechanisms. This form of stretching, performed alone or with a partner, allows for relaxation and concomitant elongation of muscle.
Self-myofascial rolling (SMR)	This is a self-induced rolling technique to inhibit overactive muscles and improve flexibility using various tools such as foam rollers, rolling balls, and sticks.
Dynamic stretching	Dynamic stretching uses a controlled movement through the full or nearly full joint range of motion.

STATIC STRETCHING

Arguably, during the last half-century, static stretching has been the most common flexibility training technique used by health and fitness professionals (Alter, 2004; Behm, 2018; Behm et al., 2016; Behm & Chaouachi, 2011; Kay & Blazevich, 2012). Static stretching represents a group of flexibility techniques used to increase the extensibility of muscle and connective tissue (lengthening), and thus the range of motion at a joint (Alter, 2004; Behm, 2018; Behm et al., 2016; Behm & Chaouachi, 2011; Kay & Blazevich, 2012).

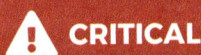 **CRITICAL**

Improvements in joint range of motion are due to several factors:

- Mechanical (muscle and tendon factors affecting elasticity or stiffness)
- Neural (effects on the central nervous system to help the muscle relax)
- Psycho-physiological (stretch tolerance)

This form of flexibility training is associated with the lowest risk for injury during the stretching routine and is deemed the safest to use because individuals can perform static stretching on their own with the slow, minimal-to-no motion required (Smith, 1994). Evidence has documented that static stretching can reduce the incidence of lower body muscle and tendon injuries, especially with high-velocity contractions and activities requiring rapid changes in direction (Behm, 2018; McHugh & Cosgrave, 2010). Additionally, although static stretching can be done with another person, it is commonly performed alone; therefore, it can easily be incorporated into any integrated exercise program (**Figure 6.2**).

PRACTICE THIS

Sit down with your knees extended and slowly reach as far as possible to your toes (or past). Hold that position for 30 seconds. Now try again and see if you can reach farther. It is likely that you can because of the multiple mechanisms at work that caused your muscles to relax.

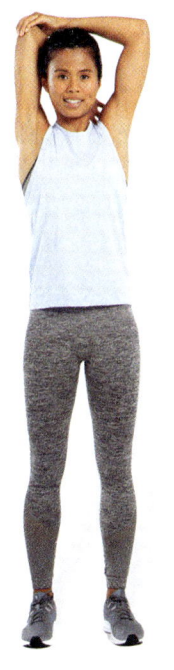

FIGURE 6.2 Static Stretching

Strength Training

Strength training, also known as resistance training, is done to improve muscular fitness. Strength training can target improvements in strength, hypertrophy, endurance, and/or power. Each aspect of muscular fitness has application to function and performance and should be included in an overall training program. Strength training is an effective method not only for building muscular fitness but also for improving health and wellness across all age groups (Borde et al., 2015; Garber et al., 2011).

TYPES OF STRENGTH TRAINING

Individuals who come to group fitness classes may have specific goals they would like to meet or certain expectations, which means offering recommendations and coaching with realistic expectations. Group fitness classes with a muscular fitness focus should involve a combination of multi-joint and single-joint exercises performed at an intensity that is appropriate for the goal and the participant. Instructors teaching a strength-based format should be familiar with a multitude of strength training exercises and be capable of demonstrating and coaching proper form. Knowledge of the muscle groups being trained (agonists) is also important, and instructors are encouraged to seek additional education to further familiarity with these exercises.

Group exercise offers several formats that include strength training, some of which include barbell classes, boot camps, circuit training, suspension training, Pilates, yoga, and many others. Newer exercisers should be encouraged to focus on learning new exercises, mastering technique, and building consistency. As they get stronger, you can challenge them with increased intensity, volume, and load. You should include some variety and options for progressions in your classes. This will help increase adherence and interest and reduce overtraining or plateaus. Common progression methods include adding weight, decreasing rest, learning more exercises, adjusting tempo, increasing complexity, and increasing the frequency of training.

Core Training

When most people think of core training, they think of training their abs with crunches and planks. Although these are common core training exercises, they are only a part of what instructors should target and plan for properly training the core. The core consists of all the muscles of the trunk, including the abdominals, muscles of the spine, and the hips. These muscles are the center of power and strength for the body and provide stability for all the body's movements. The core works to absorb and transfer forces to and from the upper and lower extremities. The core also helps to stabilize the lumbar spine, pelvis, and hips, protecting these regions from excessive stress and injury. Muscles of the core can be classified as either muscle stabilizers or those that produce movement (see **Table 6.11**; **Figures 6.3** and **6.4**).

Common goals participants will have for core training are improved aesthetics (e.g., a "six-pack"), better functional or sports performance, and preventing or managing low back pain. By understanding the different types of core exercises and what they will accomplish, you can design classes to achieve these goals and help educate and motivate participants.

TYPES OF CORE TRAINING

There are essentially three levels of core training that will help to improve the function of the core. These include stabilization, isolated strengthening to condition-specific core muscles, and integrated training to help the core work as a functional unit.

Stabilization training involves abdominal bracing (e.g., as with planks) or the drawing-in maneuver, which can be very helpful for improving stability in the core musculature. This type

TABLE 6.11 Stabilization and Movement Muscles

Stabilization Muscles of the Core	Movement Muscles of the Core
Transverse abdominis	Latissimus dorsi
Multifidus	Hip flexors
Internal oblique	Hamstring complex
Diaphragm	Quadriceps
Pelvic floor muscles	Pectoralis major
Rotator cuff	Deltoid
External obliques	Gluteus maximus
Quadratus lumborum	Triceps
Psoas major	Biceps
Rectus abdominis	Erector spinae
Gluteus medius	
Adductor complex	

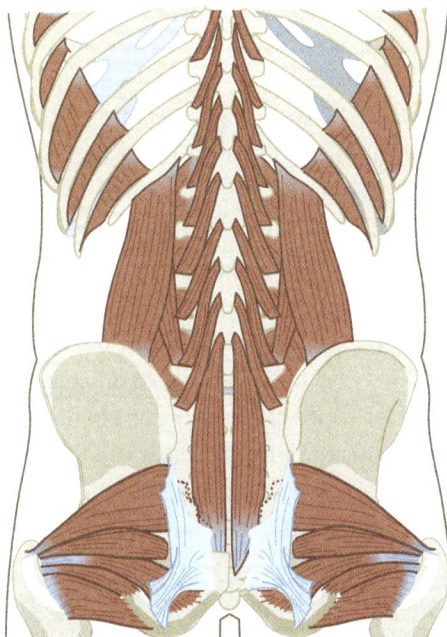

FIGURE 6.3 Local (Stabilization) Core Musculature

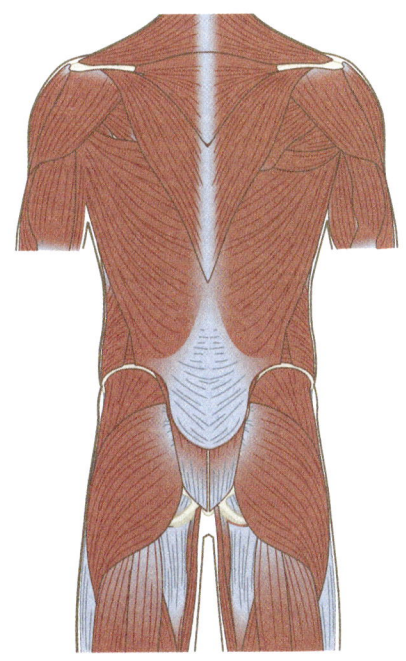

FIGURE 6.4 Global (Movement) Core Musculature

of training helps participants *feel* the muscle groups they should be training and educates them on how to stabilize their spine during movement (McGill et al., 2003). This will be helpful during exercise progression, and the instructor can refer to this idea during heavy lifts or challenging exercises during the workout. For this reason, these exercises are great choices during the movement prep portion of the class or in an introduction class.

Isolated strengthening exercises (e.g., crunches) emphasize a specific muscle group or movement and will improve strength or muscle endurance (Jørgensen et al., 2010). For example, a bridging exercise can improve strength or activation of the hip extensors. Note that it is important to consider muscle balance when training for isolated strength and to include the muscles on the posterior side of the body. For example, to improve low back strength you could include

The Drawing-in Maneuver
Stand with good posture and place your hand over your navel. Pull your navel away from your hand. You should be able to complete this without holding your breath (i.e., sucking in) and keeping your shoulders away from your ears.

lumbar spine extension exercises such as a cobra or a superman as part of core training. This could be included in a workout to give balance for lumbar spine flexion exercises such as a crunch.

Integrated core training exercises are used to train the core muscles to work in conjunction with the muscles of the lower and upper body, often involving exercises that include overhead pressing and unilateral movements (Saeterbakken & Fimland, 2012). During functional movement and several exercises, force is generated in the lower body and then transmitted through the core to the upper body. During integrated core training, exercises are included to give the nervous system the practice it needs to do these movements properly.

CORE TRAINING IN GROUP FITNESS

Core training in group fitness will depend greatly on the format you are teaching but, in general, you should make an effort to include some form of core training, when applicable. Classes such as indoor cycling will likely not have a portion dedicated to core training, but other formats will likely have the option to include time dedicated to core training. Many instructors choose to include core exercises at the end of the workout. Other instructors include low-volume core activation exercises at the beginning of class to engage the muscles and prep them for more intense work during the class. Another great option is to include some isolated or integrated exercises during the workout that will enhance the performance of exercises done in that specific format. For example, you could include a dumbbell squat to press during a strength training class and cue participants to focus on engaging their core and stabilizing the spine during the overhead press movement. This will activate the muscles of the core and improve functional performance.

Although it is tempting to jump right to the most difficult core exercise, it is important to meet participants where they are in terms of abilities and strength. An exercise can be made more difficult by increasing range of motion, exercise speed, or the length of the limb being moved or by adding weight. For example, during a crunch exercise you could add a weight plate during the crunch, focus on a specific tempo, increase how high the shoulder blades are lifted off the ground, lengthen the arms overhead, or add rotation (**Figures 6.5** through **6.7**). Each option would make the same exercise more challenging.

Static and Dynamic Balance Training

BALANCE is the body's ability to maintain the center of gravity over its base of support and is required to maintain posture and to execute all types of movement. Balance can be divided into two forms: static and dynamic. **STATIC BALANCE** refers to the ability to maintain a static equilibrium through a **PERTURBATION** while remaining still (e.g., standing on one foot). **DYNAMIC BALANCE** refers to the ability to maintain the intended path of motion following

BALANCE

Ability to maintain the body's center of gravity within its base of support.

STATIC BALANCE

Ability to maintain equilibrium in place with no external forces.

PERTURBATION

A disturbance of equilibrium; shaking.

DYNAMIC BALANCE

Ability to maintain equilibrium through the intended path of motion when external forces are present.

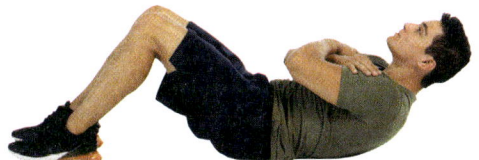

FIGURE 6.5 Floor Crunch

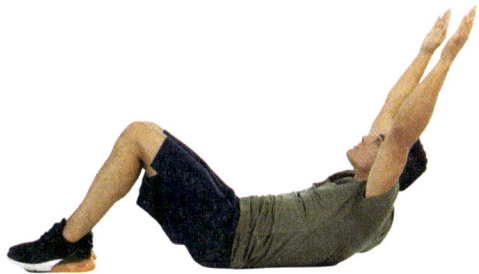

FIGURE 6.6 Long-Lever Floor Crunch

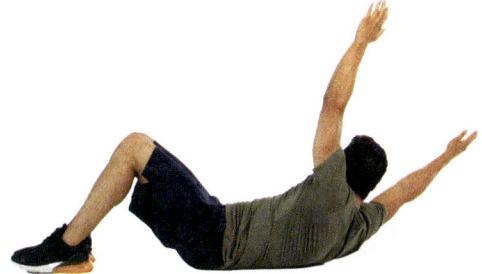

FIGURE 6.7 Long-Lever Floor Crunch with Rotation

an external perturbation or force placed on the moving body (e.g., maintaining position during a hop).

Balance training will train both the nervous system and the muscular system. A significant portion of balance comes from the nervous system recruiting the right muscle at the right time with the right amount of force. Exercises that emphasize balance will improve the coordination of the muscles used and also allow the individual to perform that movement with more ease and control. This can be helpful for a wide range of individuals. Athletes can improve performance with improved balance. A group exercise participant will be able to work at a higher intensity or lift more weight if they have better balance. Older adults will improve their ability to perform ADLs, reduce their risk of falling, and increase balance confidence.

TYPES OF BALANCE TRAINING

A balance component can be added to any workout by making the base of support less stable, such as by standing on an unstable surface or simply standing in a narrow stance or on one foot instead of two while performing upper body resistance exercises (**Table 6.12**). To emphasize static balance, you can give tasks that require the participant to maintain a posture despite a reduced base of support or a change in the center of mass (moving the upper body away from the position over the lower body). Common examples can be found in yoga classes with tree pose and other single-leg balance exercises. You can also incorporate these into resistance training exercises, having the participants perform exercises with a reduced base of support, such as with the feet close together, or on one leg, such as a standing bicep curl. Static balance exercises can also be included in the static stretching portion of class by asking participants to complete a stretch that requires a single-leg stance, such as a standing quadricep stretch.

Dynamic balance can be enhanced with movements that require a constant change in the base of support while keeping control and maintaining proper posture. Walking lunges are a common exercise that require dynamic balance and could be used in place of a squat or other lower body exercise if dynamic balance is a goal.

You can add challenge and progress exercises by giving options to reduce the base of support further or by increasing the range of movements that are done with the torso and upper body. These give the body a progressed challenge to maintain posture and control.

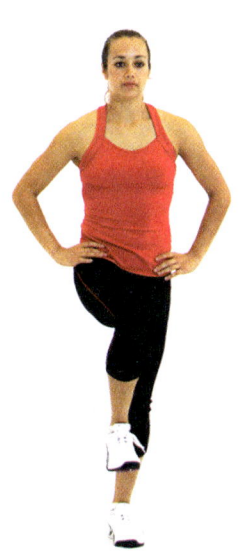

TABLE 6.12 Base of Support Progression

Proprioceptive Challenge	Surface Stability	Lower Body	Upper Body	Full Body
Foundational	Floor	Two-leg	Two arms at the same time	More points of contact with the ground
	Sport beam	Staggered stance	Alternating arms	
	Half foam roll	Single-leg	Single-arm	
	Foam pad	Two-leg (unstable surface)	Single-arm with motion (e.g., trunk rotation)	
	Balance disc	Staggered stance (unstable surface)		
Advanced	Wobble board	Single-leg (unstable surface)		Fewer points of contact with the ground

Plyometric Training

PLYOMETRIC TRAINING, at one time called reactive training, is a form of training that improves power development. Integrated plyometric training teaches the body how to respond at realistic speeds to changes in the environment encountered during functional activities. This type of training uses quick, powerful movements involving an eccentric contraction followed immediately by an explosive concentric contraction. Put simply, a person must control their landing (deceleration) and quickly accelerate under control on landing. Most high-intensity formats, such as HIIT and kickboxing, have a robust reactive component due to the frequent jumping and landing movements used.

Plyometric training is important because it develops a rapid, powerful neuromuscular response to allow safe movement at functional speeds. When done properly, plyometric training has been shown to provide benefits such as increased jumping ability and rate of force development as well as injury prevention (Arabatzi et al., 2010; Markovic & Mikulic, 2010). Plyometric training improves participants' ability to manage their bodies in their physical space and environment.

TYPES OF PLYOMETRIC TRAINING

Any type of jumping movement involves plyometric training for the lower body, including hopping, skipping, and bounding. Plyometric training can be used as part of movement prep to prepare the body for its application at greater intensities or as the primary focus of the workout in advanced classes.

When it comes to programming plyometrics, it is important to be familiar with the proper technique for each move completed, including landing technique and proper joint alignment. Instructors should cue to land "softly" or "quietly" and ensure that the knees are in line with the second and third toes as they absorb the force.

Plyometrics should be carefully progressed due to the high amount of stress on the joints, muscles, and connective tissues.

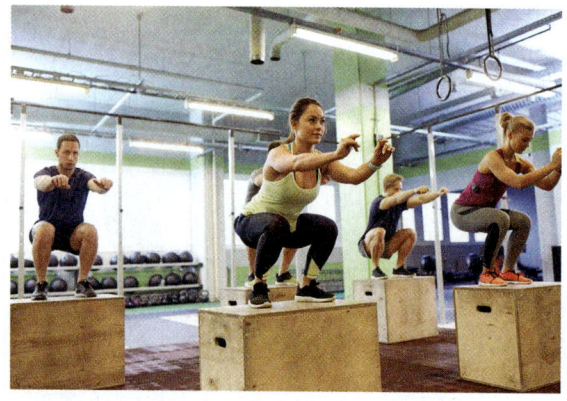

© Ground Picture/Shutterstock

Special attention should be paid to the intensity of the drill as well as the volume of impact and the frequency of training. Plyometrics are ultimately optional and should be done cautiously with participants who are untrained or overweight and are best for participants who have a base layer of strength to ensure that the tendons, ligaments, and muscles are not overstressed.

Speed, Agility, and Quickness (SAQ) Training

Integrated fitness, including **SPEED**, **AGILITY**, and **QUICKNESS** (SAQ) training, is often used to prepare athletes for the demands of their sport. Although in some instances a typical group fitness participant can benefit from SAQ training to improve their daily functioning and overall conditioning, most Group Fitness Instructors will use SAQ training sparingly based on class format. SAQ training can be used to add an element of fun and variety to training, and some drills can be used to increase heart rate when appropriate for the class.

Examples of SAQ training in group fitness include drills with a ladder or cones to teach participants to move quickly and accurately. To make these more appropriate for a group, keep moves simple and encourage participants to start slowly to learn exercises and progress speed and complexity as they master early patterns.

SUMMARY

As a Group Fitness Instructor, you can create real and meaningful changes for your participants' health and fitness. Using the training principles discussed in this chapter, you now have the guidelines that will help you plan your classes with a goal-focused approach. Your ability to plan and manipulate the acute program variables in your group fitness classes will make you a powerful leader, helping your class to improve one workout at a time. Do not forget to always think about the purpose of the class and format that you are teaching and be mindful of what you can do to make your class as effective as possible. The adaptations that you plan for will require overload and the use of variables that are specific to the goals of your class and should be progressed over time.

SPEED

The straight-ahead velocity of an individual.

AGILITY

Ability to maintain center of gravity over a changing base of support while changing direction at various speeds.

QUICKNESS

Ability to react to a stimulus with an appropriate muscular response without hesitation.

REFERENCES

Allen, H., & Coggan, A. (2010). *Training and racing with a power meter* (2nd ed.). VeloPress.

Alter, M. J. (2004). *Science of flexibility* (3rd ed.). Human Kinetics.

Anderson, L., Oldridge, N., Thompson, D. R., Zwisler, A.-D., Rees, K., Martin, N., & Taylor, R. S. (2016). Exercise-based cardiac rehabilitation for coronary heart disease: Cochrane Systematic Review and Meta-Analysis. *Journal of the American College of Cardiology*, *67*(1), 1–12. https://doi.org/10.1016/j.jacc.2015.10.044

Arabatzi, F., Kellis, E., & Saèz-Saez De Villarreal, E. (2010). Vertical jump biomechanics after plyometric, weight lifting, and combined (weight lifting + plyometric) training. *Journal of Strength & Conditioning Research*, *24*(9), 2440–2448. https://doi.org/10.1519/JSC.0b013e3181e274ab

Behm, D. G. (2018). *The science and physiology of flexibility and stretching: Implications and applications in sport performance and health*. Routledge.

Behm, D. G., Blazevich, A. J., Kay, A. D., & McHugh, M. (2016). Acute effects of muscle stretching on physical performance, range of motion, and injury incidence in healthy active individuals: A systematic review. *Applied Physiology, Nutrition, and Metabolism*, *41*(1), 1–11. https://doi.org/10.1139/apnm-2015-0235

Behm, D. G., & Chaouachi, A. (2011). A review of the acute effects of static and dynamic stretching on performance. *European Journal of Applied Physiology, 111*(11), 2633–2651. https://doi.org/10.1007/s00421-011-1879-2

Blair, S. N., & Connelly, J. C. (1996). How much physical activity should we do? The case for moderate amounts and intensities of physical activity. *Research Quarterly for Exercise and Sport, 67*(2), 193–205. https://doi.org/10.1080/02701367.1996.10607943

Borde, R., Hortobágyi, T., & Granacher, U. (2015). Dose-response relationships of resistance training in healthy old adults: A systematic review and meta-analysis. *Sports Medicine, 45*(12), 1693–1720. https://doi.org/10.1007/s40279-015-0385-9

Campos, G. E. R., Luecke, T. J., Wendeln, H. K., Toma, K., Hagerman, F. C., Murray, T. F., Ragg, K. E., Ratamess, N. A., Kraemer, W. J., & Staron, R. S. (2002, Nov.). Muscular adaptations in response to three different resistance-training regimens: Specificity of repetition maximum training zones. *European Journal of Applied Physiology, 88*(1–2), 50–60. https://doi.org/10.1007/s00421-002-0681-6

Carmichael, C., & Rutberg, J. (2012). *The time-crunched cyclist: Fit, fast, powerful in 6 hours a week* (2nd ed.). VeloPress.

Cheatham, S. W., Kolber, M. J., Cain, M., & Lee, M. (2015). The effects of self-myofascial release using a foam roll or roller massager on joint range of motion, muscle recovery, and performance: A systematic review. *International Journal of Sports Physical Therapy, 10*(6), 827–838.

Comana, F. (2019). *National Academy of Sports Medicine cardio programming.* [Unpublished Manuscript]. National Academy of Sports Medicine.

Cormie, P., McCaulley, G. O., & McBride, J. M. (2007). Power versus strength-power jump squat training: Influence on the load-power relationship. *Medicine & Science in Sports & Exercise, 39*(6), 996–1003. https://doi.org/10.1097/mss.0b013e3180408e0c

Coyle, E. F., Feiring, D. C., Rotkis, T. C., Cote, R. W., III, Roby, F. B., Lee, W., & Wilmore, J. H. (1981). Specificity of power improvements through slow and fast isokinetic training. *Journal of Applied Physiology: Respiratory, Environmental and Exercise Physiology, 51*(6), 1437–1442. https://doi.org/10.1152/jappl.1981.51.6.1437

Cronin, J. B., McNair, P. J., & Marshall, R. N. (2002). Is velocity-specific strength training important in improving functional performance? *Journal of Sports Medicine and Physical Fitness, 42*(3), 267–273.

Dantas, E. H. M., Daoud, R., Trott, A., Nodari-Junior, R. J., & de Souza Costa Conceição, M. C. (2011). Flexibility: Components, proprioceptive mechanisms and methods. *Biomedical Human Kinetics, 3*(3), 39–43. https://doi.org/10.2478/v10101-011-0009-2

De Feo, P. (2013). Is high-intensity exercise better than moderate-intensity exercise for weight loss? *Nutrition, Metabolism, and Cardiovascular Diseases, 23*(11), 1037–1042. https://doi.org/10.1016/j.numecd.2013.06.002

Del Vecchio, A., Casolo, A., Negro, F., Scorcelletti, M., Bazzucchi, I., Enoka, R., Felici, F., & Farina, D. (2019). The increase in muscle force after 4 weeks of strength training is mediated by adaptations in motor unit recruitment and rate coding. *Journal of Physiology, 597*(7), 1873–1887. https://doi.org/10.1113/JP277250

Depino, G. M., Webright, W. G., & Arnold, B. L. (2000). Duration of maintained hamstring flexibility after cessation of an acute static stretching protocol. *Journal of Athletic Training, 35*(1), 56–59.

Fahey, T. D. (Ed.). (1998). *Encyclopedia of sports medicine and science.* Internet Society for Sport Science. http://www.sportsci.org/encyc/

Folland, J. P., & Williams, A. G. (2007). The adaptations to strength training: Morphological and neurological contributions to increased strength. *Sports Medicine, 37*(2), 145–168. https://doi.org/10.2165/00007256-200737020-00004

Gabriel, D. A., Kamen, G., & Frost, G. (2006). Neural adaptations to resistive exercise: Mechanisms and recommendations for training practices. *Sports Medicine, 36*(2), 133–149. https://doi.org/10.2165/00007256-200636020-00004

Garber, C. E., Blissmer, B., Deschenes, M. R., Franklin, B. A., Lamonte, M. J., Lee, I. M., Nieman, D. C., Swain, D. P., & American College of Sports Medicine. (2011). American College of Sports Medicine position stand. Quantity and quality of exercise for developing and maintaining cardiorespiratory, musculoskeletal, and neuromotor fitness in apparently healthy adults: Guidance for prescribing exercise. *Medicine & Science in Sports & Exercise, 43*(7), 1334–1359. https://doi.org/10.1249/MSS.0b013e318213fefb

Hawley, J. A. (2002). Adaptations of skeletal muscle to prolonged, intense endurance training. *Clinical and Experimental Pharmacology & Physiology, 29*(3), 218–222. https://doi.org/10.1046/j.1440-1681.2002.03623.x

Heinrich, K. M., Patel, P. M., O'Neal, J. L., & Heinrich, B. S. (2014). High-intensity compared to moderate-intensity training for exercise initiation, enjoyment, adherence, and intentions: An intervention study. *BMC Public Health, 14*, 789. https://doi.org/10.1186/1471-2458-14-789

Hellsten, Y., & Nyberg, M. (2015). Cardiovascular adaptations to exercise training. *Comprehensive Physiology, 6*(1), 1–32. https://doi.org/10.1002/cphy.c140080

Holtermann, A., Roeleveld, K., Vereijken, B., & Ettema, G. (2007). The effect of rate of force development on maximal force production: Acute and training-related aspects. *European Journal of Applied Physiology, 99*(6), 605–613. https://doi.org/10.1007/s00421-006-0380-9

Hughes, D. C., Ellefsen, S., & Baar, K. (2018). Adaptations to endurance and strength training. *Cold Spring Harbor Perspectives in Medicine, 8*(6), a029769. https://doi.org/10.1101/cshperspect.a029769

Jørgensen, M. B., Andersen, L. L., Kirk, N., Pedersen, M. T., Søgaard, K., & Holtermann, A. (2010). Muscle activity during functional coordination training: Implications for strength gain and rehabilitation. *Journal of Strength & Conditioning Research, 24*(7), 1732–1739. https://doi.org/10.1519/JSC.0b013e3181ddf6b5

Joyner, M. J., & Coyle, E. F. (2008). Endurance exercise performance: The physiology of champions. *Journal of Physiology, 586*(Pt 1), 35–44. https://doi.org/10.1113/jphysiol.2007.143834

Kay, A. D., & Blazevich, A. J. (2012). Effect of acute static stretch on maximal muscle performance: A systematic review. *Medicine & Science in Sports & Exercise, 44*(1), 154–164. https://doi.org/10.1249/MSS.0b013e318225cb27

Kongsgaard, M., Aagaard, P., Kjaer, M., & Magnusson, S. P. (2005). Structural Achilles tendon properties in athletes subjected to different exercise modes and in Achilles tendon rupture patients. *Journal of Applied Physiology, 99*(5), 1965–1971. https://doi.org/10.1152/japplphysiol.00384.2005

Kraemer, W. J., Nindl, B. C., Ratamess, N. A., Gotshalk, L. A., Volek, J. S., Fleck, S. J., Newton, R. U., & Häkkinen, K. (2004). Changes in muscle hypertrophy in women with periodized resistance training. *Medicine & Science in Sports & Exercise, 36*(4), 697–708. https://doi.org/10.1249/01.mss.0000122734.25411.cf

Kraemer, W. J., & Ratamess, N. A. (2004). Fundamentals of resistance training: Progression and exercise prescription. *Medicine & Science in Sports & Exercise, 36*(4), 674–688. https://doi.org/10.1249/01.mss.0000121945.36635.61

Magnusson, S. P., Simonsen, E. B., Aagaard, P., Dyhre-Poulsen, P., McHugh, M. P., & Kjaer, M. (1996). Mechanical and physiological responses to stretching with and without preisometric contraction in human skeletal muscle. *Archives of Physical Medicine and Rehabilitation, 77*(4), 373–378. https://doi.org/10.1016/s0003-9993(96)90087-8

Magnusson, S. P., Simonsen, E. B., Aagaard, P., & Kjaer, M. (1996). Biomechanical responses to repeated stretches in human hamstring muscle in vivo. *American Journal of Sports Medicine, 24*(5), 622–628. https://doi.org/10.1177/036354659602400510

Magnusson, S. P., Simonsen, E. B., Aagaard, P., Sorensen, H., & Kjaer, M. (1996). A mechanism for altered flexibility in human skeletal muscle. *Journal of Physiology, 497*(Pt 1), 291–298. https://doi.org/10.1113/jphysiol.1996.sp021768

Markovic, G., & Mikulic, P. (2010). Neuro-musculoskeletal and performance adaptations to lower-extremity plyometric training. *Sports Medicine, 40*(10), 859–895. https://doi.org/10.2165/11318370-000000000-00000

Maturana, F. M., Martus, P., Zipfel, S., & Nieß, A. M. (2021). Effectiveness of HIIE versus MICT in improving cardiometabolic risk factors in health and disease: A meta-analysis. *Medicine & Science in Sports & Exercise, 53*(3), 559–573. https://doi.org/10.1249/MSS.0000000000002506

McCafferty, W. B., & Horvath, S. M. (1977). Specificity of exercise and specificity of training: A subcellular review. *Research Quarterly, 48*(2), 358–371.

McGill, S. M., Grenier, S., Kavcic, N., & Cholewicki, J. (2003). Coordination of muscle activity to assure stability of the lumbar spine. *Journal of Electromyography and Kinesiology, 13*(4), 353–359. https://doi.org/10.1016/S1050-6411(03)00043-9

McHugh, M. P., & Cosgrave, C. H. (2010). To stretch or not to stretch: The role of stretching in injury prevention and performance. *Scandinavian Journal of Medicine & Science in Sports, 20*(2), 169–181. https://doi.org/10.1111/j.1600-0838.2009.01058.x

Medeiros, D. M., Cini, A., Sbruzzi, G., & Lima, C. S. (2016). Influence of static stretching on hamstring flexibility in healthy young adults: Systematic review and meta-analysis. *Physiotherapy Theory and Practice, 32*(6), 438–445. https://doi.org/10.1080/09593985.2016.1204401

Melzack, R., & Wall, P. D. (1965). Pain mechanisms: A new theory. *Science, 150*(3699), 971–979. https://doi.org/10.1126/science.150.3699.971

National Institute on Aging. (2020, April). *Real life benefits of exercise and physical activity.* https://www.nia.nih.gov/health/real-life-benefits-exercise-and-physical-activity

Opplert, J., & Babault, N. (2018). Acute effects of dynamic stretching on muscle flexibility and performance: An analysis of the current literature. *Sports Medicine, 48*(2), 299–325. https://doi.org/10.1007/s40279-017-0797-9

Peterson, M. D., Rhea, M. R., & Alvar, B. A. (2005). Applications of the dose-response for muscular strength development: A review of meta-analytic efficacy and reliability for designing training prescription. *Journal of Strength & Conditioning Research, 19*(4), 950–958. https://doi.org/10.1519/R-16874.1

Pimenta, L. D., Massini, D. A., dos Santos, D., Vasconcelos, C. M. T., Simionato, A. R., Gomes, L. A. T., Guimarães, B. R., Neiva, C. M., & Filho, D. M. P. (2019). Bone health, muscle strength and lean mass: Relationships and exercise recommendations. *Revista Brasileira de Medicina Do Esporte, 25*(3), 245–251. https://doi.org/10.1590/1517-869220192503210258

Rhea, M. R., Alvar, B. A., Burkett, L. N., & Ball, S. D. (2003). A meta-analysis to determine the dose response for strength development. *Medicine & Science in Sports & Exercise, 35*(3), 456–464. https://doi.org/10.1249/01.MSS.0000053727.63505.D4

Saeterbakken, A. H., & Fimland, M. S. (2012). Muscle activity of the core during bilateral, unilateral, seated and standing resistance exercise. *European Journal of Applied Physiology, 112*(5), 1671–1678. https://doi.org/10.1007/s00421-011-2141-7

Sainz de Baranda, P., & Ayala, F. (2010). Chronic flexibility improvement after 12 week of stretching program utilizing the ACSM recommendations: Hamstring flexibility. *International Journal of Sports Medicine, 31*(6), 389–396. https://doi.org/10.1055/s-0030-1249082

Selye, H. (1950). Stress and the general adaptation syndrome. *British Medical Journal, 1*(4667), 1383–1392. https://doi.org/10.1136/bmj.1.4667.1383

Sherrington, C., Fairhall, N. J., Wallbank, G. K., Tiedemann, A., Michaleff, Z. A., Howard, K., Clemson, L., Hopewell, S., & Lamb, S. E. (2019). Exercise for preventing falls in older people living in the community. *Cochrane Database of Systematic Reviews, 1*(1), CD012424. https://doi.org/10.1002/14651858.CD012424.pub2

Smith, C. A. (1994). The warm-up procedure: To stretch or not to stretch. A brief review. *Journal of Orthopedic & Sports Physical Therapy, 19*(1), 12–17. https://doi.org/10.2519/jospt.1994.19.1.12

Spirduso, W. W., & Cronin, D. L. (2001). Exercise dose-response effects on quality of life and independent living in older adults. *Medicine & Science in Sports & Exercise, 33*(6 Supplement), S598–S608. https://doi.org/10.1097/00005768-200106001-00028

Sutton, B. G. (Ed.). (2022). *NASM essentials of personal fitness training* (7th ed.). Jones & Bartlett Learning.

Swain, D. P., & Franklin, B. A. (2002). Is there a threshold intensity for aerobic training in cardiac patients? *Medicine & Science in Sports and Exercise, 34*(7), 1071–1075. https://doi.org/10.1097/00005768-200207000-00003

Tesch, P. A., Thorsson, A., & Essén-Gustavsson, B. (1989). Enzyme activities of FT and ST muscle fibers in heavy-resistance trained athletes. *Journal of Applied Physiology, 67*(1), 83–87. https://doi.org/10.1152/jappl.1989.67.1.83

Thorogood, A., Mottillo, S., Shimony, A., Filion, K. B., Joseph, L., Genest, J., Pilote, L., Poirier, P., Schiffrin, E. L., & Eisenberg, M. J. (2011). Isolated aerobic exercise and weight loss: A systematic review and meta-analysis of randomized controlled trials. *The American Journal of Medicine, 124*(8), 747–755. https://doi.org/10.1016/j.amjmed.2011.02.037

Warburton, D. E. R., Nicol, C. W., & Bredin, S. S. D. (2006). Health benefits of physical activity: The evidence. *Canadian Medical Association Journal, 174*(6), 801–809. https://doi.org/10.1503/cmaj.051351

Wernbom, M., Augustsson, J., & Thomeé, R. (2007). The influence of frequency, intensity, volume and mode of strength training on whole muscle cross-sectional area in humans. *Sports Medicine, 37*(3), 225–264. https://doi.org/10.2165/00007256-200737030-00004

Wilson, J. M., Loenneke, J. P., Jo, E., Wilson, G. J., Zourdos, M. C., & Kim, J.-S. (2012). The effects of endurance, strength, and power training on muscle fiber type shifting. *Journal of Strength & Conditioning Research, 26*(6), 1724–1729. https://doi.org/10.1519/JSC.0b013e318234eb6f

CHAPTER 7

A SUPPORTIVE APPROACH TO GROUP FITNESS

LEARNING OBJECTIVES

The intent of this chapter is to make group fitness available to and safe for all participants through inclusivity and by adjusting external environmental variables.

After reading this content, students should be able to demonstrate the following objectives:

- **Identify** considerations and approaches that support an inclusive group fitness experience.

- **Identify** environmental responses and considerations for the group fitness setting.

Lesson 1: Individual Health Considerations

Introduction

Being a Group Fitness Instructor means that you will be working to improve health and fitness for individuals with unique needs and considerations. No matter who walks into class, it is important that they feel welcome, comfortable, and that they belong. One of the best ways you can create this environment is by being comfortable with and capable of working with a spectrum of fitness levels and health conditions.

This chapter will introduce some common health conditions and other considerations that may affect participants in group fitness classes. Consider this to be a starting point for learning, and recognize that you will need to build additional knowledge about the specific needs of individual class participants. Knowledge about how

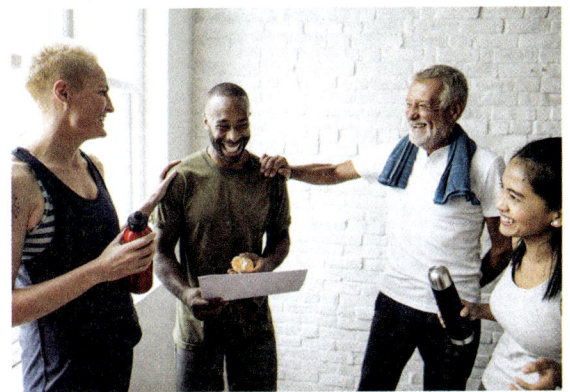
© Rawpixel.com/Shutterstock

common conditions may affect a participant's experience and their movement quality will aid you in designing classes for individuals of all levels. Regardless of a participant's fitness level, you will be able to meet them where they are and help them feel successful in your class.

To be a supportive and empowering instructor, you should have the mindset that exercise is essential and accessible for everyone.

INSTRUCTOR TIP

Not everyone likes attention! Although you want to be prepared with options and modifications for exercises, not all participants feel comfortable having the attention of the class on them. Some may also feel embarrassed if they are pointed out with a specific option. To avoid this, practice offering and demonstrating options that anyone could take for the exercise to the entire class without pointing out the individual that may need that choice.

Individual Considerations

Although your classes will include people of varying backgrounds, ages, and fitness levels, this section focuses on certain populations and conditions that you are likely to encounter when teaching. People often attend group fitness classes because of the motivation and guidance provided, and it is the Group Fitness Instructor's goal to help people move more. When instructors show that they have knowledge of various health conditions, it can inspire confidence and security among participants, which will hopefully lead to increased motivation and adherence to the exercise program. Use the guidelines provided in this section to ensure that your classes are inclusive and effective for a wide variety of individuals. Note that it is also important that you stay within your scope of practice as a fitness professional and follow the guidelines consistent with your training and licensure (or lack thereof).

⚠ CRITICAL

Fitness professionals must remain within their scope of practice when working with participants who have medical conditions. Safely working within the scope of practice requires proper screening and healthcare referral of participants when necessary. Always defer to the participant's limitations and healthcare provider recommendations when coaching in class.

Medical or Orthopedic Conditions

Oftentimes, individuals in group fitness classes are managing chronic health conditions that may affect their movement quality and functional capacity during class (**Table 7.1**). Each condition will affect different aspects of the body, and the effects can vary greatly between individuals. As an instructor, you can make your classes more approachable if you understand the basic systems that are affected by medical or orthopedic conditions, communicate with individuals to understand their limitations and goals, and provide options that are appropriate for their unique needs. Keep in mind that you should follow the recommendations set forth by any healthcare professionals the participants are working with and refer them to a medical professional for guidance, as needed.

TABLE 7.1 Common Medical Conditions and Classifications

Condition/Classification	Description
Obesity	A chronic low-grade inflammatory disease associated with a body mass index (BMI) of 30 or above.
Hypertension	Chronically high blood pressure defined as a systolic pressure above 130 mm Hg and/or a diastolic blood pressure above 80 mm Hg.
Coronary heart disease	The heart's blood supply becomes narrowed due to fatty deposits along the walls of its arteries.
Congestive heart failure	A chronic condition defined by impairment of the heart muscle's pumping power.
Atherosclerosis	Narrowing of the arteries due to a build-up of plaque along their walls.
Peripheral artery disease	Condition in which blood flow to the extremities is reduced due to the narrowing of arteries.
Stroke	An acute condition in which blood supply to the brain, or areas of the brain, is greatly reduced or interrupted. Individuals who have suffered a stroke may be left with chronic paralysis or physical dysfunction.
Cancer	Abnormal, invasive growth of cells within the body.
Osteoporosis	Bones become thin, fragile, and prone to fracture.

HYPERTENSION

HYPERTENSION, also known as high blood pressure, is a common chronic condition of the cardiovascular system that affects nearly one out of two American adults (Centers for Disease Control & Prevention [CDC], 2022). Exercise is recommended for the prevention and reduction of hypertension, and group fitness can be an effective method to achieve this (Cornelissen & Fagard, 2005; Fagard, 2001; Kelley & Kelley, 2000; Li et al., 2015; Wallace, 2003; Whelton et al., 2002). Due to how common this condition is, you are almost guaranteed to have hypertensive individuals in your group fitness classes; therefore, you should be familiar with how it may affect performance in a fitness setting.

The recommendation is that hypertensive individuals participate in aerobic fitness and/or muscular fitness exercise on most or preferably all days of the week (**Table 7.2**). Regular participation in cardiorespiratory exercise reduces blood pressure and risk of hypertension because it increases stroke volume, thus decreasing the workload on the heart (Faselis et al., 2014; Kokkinos & Myers, 2010). Resistance training, once considered something hypertensive patients should avoid, has been found to be useful as a supplement to cardiorespiratory exercise in order to improve functional capacity; it does not exacerbate high blood pressure and may help lower blood pressure in some individuals (Cornelissen et al., 2011; Li et al., 2015; Wallace, 2003). With any form of exercise, caution is warranted to avoid excessive increases in blood pressure (Le et al., 2008).

Individuals who have been diagnosed with hypertension may be prescribed lifestyle modifications and/or medications to help control their condition. Several prescription medications can affect the way the body responds to exercise, such as a drop in blood pressure during activity, stabilizing the heart rate, or feelings of fatigue. As an instructor, you should cue participants

HYPERTENSION

Chronically high blood pressure as defined by a systolic pressure above 130 mm Hg and/or a diastolic blood pressure above 80 mm Hg.

TABLE 7.2 Exercise Recommendations for Participants with Hypertension

Frequency	■ Aerobic: 5–7 days per week ■ Muscular fitness: 2–3 days per week ■ Flexibility: 2–3 days per week
Intensity	■ Aerobic: Moderate intensity ■ Muscular fitness: Moderate load
Time	■ Aerobic: Work up to 30 minutes per day ■ Muscular fitness: 2–4 sets of 8–12 reps
Type	■ Aerobic or resistance training exercise alone or combined, as well as flexibility exercises incorporating yoga or tai chi
Special considerations	■ Cue to breathe regularly and avoid the Valsalva maneuver. ■ Give adequate time for the warm-up and cool-down. ■ Progression should be gradual. ■ Monitor for signs of heat intolerance. ■ Modify tempo to avoid extended isometric and concentric muscle actions. ■ Avoid lying down. ■ Allow participants to stand up slowly to avoid possible dizziness.

VALSALVA MANEUVER

Exhaling against a closed glottis.

to breathe regularly and avoid the **VALSALVA MANEUVER** and ensure that hypertensive participants take the time to adequately warm up and cool down after exercising to prevent the sharp decrease in blood pressure that can result from abruptly halting aerobic exercise (Mar et al., 2016; Riebe et al., 2018).

⚠ CRITICAL

Certain anti-hypertensive medications slow the heart rate, which may prevent a participant from reaching their estimated training zone target. Participants taking these medications should instead rely on ratings of perceived exertion (RPE) or a talk test to gauge intensity.

CARDIOVASCULAR DISEASE

Cardiovascular disease (CVD) encompasses a group of chronic conditions that affect the heart and the blood vessels. Coronary heart disease, congestive heart failure, atherosclerosis, and peripheral artery disease are all forms of CVD that impair physical function, increase risk of mortality, and are leading causes of disability. Exercise such as group fitness in the proper amounts can improve cardiorespiratory and muscular fitness, decrease morbidity and mortality, positively influence conditions such as obesity and hypertension, and enhance overall quality of life (Benton, 2005; Brogårdh & Lexell, 2012; Pinckard et al., 2019; Roitman & LaFontaine, 2006; Tran, 2005; Williams et al., 2007).

Light to moderate cardiorespiratory exercise can provide individuals with CVD the appropriate level of stress for the cardiovascular system, resulting in improved function (Pinckard et al., 2019; Tran, 2005). Resistance training complements cardiorespiratory exercise because improved muscular fitness contributes to the ability to perform and sustain exercise and prevents age-related muscle loss, which can also be a risk factor for developing CVD (Fiuza-Luces et al., 2018; Williams et al., 2007). An individual who exhibits **DYSPNEA** (i.e., difficult or troubled breathing) during exercise should take longer breaks and train with reduced loads. Exercise must be ceased immediately if chest pain, nausea, dizziness, or **HEART PALPITATIONS** result. Keep an eye on these participants in your classes and help cue them when they need to decrease intensity or take longer recovery time between exercises. **Table 7.3** provides some basic exercise guidelines and acute variables for individuals suffering from CVD (Tran, 2005).

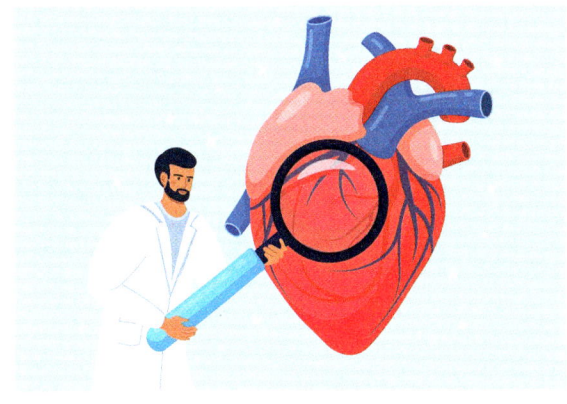

© Buravleva stock/Shutterstock

TABLE 7.3 Exercise Recommendations for Participants with CVD

Frequency	■ Aerobic: 5–7 days per week ■ Muscular fitness: 2–3 days per week ■ Flexibility: 2–3 days per week
Intensity	■ Aerobic: Light to moderate intensity ■ Muscular fitness: Moderate load
Time	■ Aerobic: 20–60 minutes per day ■ Muscular fitness: 1–3 sets with 10–15 reps
Type	■ Low impact exercise that is comfortable and safe for the individual to use
Special considerations	■ Use adequate time (5–10 minutes) for movement prep and for the transition after the workout. ■ Watch for any sign/symptom of a medical emergency. ■ Follow medical advice and recommendations. ■ Progress slowly. ■ Achieve a body weight consistent with reduced risk.

OBESITY

OBESITY is a common condition in the United States, with roughly 42% of the population classified as obese (CDC, 2022). Obesity is a chronic low-grade inflammatory disease and is characterized by an excessive amount of body fat, often indicated by a **BODY MASS INDEX (BMI)** greater than 30.0 kg/m^2 (Uranga & Keller, 2019).

Obesity is associated with a diverse set of complications, including CVD, type 2 diabetes, musculoskeletal problems, and hypertension (CDC, 2022). The increased weight of people in larger bodies can place additional pressure on the musculoskeletal system, which may make exercise and physical activity more fatiguing.

DYSPNEA

Difficulty or trouble breathing.

HEART PALPITATIONS

Heart flutters or rapid heartbeat.

OBESITY

A complex, chronic noncommunicable disease involving an excessive amount of body fat; classified by a body mass index (BMI) of 30 or greater.

BODY MASS INDEX (BMI)

Formula for screening weight categories in which an individual's weight (in kg) is divided by the square of their height (in meters).

Exercise and physical activity are part of a healthy lifestyle that can help individuals manage their body composition, improve mental and emotional health, decrease chronic disease risk, and improve fitness levels. Group fitness can help all people achieve their physical activity goals in a welcoming and encouraging environment. As an instructor, you can offer a group fitness class that participants will enjoy and stick with, helping to form positive associations with physical activity and a lifestyle habit that can be maintained.

At the start of a fitness program, those in larger bodies may need to begin with low-impact activities, such as water aerobics, or low-impact cardio classes to decrease the load on their joints. Over time, as their conditioning improves, they can transition to higher-intensity activities as desired. Although the target duration for activity is 45–60 minutes per day of moderate-intensity activity (**Table 7.4**), you should encourage these participants to start small and progress slowly to reduce injury risk and improve motivation. You should be prepared to offer options for exercises that will help participants feel engaged and comfortable, without making them feel singled out or embarrassed. For example, some participants may find it difficult or uncomfortable to get down to the ground or onto a mat. You could offer standing options to help avoid discomfort or embarrassment during these phases of class. It is important not to single them out when providing options. Offer alternatives to the class as a whole without directing progressions to an individual.

TABLE 7.4 Exercise Recommendations for Participants in Larger Bodies

Frequency	5 days per week as an ultimate goal, but start with whatever frequency is comfortable
Intensity	60–80% of maximum heart rate as a general guideline. Training ranges can be adjusted to 40–70% as desired.
Time	40–60 minutes per day or 20- to 30-minute sessions twice each day of cardiorespiratory training
Type	Classes such as low-impact cardio, dance, resistance, or aquatics
Special considerations	■ Make sure the participant is comfortable. ■ Exercise should be performed in a standing or seated position when possible. ■ Due to increased fatigue, participants may require longer rest periods or shorter durations. ■ The participant may have other chronic diseases. In these cases, a medical release should be obtained from the individual's physician. The recommendations above are only guidelines, not must-dos. Finding the right mix of activity that matches the lifestyle, personal preferences, and needs of the participant is more important than hitting specific targets.

CANCER

Group fitness classes may also have individuals who are undergoing treatment for various forms of cancer or returning to exercise after treatment. Some unique side effects they may experience include fatigue, cognitive problems, pain, trouble sleeping, anxiety, depression, and physical dysfunction (Mustian et al., 2012). Cancer-related fatigue commonly interferes with normal functioning and contributes to muscle wasting, declines in cardiorespiratory fitness, negative changes in body composition, and depression (Cramp et al., 2010; Strasser et al., 2013). Research has shown that cardiorespiratory exercise and resistance training may counteract many of the side effects of cancer treatments and, with some forms of early stage cancer, may decrease the risk of cancer-specific mortality (Cramp et al., 2010; Friedenreich et al., 2016; Hayes et al., 2009; Lønbro, 2014; Meneses-Echávez et al., 2015; Paramanandam & Roberts, 2014; Puetz & Herring, 2012; Strasser et al., 2013).

During group fitness classes, you should monitor the individual's reaction to activity and provide modifications when necessary. Exercise should be avoided during periods of increased infection risk, **ATAXIA**, or dizziness or during wound recovery from surgery (Lønbro, 2014). Keeping these participants engaged and building community in your classes will help them stay consistent with their workouts on days when it might be challenging for them to do so. **Table 7.5** shows some basic exercise guidelines and acute variables for individuals being treated for cancer (Cramp et al., 2010; Lønbro, 2014; Meneses-Echávez et al., 2015).

TABLE 7.5 Exercise Recommendations for Participants with Cancer

Frequency	■ Aerobic: 3–5 days per week ■ Muscular fitness: 2–3 days per week ■ Flexibility: 2–3 days per week
Intensity	■ Aerobic: Moderate intensity ■ Muscular fitness: Moderate load
Time	■ Aerobic: 20–60 minutes per day ■ Muscular fitness: 1–3 sets with 6–15 reps
Type	■ Combination of aerobic, muscular fitness, balance, and flexibility training
Special considerations	■ May need to lower intensity and duration if undergoing treatment. ■ Engage in physical activity when able. ■ Start and progress slowly. ■ Allow for adequate rest.

OSTEOPOROSIS

OSTEOPOROSIS is a skeletal condition of decreased bone mass and increased risk of fracture commonly found in older women. Exercise has been shown to reduce bone mass loss and increase bone mineral density (Waltman et al., 2010; Zhao et al., 2015). For those with osteoporosis, exercise can be a valuable tool for improving physical function, decreasing risk of falls and fractures, and improving quality of life (Giangregorio et al., 2014). Some of the most effective exercise methods for building bone include weight-bearing aerobic activity and resistance training, with both requiring adequate mechanical loading of the bones and very site-specific adaptations (Benedetti et al., 2018). The greatest exercise risk for those suffering from osteoporosis is bone fracture, either caused by excessive weight or falls during exercise. Instructors should do all they can to help prevent a fracture from occurring and should also include some balance exercises to improve function and decrease fall risk (Benedetti et al., 2018; Buranarugsa et al., 2012). **Table 7.6** shows some basic exercise guidelines and acute variables for individuals with osteoporosis (Waltman et al., 2010; Zhao et al., 2015).

TABLE 7.6 Exercise Recommendations for Participants with Osteoporosis

Frequency	■ Aerobic: 4–5 days per week ■ Muscular fitness: Start with 1–2 days per week. Can progress to 2–3 days per week. ■ Flexibility: 5–7 days per week
Intensity	■ Aerobic: Moderate intensity ■ Muscular fitness: Progress to high intensity and power training when tolerated.
Time	■ Aerobic: 20–60 minutes per day or multiple 8–10 minute bouts ■ Muscular fitness: 1–2 sets with 8–12 reps
Type	■ Low-impact exercise that is comfortable and safe for the individual to avoid falls
Special considerations	■ Progression should be slow and well-monitored. ■ Exercises should be progressed toward free sitting (no back support) or standing. ■ Participants should breathe in a normal manner and avoid holding their breath as in a Valsalva maneuver. ■ If a participant cannot tolerate self-myofascial rolling or static stretches due to other conditions, perform slow rhythmic active or dynamic stretches. ■ Twisting motions should be performed slowly, if at all.

Older Adults

Older adults, generally identified as those 60 years of age or older, make a up a large segment of the U.S. population and are well represented in group fitness settings. According to the U.S. Department of Health and Human Services, older adults made up 16% of the American population in 2019, a 36% increase over a 10-year period (Administration for Community Living, 2021).

© BearFotos/Shutterstock

This growing population has unique needs in a group fitness setting but has the potential to gain tremendous health benefits from regular participation in exercise and physical activity.

Most older adults have at least one chronic condition, such as arthritis (48%), coronary artery disease (14%), or diabetes (29%), and many have multiple conditions (Administration for Community Living, 2021). These conditions can affect an individual's ability to participate fully in group fitness classes, and your ability to help them adapt and feel successful will be imperative to keep them coming back.

The human movement system changes in several ways with age that will affect function and performance. These include changes to the cardiorespiratory, musculoskeletal, and nervous systems.

Research suggests that aerobic capacity begins to decrease after the age of 20, with the rate of decline becoming more severe in older decades (Fleg et al., 2005; Inbar et al., 1994). This reduced cardiorespiratory function can make everyday activities more strenuous for older adults. The loss in aerobic capacity is attributed to a decrease in physical activity as well as physiological changes to the cardiorespiratory system, such as a decrease in maximal heart rate in older adults (Christou & Seals, 2008; Heath et al., 1981).

Muscular strength decreases with age as a result of **SARCOPENIA**, or age-related muscle loss, with a specific loss in the powerful Type II muscle fibers. This decrease in strength can make it difficult to execute **ACTIVITIES OF DAILY LIVING (ADL)**. It will also often result in further reduction in physical activity, decreasing resting metabolic rate and increasing the risk for type 2 diabetes.

Along with these changes, older adults will often have decreased balance control, which can result in a loss of balance or a fall. Combined with a possible decrease in bone density, decreased balance can lead to injuries that affect independence and function.

GETTING TECHNICAL

Aging is associated with a loss of Type II muscle fibers, which are responsible for fast, powerful muscle actions (such as catching yourself from a loss of balance). This selective loss of the fast-twitch muscle fibers can result in reduced ability to perform ADLs and also to respond to a sudden change in balance. However, these Type II muscle fibers can be trained by using heavier loads (relative to the individual) and fast/powerful movements, leading to preservation or even further improvements in these important functional muscles. Remember that strength and power movements are important for older adults and what is heavy or fast will be relative to their current capacity and abilities. Never lose sight of safety being your first priority as a Group Fitness Instructor.

SARCOPENIA

Age-related loss of muscle mass and strength.

ACTIVITIES OF DAILY LIVING (ADL)

The fundamental tasks needed to manage basic self-care activities, such as bathing, dressing, grooming, meal preparation and feeding, and homemaking.

BENEFITS FROM EXERCISE AND PHYSICAL ACTIVITY

It is easy to assume that age-related declines in fitness are an inevitable part of getting older. Fortunately, exercise and physical activity can have a dramatic effect on the work capacity of the older population. Exercise, such as group fitness, has been found to help improve aerobic function, build muscle mass and strength, and preserve bone density in older adults (Behnke et al., 2012; Seguin & Nelson, 2003). These improvements can have a meaningful influence on older adults by decreasing the risk of disability and helping them to maintain independence for an active life. Regular participation in exercise and physical activity will also help older adults increase self-efficacy, manage and prevent the progression of chronic disease, and improve overall health and wellness.

PROGRAMMING CONSIDERATIONS

Although it is common to see decreased performance and chronic conditions with older exercisers, this population is diverse and has varying health and fitness levels. In a group fitness class, you can use coaching, cues, and feedback with these participants to help them find the exercises and intensities that are appropriate for them.

When working with older clients, you should ensure that you are still working to find the relative intensity that will provide progressive overload. Note that an older adult may not be able to complete the same exercises as a younger participant; thus, you should plan to have options that will allow them to feel included, challenged, and successful during the workout. Balance may be diminished, so exercises that challenge balance may be more difficult. For example, lunges involve a decreased base of support and may be more difficult to control for an older adult. You might want to provide the option to hold on to a chair, wall, or other device to provide assistance.

You should consider the specificity principle and prioritize exercises that will enhance daily function and the performance of ADLs such as stair climbing and picking up objects. You can also help increase motivation by relating exercises to the movements that they will develop.

When it comes to programming, strength training is imperative for older adults, because strength is necessary to allow the older adult to be active enough to improve other components of fitness (**Table 7.7**). For example, if the individual cannot stand up, they will not be able to walk to improve cardiorespiratory fitness.

TABLE 7.7 Exercise Guidelines for Older Adults

Frequency	Aerobic: 3–4 days per week Muscular fitness: 2 days on non-consecutive days Flexibility: 2–7 days per week
Intensity	Light to moderate intensity (relative to the individual) Muscular fitness: 10–15 reps for beginners; work up to 8–10 reps (heavier load, fewer reps)
Time	20–30 minutes per day (cumulative 150 minutes per week). May need to start with 5- to 10-minute bouts and work up to meet recommendations.
Type	Cardiorespiratory: ■ Rhythmic, continuous, large muscle group ■ Low risk of falling Muscular: ■ Full body with an emphasis on functional movements to enhance ADLs (walking, carrying groceries, climbing stairs, etc.) Flexibility: ■ Slow static stretching
Special considerations	■ Balance training should be included to prevent falls. ■ Focus on building bone mineral density (BMD) with heavy resistance training (8–10 reps) for major muscle groups. ■ Medications can have a drastic effect on performance and will have side effects that can affect performance (balance, heart rate, etc.). ■ Include socialization and emphasize sense of safety and community.

Pre- and Post-Natal

POST-NATAL

The period just after delivery of a baby.

No matter what formats you teach, you will likely have pregnant or **POST-NATAL** individuals in your classes. It is important that we encourage people to be active during all stages of life. A basic knowledge of the guidelines regarding pregnancy will help you to accommodate pregnant and post-natal participants and welcome them to your classes with confidence.

Pregnancy results in several anatomical and physiological changes to the body that place large demands on the human movement system. Despite these changes, for healthy people with uncomplicated pregnancies, the risk of exercise participation is minimal, and exercise has been shown to have a protective factor for established pregnancies (American College of Obstetricians and Gynecologists, 2020; Thorell et al., 2015).

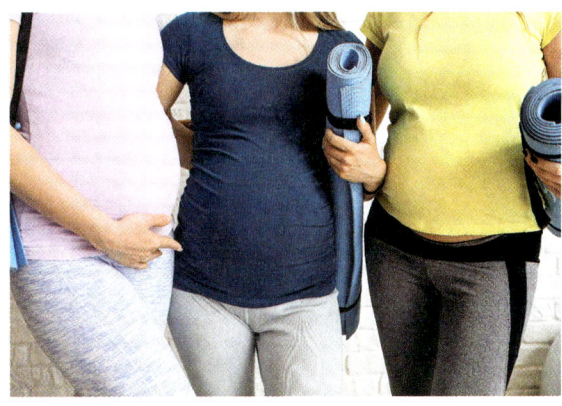

© Pixel-Shot/Shutterstock

BENEFITS FROM EXERCISE AND PHYSICAL ACTIVITY

Individuals should be active during pregnancy because exercise is safe and beneficial for the mother and the baby; both can experience benefits during pregnancy, during birth, and after delivery. Those who are more physically active during pregnancy have been found to be at less risk for excessive weight gain, development of gestational diabetes, Cesarean birth, and postpartum depression. They also have shorter labors and improved postpartum recovery times (American College of Obstetricians and Gynecologists, 2020; Dipietro et al., 2019). As pregnancy progresses, physical fitness parameters tend to decrease, but those who are more physically active can prevent severe decreases in cardiorespiratory and muscular fitness levels, as well as decrease low back pain (American College of Obstetricians and Gynecologists, 2020). Group fitness can be a great avenue to help people to maintain fitness and remain physically active during pregnancy, and, with sound guidance, you can keep these participants safe and motivated.

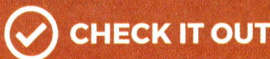 **CHECK IT OUT**

Benefits of physical activity and exercise during pregnancy:

- Improves psychological well-being and mood
- Decreases fatigue
- Prevents excessive weight gain
- Prevents low back pain and improves posture
- Improves the health of the fetus and infant following birth
- Promotes shorter and easier delivery
- Reduces risk of gestational diabetes
- Reduces decreases in cardiorespiratory and muscular fitness

PROGRAMMING CONSIDERATIONS

When a pregnant person is starting an exercise program, you should recommend that they see their physician for a health screening to rule out contraindications and be cleared for usual exercise-based physical activity. You can then help them follow any guidelines set by their physician, if any. Generally, pregnancy is not the time to start novel, higher-intensity exercise programs if that is not what a participant has been accustomed to. The individual should exercise in a manner they have been used to leading up to pregnancy. Group Fitness Instructors should know the basic guidelines for exercise during pregnancy and be aware of the signs and symptoms that indicate that exercise should be ceased immediately.

Due to physiological changes experienced during pregnancy, special attention should be paid to ensuring that pregnant individuals avoid heat injury and that they ingest adequate water during workouts (Artal et al., 2003). Workouts in hot environments should be avoided, such as hot yoga or exercise in rooms without sufficient cooling and ventilation. Clothing that allows for proper cooling should also be recommended.

The Group Fitness Instructor should offer modifications to the exercise routine to account for increased secretion of relaxin, a hormone that relaxes joints during pregnancy, postpartum, and for as long as the parent is nursing, if they choose to do so. Because this hormone will cause joints to become less stable, you should emphasize to the participant that loads must be controlled and that proper exercise technique be strictly adhered to (Artal et al., 2003). High-impact, reactive exercises should be replaced with exercises that present less stress on the joints. Additionally, participants should be advised to avoid excessive range of motion in flexibility exercises and perform static stretches slowly and under control.

Resistance training exercises should emphasize posture and core strength to help prevent low back pain during pregnancy; they have been shown to have a positive effect on labor (Hall & Kaufmann, 1987). Strength training exercises for posture and the upper body can also help to strengthen the muscle groups that will help the postpartum parent hold their infant after birth (**Table 7.8**).

Exercise can also be an effective way to improve health and fitness following the birth of the baby. Postpartum exercise has garnered a great deal of attention in the research literature as well, showing significant benefits, including (O'Connor et al., 2011):

- Body fat loss
- Improved cardiorespiratory and muscular fitness
- Improved bone health
- Enhanced mood

The timing of return to exercise following delivery should be at the discretion of the individual in consultation with their primary care physician, but it typically ranges from 6 to 12 weeks after delivery. Low-intensity resistance training can be added to focus on core and total-body muscular endurance, within the following guidelines:

- Frequency: 2–3 days per week
- Volume: 1–3 sets per exercise (no more than 8–10 exercises per session)
- Repetitions: 10–15 per set
- Intensity: Less than 50% of one-repetition maximum (1RM)

TABLE 7.8 Exercise Guidelines for Participants with Healthy, Uncomplicated Pregnancies

Frequency	5–7 days per week
Intensity	Light to moderate intensity (monitored by either talk test or RPE) Those diagnosed as overweight or who were previously inactive should use low/light intensity.
Time	20–30 minutes per day (150 minutes per week)
Type	Cardiorespiratory: ■ Rhythmic, continuous, large muscle groups ■ Consider what is comfortable for the woman. ■ Low risk of falling or impact Muscular: ■ Moderate intensity (12 reps or more) ■ Avoid the Valsalva maneuver. ■ Avoid extensive isometric holds. ■ Avoid heavy lifting. Flexibility: ■ Slow static stretching
Special considerations	■ Avoid exercises in a prone or supine position after 12 weeks of pregnancy. ■ Avoid SMR on varicose veins and areas of swelling. ■ Obtain physician clearance before any self-myofascial techniques or other techniques that place direct pressure on trigger points, as some may induce labor contractions. ■ Plyometric movement is not advised in the second and third trimesters.

Bodyweight exercises can be excellent choices to produce improvements in muscular fitness, stability, and muscle coordination immediately following pregnancy.

Participants with Special Circumstances

According to the U.S. Census Bureau, as of 2020, nearly 1 in 4 people in the United States have a disability (CDC, 2020). Of the over 61 million people (approximately 26% of the population) affected, many individuals with disabilities indicate that they get no physical activity whatsoever (Spicer, 2004). This same population is three times more likely to have a chronic health condition, such as heart disease, cancer, and diabetes, than those without disabilities (CDC, 2021).

Consider the following tips to promote inclusivity:

- Introduce yourself and make eye contact as you would with any other participant.
- Connect with and acknowledge the individual's presence.
- Respond to all communicative attempts by observing body language.
- Do not refer to an individual as *handicapped* or *disabled*. They are a person *with* a disability or medical diagnosis.
- Understand that a person's wheelchair or other mobility device is an extension of their body. Respect personal space and never move a wheelchair out of its user's reach.
- Use clear and concise instructions and demonstrate whenever possible.
- Encourage participants to keep working on accomplishing tasks rather than rewarding false wins.

The Americans with Disabilities Act (ADA) "prohibits discrimination against people with disabilities in employment, transportation, public accommodations, communications, access to state and local government's programs and services" (U.S. Department of Labor, n.d.). This includes gyms and other fitness services. When developing programs and classes, Group Fitness Instructors and management must keep these guidelines in mind.

Regardless of experience level with disability issues, opportunities exist to "remove the obstacles that traditionally get in the way of gym participation" (Spicer, 2004). To be compliant with the law, fitness and recreational facilities must provide general access and reasonable accommodations for people with disabilities.

📋 INSTRUCTOR TIP

Fitness professionals should adopt the following practices of inclusion (Spicer, 2004):

- **Show enthusiasm.** Creative opportunities for inclusion should be offered with positivity and energy without being condescending.
- **Make accommodations.** Even without special modifications, some programs and equipment can be adapted.
- **Keep activities age appropriate.** Avoid perpetuating the myth that persons with disabilities are different by using childlike games, toys, or rewards. Whenever possible, participants with disabilities should learn by the same rules as a person without disabilities.

Lesson 2: Environmental Considerations

Environmental Physiology

The exercise environment can have a dramatic influence on function and performance. Any elite-level athlete will say that they must consider the location of their competition when preparing to maximize performance. In group fitness, you should understand the effects that the environment can have on your participants and be able to give recommendations to those who are not accustomed to the conditions in which you teach and to ensure that the group exercise space is safe for all participants. If you know that the conditions have changed for a class, you should make adjustments to the workout plan, cue your class on how to remain healthy and safe, and understand when and if exercise should be minimized or avoided.

THERMOREGULA-TION

The ability to maintain body temperature within a healthy range despite the surrounding environment.

Temperature

The temperature during exercise will affect participants' ability to thermoregulate. **THERMOREGULATION** affects both the safety and performance of physical activity. Temperature-related emergencies are due to overexposure to heat or cold, and most are preventable. By wearing appropriate clothing for the external conditions and maintaining proper hydration and electrolyte balance, individuals can easily avoid environmentally induced injury or illness. The signs, symptoms, and response protocols for hot and cold weather injuries should be fully understood.

A reasonable temperature for an exercise class is between 68°F and 72°F (20–22°C), but note that participants living in different climates will have different levels of temperature acclimation. Age and gender also factor into an individual's hot or cold tolerance (Powers & Howley, 2011).

Should inclement weather or temperature make exercise outdoors dangerous, instructors should be prepared to do the following:

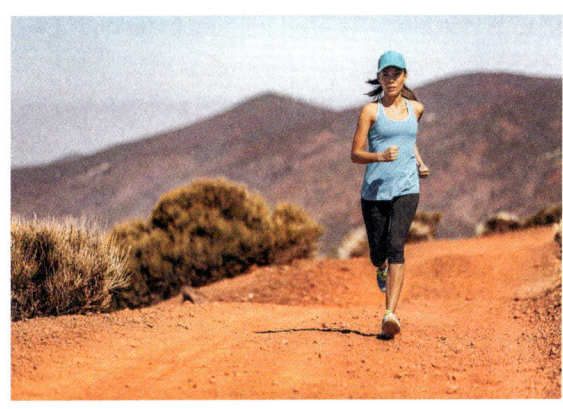
© Maridav/Shutterstock

- Move class to a climate-controlled indoor space.
- Minimize time in extreme weather.
- Actively alter exercise sessions if signs of weather-related stress are observed.
- Have appropriate emergency equipment available (e.g., ice, cold water, cold packs, and mobile phone).

HEAT AND EXERCISE

Heat will affect the health and safety of exercise participants. It can decrease exercise performance and make exercise feel difficult and uncomfortable. When exercising in hot environments, it is important to promote thermoregulation to avoid an increase in core temperature and dehydration. Exercising muscles generate heat. The body will dissipate that heat in various ways, the most common being evaporation via sweating. The amount of heat produced during exercise is directly related to exercise intensity; thus, if exercising in a hot environment, it may be a good idea to adjust the intensity of the workout to avoid heat-related injuries (**Table 7.9**).

TABLE 7.9 Heat-Related Injuries

Heat-Related Injury	Description	Common Signs and Symptoms	Response Protocols
Heat cramps	Heat cramps are painful muscle spasms. They could be a warning signal or sign of a heat-related emergency.	Painful muscle spasms in the legs or abdominal region	- Rest the individual in a cool place. - Provide cool water. - Do not give salt tablets or saltwater to drink.
Heat exhaustion	More severe than heat cramps and usually occurring after a long period of strenuous exercise or work in the heat and/or humidity	- Cool, moist, pale, or red skin - Headache or dizziness - Nausea - Normal or below normal body temperature - Weakness and/or exhaustion	- Get the individual out of the heat and call emergency services immediately. - Attempt to reduce body temperature with cool, wet cloths or towels. - Loosen all tight clothing. - If the individual is able to swallow, give cool water to drink (slowly). - Monitor vital signs and wait for EMS.

(continues)

TABLE 7.9 Heat-Related Injuries (*continued*)

Heat-Related Injury	Description	Common Signs and Symptoms	Response Protocols
Heat stroke	The least common, but the most severe heat emergency. Usually occurs after the signals of heat exhaustion are ignored. In heat stroke, dangerously elevated internal temperatures cause vital body systems to fail.	■ Change in consciousness ■ Rapid, shallow breathing ■ Rapid, weak pulse ■ Red, hot, and dry skin	■ Call emergency services immediately. ■ Get the individual out of the heat. ■ Cool the body with cool, wet cloths or towels. ■ Loosen all tight clothing. ■ Do not give anything by mouth. ■ Monitor vital signs and wait for EMS.

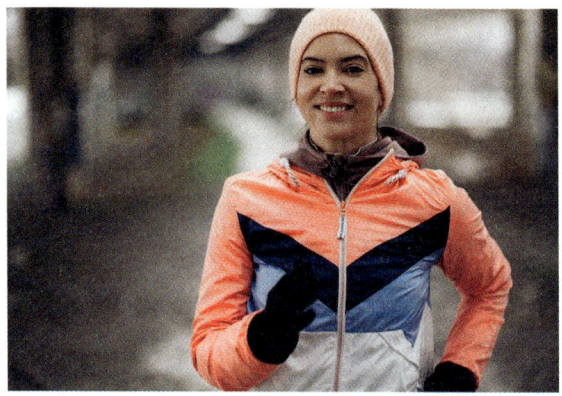

© Zamrznuti tonovi/Shutterstock

The following are tips to help keep exercise safe and healthy for group fitness participants:

- Avoid prolonged exercise in the heat.
- Be aware of predisposing factors to heat injury:
  - Older adults
  - Participants with obesity
  - Pregnancy
- Adjust exercise intensity.

COLD AND EXERCISE

Unlike exercise in hot environments, exercise in the cold is usually not a barrier to physical activity, but Group Fitness Instructors should be aware of how the cold can affect some participants and should recognize when conditions meet the criteria for increasing the risk of cold-related injuries (**Table 7.10**). Individuals who are at risk for cold-related complications from the environment include older adults, individuals with low body fat, and those with CVD, asthma, or hypoglycemia.

TABLE 7.10 Cold-Related Injury

Cold-Related Injury	Description	Common Signs and Symptoms	Response Protocols
Hypothermia	Hypothermia occurs when the body can no longer generate enough heat to maintain normal body temperature. Core body temperature drops to ≤ 95°F (35°C).	■ Apathy and decreased levels of consciousness ■ Numbness or glassy stare ■ Shivering (could be absent in latter stages) ■ Slow, irregular pulse ■ Pale, cool skin ■ Patches of cyanosis (blue color) to lips and skin	■ Call emergency services immediately. ■ Remove wet clothing and dry the individual (if applicable). ■ Gradually warm the body with blankets and dry clothes. ■ Move to a dry, warmer environment. ■ Do not warm too quickly as this could lead to shock. ■ Monitor vital signs and wait for EMS.

Cold temperatures can present a danger for those who have predisposing factors and can increase the risk of respiratory exercise-induced complications, such as bronchoconstriction and acute upper respiratory tract infections. Conditions such as cold air temperature, wind speed, and the wetness of the environment will all determine the risk of cold-related respiratory complications.

When exercising in the cold, always make sure skin is adequately covered. Wind chill should also be taken into consideration. For this reason, it is highly recommended to dress in multiple thin layers of clothing that can be progressively removed (outer garments first), or placed back on, throughout the duration of a cold-weather exercise session to maintain comfort and safety. A head covering is also recommended, as it can be removed or replaced easily to accommodate the temperature.

Humidity

Humidity can affect the body's ability to cool itself through evaporation, increasing the risk of heat injury or dehydration. High relative humidity will cause a decrease in performance and can make exercise feel more difficult. If the air is humid, the water in sweat does not evaporate into the surrounding air as readily, decreasing sweat's ability to remove heat from the body and increasing the chance of overheating. When relative humidity is high, it is important to have adequate air flow to allow more efficient evaporation through sweat. Participants should also be encouraged to rest often and as needed to avoid overheating. High levels of caution should be taken when exercising in hot and humid conditions.

⊘ CHECK IT OUT

Relative Humidity

Figure 7.1 shows how the combination of air temperature and humidity creates the sensation of how hot the environment feels to the participant. This is called the heat index.

Temperature (°F)

Relative Humidity (%)	80	82	84	86	88	90	92	94	96	98	100	102	104	106	108	110
40	80	81	83	85	88	91	94	97	101	105	109	114	119	124	130	136
45	80	82	84	87	89	93	96	100	104	109	114	119	124	130	137	
50	81	83	85	88	91	95	99	103	108	113	118	124	131	137		
55	81	84	86	89	93	97	101	106	112	117	124	130	137			
60	82	84	88	91	95	100	105	110	116	123	129	137				
65	82	85	89	93	98	103	108	114	121	128	136					
70	83	86	90	95	100	105	112	119	126	134						
75	84	88	92	97	103	109	116	124	132							
80	84	89	94	100	106	113	121	129								
85	85	90	96	102	110	117	126	135								
90	86	91	98	105	113	122	131									
95	86	93	100	108	117	127										
100	87	95	103	112	121	132										

Likelihood of Heat Disorders with Prolonged Exposure of Strenuous Activity

Caution   Extreme Caution   Danger   Extreme Danger

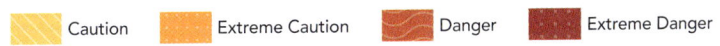

FIGURE 7.1 Heat Index

National Weather Service. (n.d.). *What is the heat index?* https://www.weather.gov/ama/heatindex

Altitude

Altitude affects exercise performance, and the impact is more pronounced as altitude becomes more extreme. As altitude increases, atmospheric pressure decreases, reducing the concentration of oxygen molecules. This means that the same breath of air at high altitude will contain less oxygen than one at low altitude, and red blood cells will become less saturated with oxygen. The heart, therefore, must pump more liters of blood per minute to maintain oxygenation; for example, VO_{2max} has been shown to be reduced by up to 27% at 4,000 meters of elevation (Powers & Howley, 2011). Some decreases in performance can be noted as low as 1,500 meters of elevation (Buskirk et al, 1967; Levine & Stray-Gundersen, 1997). Aerobic exercise is the most dramatically affected by altitude, and duration and intensity of exercise may need to be adjusted while the individual is not acclimated to the altitude. Group fitness instructors who teach at high altitudes should encourage new or visiting participants to hydrate well, decrease intensity and duration, and progress slowly.

Pollution

Poor air quality also affects outdoor exercise by reducing oxygen levels. Ozone has been shown to decrease VO_{2max} and other respiratory values. Sulfur dioxide can cause bronchoconstriction in people with asthma. Carbon monoxide binds hemoglobin, thus reducing oxygen transport in a manner similar to altitude (Powers & Howley, 2011). Dust and smoke are also highly irritating to the cardiorespiratory system.

The U.S. Environmental Protection Agency (n.d.) developed the Air Quality Index (AQI), with values ranging from good to hazardous (**Table 7.11**). Exercise should not take place when the AQI is greater than 150; those sensitive to air pollution should avoid exposure to values greater than 100.

Group Fitness Instructors should listen to health officials and recommendations for activity levels and adjust accordingly. Also, those who teach outdoors should make efforts to locate exercise areas away from areas of high traffic and other pollutants. Despite the negative effects of poor air quality, the risks associated with an inactive lifestyle are more severe.

TABLE 7.11 EPA Air Quality Index (AQI)

AQI	Level of Concern	Daily AQI Color
0–50	Good	Green
51–100	Moderate	Yellow
101–150	Unhealthy for sensitive persons	Orange
151–200	Unhealthy	Red
201–300	Very unhealthy	Purple
301–500	Hazardous	Maroon

Note: Values above 500 are considered beyond the AQI. Follow recommendations for the Hazardous category.

Environmental Protection Agency. (n.d.). Air Quality Index (AQI) Basics. https://www.airnow.gov/aqi/aqi-basics/

SUMMARY

Inclusive instruction requires the Group Fitness Instructor to understand the abilities, goals, and limitations of participants in their classes and to be prepared to provide modifications to help each participant feel successful. Participant-centered instruction requires an understanding of the complex behavioral factors that motivate or discourage individuals, and instructors can cue in a manner that is inclusive of all, regardless of race, gender, age, or ability.

REFERENCES

Administration for Community Living. (2021, May). 2020 *Profile of older Americans*. https://acl.gov/sites/default/files/Aging%20and%20Disability%20in%20America/2020ProfileOlderAmericans.Final.pdf

American College of Obstetricians and Gynecologists. (2020). Physical activity and exercise during pregnancy and the postpartum period: ACOG committee opinion, Number 804. *Obstetrics and Gynecology, 135*(4), e178–e188. https://doi.org/10.1097/AOG.0000000000003772

Artal, R., O'Toole, M., & White, S. (2003). Guidelines of the American College of Obstetricians and Gynecologists for exercise during pregnancy and the postpartum period. *British Journal of Sports Medicine, 37*(1), 6–12. https://doi.org/10.1136/bjsm.37.1.6

Behnke, B. J., Ramsey, M. W., Stabley, J. N., Dominguez, J. M., 2nd, Davis, R. T., 3rd, McCullough, D. J., Muller-Delp, J. M., &. Delp, M. D. (2012). Effects of aging and exercise training on skeletal muscle blood flow and resistance artery morphology. *Journal of Applied Physiology, 113*(11), 1699–1708. https://doi.org/10.1152/japplphysiol.01025.2012

Benedetti, M. G., Furlini, G., Zati, A., & Letizia Mauro, G. (2018). The effectiveness of physical exercise on bone density in osteoporotic patients. *BioMed Research International, 2018*, 4840531. https://doi.org/10.1155/2018/4840531

Benton, M. J. (2005). Safety and efficacy of resistance training in patients with chronic heart failure: Research-based evidence. *Progress in Cardiovascular Nursing, 20*(1), 17–23. https://doi.org/10.1111/j.0889-7204.2005.03888.x

Brogårdh, C., & Lexell, J. (2012, Nov.). Effects of cardiorespiratory fitness and muscle-resistance training after stroke. *PM & R, 4*(11), 901–907. https://doi.org/10.1016/j.pmrj.2012.09.1157

Buranarugsa, R., Oliveira, J., & Maia, J. (2012). Strength training in youth (resistance, plyometrics, complex training): An evidence-based review. *Revista Portuguesa de Ciências do Desporto, 12*(1), 87–115. https://doi.org/10.5628/rpcd.12.01.87

Buskirk, E. R., Kollias, J., Akers, R. F., Prokop, E. K., & Reategui, E. P. (1967). Maximal performance at altitude and on return from altitude in conditioned runners. *Journal of Applied Physiology, 23*(2), 259–266. https://doi.org/10.1152/jappl.1967.23.2.259

Centers for Disease Control and Prevention. (2020, September). *Disability and health promotion. Disability impacts all of us*. https://www.cdc.gov/ncbddd/disabilityandhealth/infographic-disability-impacts-all.html

Centers for Disease Control and Prevention. (2021, August). *Disability and health promotion. Increasing physical activity among adults with disabilities*. https://www.cdc.gov/ncbddd/disabilityandhealth/pa.html

Centers for Disease Control and Prevention. (2022, May). *Overweight & obesity. Adult obesity facts*. https://www.cdc.gov/obesity/data/adult.html

Christou, D. D., & Seals, D. R. (2008). Decreased maximal heart rate with aging is related to reduced {beta}-adrenergic responsiveness but is largely explained by a reduction in intrinsic heart rate. *Journal of Applied Physiology, 105*(1), 24–29. https://doi.org/10.1152/japplphysiol.90401.2008

Cornelissen, V. A., & Fagard, R. H. (2005). Effect of resistance training on resting blood pressure: A meta-analysis of randomized controlled trials. *Journal of Hypertension, 23*(2), 251–259. https://doi.org/10.1097/00004872-200502000-00003

Cornelissen, V. A., Fagard, R. H., Coeckelberghs, E., & Vanhees, L. (2011). Impact of resistance training on blood pressure and other cardiovascular risk factors: A meta-analysis of randomized, controlled trials. *Hypertension, 58*(5), 950–958. https://doi.org/10.1161/HYPERTENSIONAHA.111.177071

Cramp, F., James, A., & Lambert, J. (2010). The effects of resistance training on quality of life in cancer: A systematic literature review and meta-analysis. *Supportive Care in Cancer, 18*(11), 1367–1376. https://doi.org/10.1007/s00520-010-0904-z

Dipietro, L., Evenson, K. R., Bloodgood, B., Sprow, K., Troiano, R. P., Piercy, K. L., Vaux-Bjerke, A., &. Powell, K. E. (2019). Benefits of physical activity during pregnancy and postpartum: An umbrella review. *Medicine & Science in Sports & Exercise, 51*(6), 1292–1302. https://doi.org/10.1249/MSS.0000000000001941

Environmental Protection Agency. (n.d.). *Air quality index (AQI) basics.* https://www.airnow.gov/aqi/aqi-basics/

Fagard, R. H. (2001). Exercise characteristics and the blood pressure response to dynamic physical training. *Medicine & Science in Sports & Exercise, 33*(6 Supplement), S484–S492. https://doi.org/10.1097/00005768-200106001-00018

Faselis, C., Doumas, M., Pittaras, A., Narayan, P., Myers, J., Tsimploulis, A., & Kokkinos, P. (2014). Exercise capacity and all-cause mortality in male veterans with hypertension aged ≥70 years. *Hypertension, 64*(1), 30–35. https://doi.org/10.1161/HYPERTENSIONAHA.114.03510

Fiuza-Luces, C., Santos-Lozano, A., Joyner, M., Carrera-Bastos, P., Picazo, O., Zugaza, J. L., Izquierdo, M., Ruilope, L. M., & Lucia, A. (2018). Exercise benefits in cardiovascular disease: Beyond attenuation of traditional risk factors. *Nature Reviews. Cardiology, 15*(12), 731–743. https://doi.org/10.1038/s41569-018-0065-1

Fleg, J. L., Morrell, C. H., Bos, A. G., Brant, L. J., Talbot, L. A., Wright, J. G., & Lakatta, E. G. (2005). Accelerated longitudinal decline of aerobic capacity in healthy older adults. *Circulation, 112*(5), 674–682. https://doi.org/10.1161/CIRCULATIONAHA.105.545459

Friedenreich, C. M., Neilson, H. K., Farris, M. S., & Courneya, K. S. (2016). Physical activity and cancer outcomes: A precision medicine approach. *Clinical Cancer Research, 22*(19), 4766–4775. https://doi.org/10.1158/1078-0432.CCR-16-0067

Giangregorio, L. M., Papaioannou, A., Macintyre, N. J., Ashe, M. C., Heinonen, A., Shipp, K., Wark, J., McGill, S., Keller, H., Jain, R., Laprade, J., & Cheung, A. M. (2014). Too fit to fracture: Exercise recommendations for individuals with osteoporosis or osteoporotic vertebral fracture. *Osteoporosis International, 25*(3), 821–835. https://doi.org/10.1007/s00198-013-2523-2

Hall, D. C., & Kaufmann, D. A. (1987). Effects of aerobic and strength conditioning on pregnancy outcomes. *American Journal of Obstetrics and Gynecology, 157*(5), 1199–1203. https://doi.org/10.1016/s0002-9378(87)80294-6

Hayes, S. C., Spence, R. R., Galvão, D. A., & Newton, R. U. (2009). Australian Association for Exercise and Sport Science position stand: Optimising cancer outcomes through exercise. *Journal of Science and Medicine in Sport, 12*(4), 428–434. https://doi.org/10.1016/j.jsams.2009.03.002

Heath, G. W., Hagberg, J. M., Ehsani, A. A., & Holloszy, J. O. (1981). A physiological comparison of young and older endurance athletes. *Journal of Applied Physiology: Respiratory, Environmental and Exercise Physiology, 51*(3), 634–640. https://doi.org/10.1152/jappl.1981.51.3.634

Inbar, O., Oren, A., Scheinowitz, M., Rotstein, A., Dlin, R., & Casaburi, R. (1994). Normal cardiopulmonary responses during incremental exercise in 20- to 70-yr-old men. *Medicine & Science in Sports & Exercise, 26*(5), 538–546.

Kelley, G. A., & Kelley, K. S. (2000). Progressive resistance exercise and resting blood pressure: A meta-analysis of randomized controlled trials. *Hypertension, 35*(3), 838–843. https://doi.org/10.1161/01.hyp.35.3.838

Kokkinos, P., & Myers, J. (2010). Exercise and physical activity: Clinical outcomes and applications. *Circulation, 122*(16), 1637–1648. https://doi.org/10.1161/CIRCULATIONAHA.110.948349

Le, V.-V., Mitiku, T., Sungar, G., Myers, J., & Froelicher, V. (2008). The blood pressure response to dynamic exercise testing: A systematic review. *Progress in Cardiovascular Diseases, 51*(2), 135–160. https://doi.org/10.1016/j.pcad.2008.07.001

Levine, B. D., & Stray-Gundersen, J. (1997). "Living high-training low": Effect of moderate-altitude acclimatization with low-altitude training on performance. *Journal of Applied Physiology, 83*(1), 102–112. https://doi.org/10.1152/jappl.1997.83.1.102

Li, Y., Hanssen, H., Cordes, M., Rossmeissl, A., Endes, S., & Schmidt-Trucksäss, A. (2015). Aerobic, resistance and combined exercise training on arterial stiffness in normotensive and hypertensive adults: A review. *European Journal of Sport Science, 15*(5), 443–457. https://doi.org/10.1080/17461391.2014.955129

Lønbro, S. (2014). The effect of progressive resistance training on lean body mass in post-treatment cancer patients—a systematic review. *Radiotherapy and Oncology, 110*(1), 71–80. https://doi.org/10.1016/j.radonc.2013.07.008

Mar, P. L., Nwazue, V., Black, B. K., Biaggioni, I., Diedrich, A., Paranjape, S. Y., Loyd, J. E., Hemnes, A. R., Robbins, I. M., Robertson, D., Raj, S. R., & Austin, E. D. (2016). Valsalva maneuver in pulmonary arterial hypertension: Susceptibility to syncope and autonomic dysfunction. *Chest, 149*(5), 1252–1260. https://doi.org/10.1016/j.chest.2015.11.015

Meneses-Echávez, J. F., González-Jiménez, E., & Ramírez-Vélez, R. (2015). Supervised exercise reduces cancer-related fatigue: A systematic review. *Journal of Physiotherapy, 61*(1), 3–9. https://doi.org/10.1016/j.jphys.2014.08.019

Mustian, K. M., Sprod, L. K., Janelsins, M., Peppone, L. J., & Mohile, S. (2012). Exercise recommendations for cancer-related fatigue, cognitive impairment, sleep problems, depression, pain, anxiety, and physical dysfunction: A review. *Oncology & Hematology Review, 8*(2), 81–88. https://doi.org/10.17925/ohr.2012.08.2.81

National Weather Service. (n.d.). *What is the heat index?* https://www.weather.gov/ama/heatindex

O'Connor, P. J., Poudevigne, M. S., Cress, M. E., Motl, R. W., & Clapp, J. F., 3rd. (2011). Safety and efficacy of supervised strength training adopted in pregnancy. *Journal of Physical Activity & Health, 8*(3), 309–320. https://doi.org/10.1123/jpah.8.3.309

Paramanandam, V. S., & Roberts, D. (2014, Sept.). Weight training is not harmful for women with breast cancer-related lymphoedema: A systematic review. *Journal of Physiotherapy, 60*(3), 136–143. https://doi.org/10.1016/j.jphys.2014.07.001

Pinckard, K., Baskin, K. K., & Stanford, K. I. (2019). Effects of exercise to improve cardiovascular health. *Frontiers in Cardiovascular Medicine, 6*, 69. https://doi.org/10.3389/fcvm.2019.00069

Powers, S. K., & Howley, E. T. (2011). *Exercise physiology: Theory and application to fitness and performance* (8th ed.). McGraw-Hill Education.

Puetz, T. W., & Herring, M. P. (2012). Differential effects of exercise on cancer-related fatigue during and following treatment: A meta-analysis. *American Journal of Preventive Medicine, 43*(2), e1–e24. https://doi.org/10.1016/j.amepre.2012.04.027

Riebe, D., Ehrman, J. K., Liguori, G., & Magal, M. (Eds.). (2018). *ACSM's guidelines for exercise testing and prescription* (10th ed.). Wolters Kluwer.

Roitman, J. L., & LaFontaine, T. (2006). Exercise, atherosclerosis, and the endothelium: Where the action is (Part II). *Strength and Conditioning Journal, 28*(1), 75–77. https://doi.org/10.1519/00126548-200602000-00013

Seguin, R., & Nelson, M. E. (2003). The benefits of strength training for older adults. *American Journal of Preventive Medicine, 25*(3 Supplement 2), 141–149. https://doi.org/10.1016/s0749-3797(03)00177-6

Shmerling, R. H. (2020). *How useful is the body mass index (BMI)?* Harvard Health Publishing. https://www.health.harvard.edu/blog/how-useful-is-the-body-mass-index-bmi-201603309339

Spicer, P. M. (2004). *Exercise is for everyone!* IDEA. https://www.ideafit.com/uncategorized/for-everyone/

Strasser, B., Steindorf, K., Wiskemann, J., & Ulrich, C. M. (2013). Impact of resistance training in cancer survivors: A meta-analysis. *Medicine & Science in Sports & Exercise, 45*(11), 2080–2090. https://doi.org/10.1249/MSS.0b013e31829a3b63

Thorell, E., Goldsmith, L., Weiss, G., & Kristiansson, P. (2015). Physical fitness, serum relaxin and duration of gestation. *BMC Pregnancy and Childbirth, 15*(1), 168. https://doi.org/10.1186/s12884-015-0607-z

Tran, Q. T. (2005). Resistance training and safety considerations for chronic heart failure patients. *Strength and Conditioning Journal, 27*(6), 71–72. https://doi.org/10.1519/00126548-200512000-00010

Uranga, R. M., & Keller, J. N. (2019). The complex interactions between obesity, metabolism and the brain. *Frontiers in Neuroscience, 13*, 513. https://doi.org/10.3389/fnins.2019.00513

U.S. Department of Labor. (n.d.). *Americans with Disabilities Act.* https://www.dol.gov/general/topic/disability/ada

Wallace, J. P. (2003). Exercise in hypertension. A clinical review. *Sports Medicine, 33*(8), 585–598. https://doi.org/10.2165/00007256-200333080-00004

Waltman, N. L., Twiss, J. J., Ott, C. D., Gross, G. J., Lindsey, A. M., Moore, T. E., Berg, K., & Kupzyk, K. (2010). The effect of weight training on bone mineral density and bone turnover in postmenopausal breast cancer survivors with bone loss: A 24-month randomized controlled trial. *Osteoporosis International, 21*(8), 1361–1369. https://doi.org/10.1007/s00198-009-1083-y

Whelton, S. P., Chin, A., Xin, X., & He, J. (2002). Effect of aerobic exercise on blood pressure: A meta-analysis of randomized, controlled trials. *Annals of Internal Medicine, 136*(7), 493–503. https://doi.org/10.7326/0003-4819-136-7-200204020-00006

Williams, M. A., Haskell, W. L., Ades, P. A., Amsterdam, E. A., Bittner, V., Franklin, B. A., Gulanick, M., Laing, S. T., & Stewart, K. J. (2007). Resistance exercise in individuals with and without cardiovascular disease: 2007 update: A scientific statement from the American Heart Association Council on Clinical Cardiology and Council on Nutrition, Physical Activity, and Metabolism. *Circulation, 116*(5), 572–584. https://doi.org/10.1161/CIRCULATIONAHA.107.185214

Zhao, R., Zhao, M., & Xu, Z. (2015). The effects of differing resistance training modes on the preservation of bone mineral density in postmenopausal women: A meta-analysis. *Osteoporosis International, 26*(5), 1605–1618. https://doi.org/10.1007/s00198-015-3034-0

SECTION 3

CLASS DESIGN AND PLANNING

CHAPTER 8

DEFINING YOUR CLASS

LEARNING OBJECTIVES

The intent of this chapter is to explore your vision and desired objectives for your class and connect them with other class considerations to ensure that your class meets your participants' needs.

After reading this content, students should be able to demonstrate the following objectives:

- **Define** *class vision* and *objectives*.
- **Identify** other considerations in designing a group fitness class.
- **Discuss** the five components of a group fitness class in the context of class design and planning.
- **Explain** the value of flow in designing a group fitness class.

Lesson 1: Class Basics

Introduction

Before planning a workout, an instructor considers multiple variables that will influence how they prepare to teach the class and what they choose to incorporate into the class experience. If you were to compare planning a class to building a house, the class type/format, class vision and objectives, and the physical environment provide the foundation. The five components of the class (intro, movement prep, body of the workout, transition, and outro) comprise the structure that is built on top of that foundation. Finally, the details of what each of those five components will entail, along with how the class will flow from one component to the next, are the unique designs and decorations that make the house feel like a home.

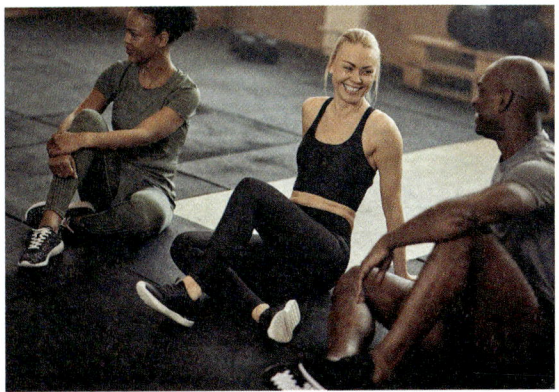

© Ground Picture/Shutterstock

Class Types and Formats

A variety of class types and formats are possible. How you will prepare to teach a class depends on the format being used: pre-choreographed, pre-formatted, or freestyle. In most pre-choreographed classes, the instructor receives a workout that is already designed and is often accompanied with a full music playlist. The instructor's primary responsibility with a pre-choreographed class is to study and rehearse the class until they are confident in their ability to deliver it. For pre-formatted classes, the instructor is usually given a template that they are responsible for plugging exercises into. They may select specific exercises that fit within prescribed sections of the workout. With freestyle formats, the instructor has the freedom and responsibility to create the class template, and then plug in exercises for each new workout. Aerobic exercise classes became very popular in the 1980s, and people enjoyed matching their movements to the music in pre-choreographed formats such as step aerobics and cardio dance classes. Over time, the benefits of resistance training in a group setting became clear, and workouts that prioritized building strength grew in popularity. Some of those resistance training classes stuck with the traditional experience of a pre-choreographed class that matches movements to music, whereas others let the music become a background detail as they experimented with pre-formatted and freestyle classes.

Some instructors prefer teaching pre-choreographed classes because of the unique energy they create, and because they allow instructors to focus on teaching and cueing. Other instructors prefer teaching pre-formatted and freestyle formats because those classes give them the opportunity to create a unique experience. Those class types require the instructor to have a solid understanding of exercise physiology to ensure that they will create safe and effective workouts. Regardless of the class format and preparation process, the instructor's style and personality will always shine. You will create a unique impression with every class you teach!

Pre-Choreographed

Pre-choreographed classes are often written by a specific brand in which the instructor holds a credential (e.g., Latin dance–based or group barbell workouts). The brand will often release new choreography at regular intervals, complete with exercise/movement selection and a full playlist. In this case, the instructor prepares to teach the class by studying and rehearsing the material the brand has provided. Although the instructor will not design the workout, they are responsible for delivering a class experience that upholds the standards of the brand they represent and are often licensed by. The amount of time dedicated to studying and rehearsing will vary depending on the class format and the complexity of the choreography.

Pre-choreographed classes provide a variety of benefits for the instructor, the class participants, and the facility where they are offered, but they come with their tradeoffs, too. For the instructor, receiving a workout that is designed and tested by the brand eliminates the pressure to create an effective workout from scratch. Another benefit of teaching pre-choreographed classes is that once they get comfortable with teaching new material, instructors can really focus on developing their coaching skills and delivering an exceptional class experience. For participants, each time they repeat the class, they become more familiar and comfortable with the movements, allowing them to feel more successful each time they attend. For facilities, incorporating pre-choreographed classes that are created by established brands into their schedule can provide structure and quality control. Although the repetitive nature of pre-choreographed classes offers many benefits, workouts can eventually become stale for the instructor and participants alike, especially for an instructor with the desire to get creative and build new class experiences regularly.

Pre-Formatted

For pre-formatted classes, the instructor is usually given a class template (**Figure 8.1**) and will choose exercises to plug into that template. The template, or signature program, is usually created by the facility in an effort to provide its membership with consistent class experiences and a structured class schedule. Although the instructor will not design the fundamental structure of the workout, they are responsible for choosing appropriate exercises and putting them in an order that will ultimately meet the class vision and objectives. The instructor will also need to update the exercises they are using on a regular basis. Pre-formatted classes generally require less time spent studying and rehearsing than pre-choreographed classes, but it is still important for the instructor to be familiar with the template and remember the exercises they choose. The less time the instructor spends consulting their notes throughout a class, the more time they can dedicate to coaching, motivating, and connecting with the participants.

Pre-formatted classes also have pros and cons. For the instructor, receiving a template that is designed and tested by the brand/facility provides them with guidance to ensure that they meet the expectations of the brand while also giving them the freedom to be creative and incorporate their own style into the workout. This may be seen as the best of both worlds of creative freedom and structure by many instructors. For members, the consistency of the structure provides them with a certain level of comfort and familiarity for each class they attend, even if the workout or instructor is new to them. Lastly, for the facility, providing instructors with a template helps

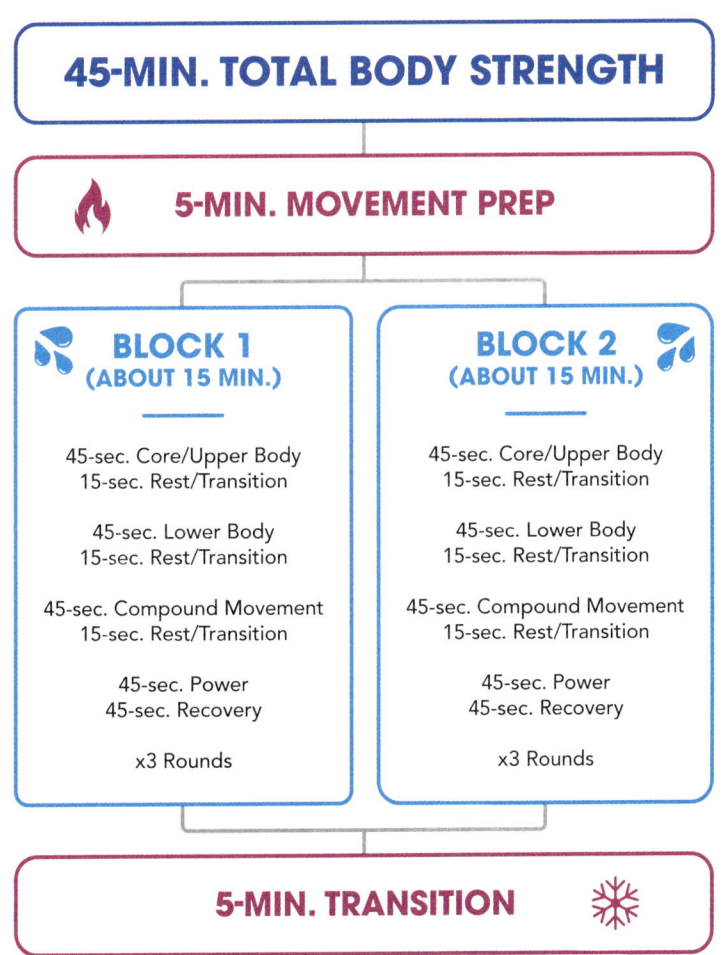

FIGURE 8.1 Sample Total-Body Strength Class Template

them build their brand recognition while ensuring that each individual class offered is of similar quality because every instructor is using the same fundamental structure. It is worth noting, however, that although pre-formatted classes give instructors the freedom to be creative, this requires regular observation and auditing by the facility to ensure that the workouts delivered to their members adequately represent the brand.

Freestyle

With freestyle class formats, instead of being provided with a template of the class structure, the instructor is responsible for creating that template and selecting all the exercises that go into it. Freestyle formats are a great opportunity for experienced and educated instructors to shine, but they could leave less experienced instructors with inadequate direction. When designing the template for a class, it is important to have a clear understanding of the desired outcomes. Establishing the outcomes will identify and clarify both the vision and objectives for the class, which will ultimately inform the decisions the instructor makes as they design the class template and choose the appropriate exercises to plug into it. After testing and revising the template design, the instructor will likely create a format they want to use long term; then, that class and the process of preparing to teach it will mimic those of pre-formatted classes.

The vision and objectives are usually already defined for pre-choreographed and pre-formatted classes; thus, most of the following information is primarily applicable to planning freestyle-format classes. However, note that several elements from the following section can be used to elevate the experience instructors provide in pre-choreographed and pre-formatted classes.

Formats

In group fitness, format refers to the base organizational structure that connects the components of a class with a particular outcome. A format may differentiate itself by moves, music, teaching style, class size, modality, equipment, and even wardrobe. Eight basic formats are prevalent in the group fitness arena today, utilizing foundational exercise-science principles and training guidelines for cardiorespiratory, strength, and flexibility improvement:

- **Strength and resistance:** Offer participants the opportunity to increase muscular strength and endurance using an opposing force for resistance.
- **Interval:** Involve alternating work periods of higher intensities with recovery periods performed at moderate to low intensities. High-intensity interval training (HIIT) workouts are typically shorter in duration, but extremely challenging.
- **Boot camp:** Include a combination of resistance and cardio elements, with the goal of providing a total-body workout, with a military-style presentation.
- **Mind–body:** Include practices such as yoga, Pilates, tai chi, and more. These formats feature slow, controlled movements that combine strength, stability, flexibility, balance, and breathing techniques. For the purpose of this program, and due to its popularity, yoga will be the primary focus when discussing mind–body group fitness formats.
- **Cycling:** Participants ride stationary bicycles designed to simulate an outdoor cycling experience.
- **Specialty formats:** Because some formats require additional certification or training, these will be covered only in brief:
  - **Dance oriented:** Designed to make cardiorespiratory training more interesting and fun. Classes rely on exhilarating, energizing moves specifically choreographed to match popular or thematic music.

- **Aquatics:** Consist of cardio, strength, and stability movements taught in shallow or deep pools and offer benefits for populations ranging from the overweight and deconditioned to elite athletes.
- **Active, aging adults:** Focus on basic functional movements, often through the use of chairs, step decks, water, and lighter resistance.
- **Discipline-specific:** Formats specific to certain disciplines or sports, such as martial arts or cardio tennis.
- **Equipment driven:** Focus on a particular modality, such as suspension training systems or kettlebells.
- **Hybrid:** A combination of two or more formats, such as yogalates, to accomplish more than one outcome.

An instructor is advised to learn and develop skills in one of the eight central formats before specializing further. Specialty formats are created and managed by businesses, education providers, corporate club chains, private studios, and even individual instructors. Common examples of specialty programs include martial arts, cardio kickboxing, barre, Pilates, yoga, athletic performance, injury prevention, and many more that may require experience with specific equipment (e.g., treadmill, rower, balance plate).

Class Vision and Objectives

The **CLASS VISION** identifies an intention for the overall class experience and guides the specific decisions an instructor makes as they prepare to teach it. The vision is not always easy to track or measure, especially if it centers on participants' mental and emotional responses to the class (e.g., empowering, energizing, relaxing, etc.). A **CLASS OBJECTIVE** is one of multiple, specific goals that, when combined, create a clear path for the participants to achieve the desired outcome. Like most journeys, there are many steps to the ultimate destination, so it is common to pursue multiple objectives in the same class (**Figure 8.2**). It is also common for objectives to start out broad and evolve into something more specific (e.g., clarifying that an upper body workout will specifically target the deltoids). To achieve the desired outcome, the vision and objectives will complement and align with one another. For example, if the vision is to create a challenging and empowering experience for participants, objectives such as muscular strength and cardio conditioning better align with that vision than an objective such as a meditative practice.

CLASS VISION

A broad intention that guides the specific decisions the instructor makes as they plan the class.

CLASS OBJECTIVE

A specific, clearly defined milestone that acts as a stepping stone along the journey toward achieving the desired outcome.

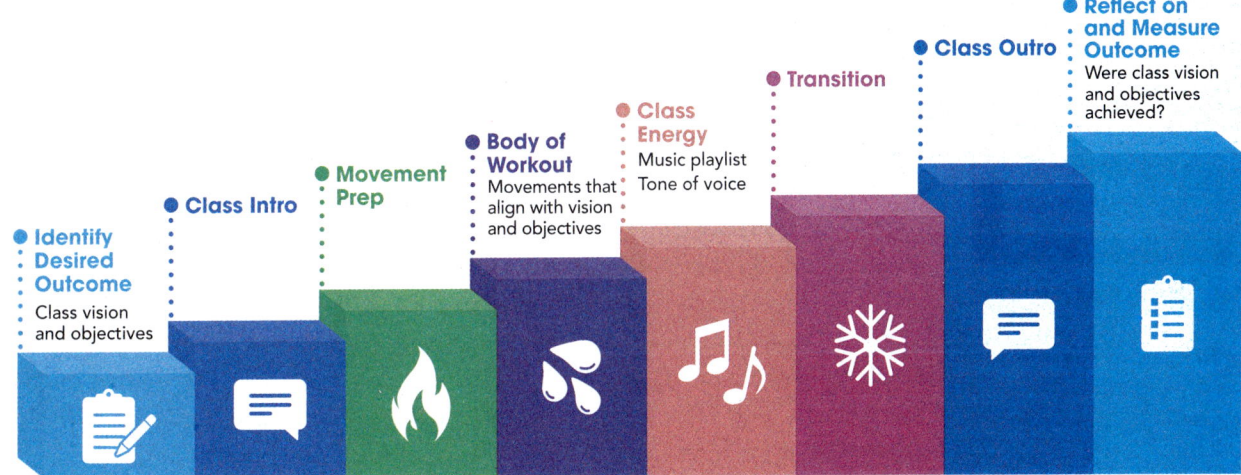

FIGURE 8.2 The Journey to Achieving the Class Vision and Objectives

Creating a Vision

In some cases, the instructor is told what objectives to pursue, leaving them to create a vision for the overall class experience. Say an instructor at a large, commercial facility is scheduled to teach a weekly class called Total Body Strength. Both the class name and the written description will provide insight into the class objectives, which will guide the instructor as they create a vision that aligns with those objectives. The vision can even change from class to class to keep things fresh and interesting. In one class, the instructor's vision may be to inspire participants to find the kid inside by creating a fun, playful environment; in the next class, their vision may be to encourage participants to unleash their inner beast by creating an intense, challenging environment. In a mind–body format, an instructor's vision for one class could be to reduce both physical and mental stress for attendees; in the next class, their vision could be to foster a positive mindset and energize the attendees. When first creating a vision, it is useful to find inspiration in the classes of other instructors and mentors. Speak with them about what features they incorporate into their class design to emotionally connect their participants to the workout.

Determining Class Objectives

In other cases, the vision is already defined, leaving the instructor to determine the appropriate objectives. Say an instructor is asked to teach a weekly class during the lunch break at a corporate office. The company wants to offer their employees a class that will help combat the high-stress, fast-paced office environment, but that will not make participants sweat too much, because there is not enough time to shower before returning to their desks. Knowing that the desired outcome is to reduce stress and that the class cannot be too strenuous, the instructor will probably stick to objectives such as mindfulness and flexibility. The objectives can also change from class to class. Maybe the employees will express an interest in alternating between a mindfulness and meditation session one week and then a stretching and mobility class the next week.

Getting Specific About Class Objectives

Class objectives can start out fairly broad and then evolve into something more dialed in and specific. The written description usually identifies the **BROAD OBJECTIVES** for a class, which can guide the instructor as they decide on the different **SPECIFIC OBJECTIVES** they will pursue each time they teach it. Continuing with the example of the Total Body Strength class, the description could read: "Get ready to feel the burn! This 45-minute class includes a variety of bodyweight, dumbbell, medicine ball, and kettlebell exercises and is designed to improve muscular strength, muscular endurance, and core stability." Examples of objectives are provided in **Table 8.1**. Although they are expected to execute the broad objectives of improving muscular strength, muscular endurance, and core stability every time they teach the class, the instructor can still craft a unique experience with each workout they teach by switching up the specific objectives they pursue. For example, one week the instructor's specific objectives may include targeting the **POSTERIOR CHAIN** by working the hamstrings, glutes, and back while also incorporating rotational movements; the next week, their specific objectives may be to incorporate **COMPOUND MOVEMENTS**, exercises that work multiple muscle groups at once while also challenging the participants' balance.

BROAD OBJECTIVES

Class objectives that are open-ended and vague, usually referenced in the written description.

SPECIFIC OBJECTIVES

Class objectives that are clear, explicit, and often change for each individual class.

POSTERIOR CHAIN

Group of coordinating muscles along the back of the body (i.e., the hamstrings, glutes, and back).

COMPOUND MOVEMENT

An exercise in which multiple joint segments and muscle groups are engaged during the exercise.

TABLE 8.1 Choosing Specific Class Objectives That Align with the Broad Class Objectives

Broad Objective	Specific Objectives	Modality/Equipment Used
Cardiovascular endurance	Equipment-based drills Athletic drills Interval training Steady-state training Low-impact exercises Plyometrics	Cycling Running Rowing Boxing Athletic drills
Strength and conditioning	Intervals for time Specific rep and set counts Total-body exercises Exercises targeting specific muscle groups Compound movements Plyometrics Speed, agility, and quickness (SAQ) exercises	Bodyweight Free weights Kettlebells Suspension straps Resistance bands Medicine balls Athletic equipment such as agility ladders, hurdles, or cones
Mobility and flexibility	Flexibility techniques (dynamic and static) Myofascial rolling techniques	Various stretching techniques Yoga straps Yoga blocks Myofascial rolling tools
Mind–body	Meditation versus movement	Guided meditation Yoga flow Pilates formats

⚙ PRACTICE THIS

Read the description of a group fitness class you love to attend.

1. Identify the broad objectives.
2. Create an appropriate class vision for two to three different classes.
3. Choose at least two specific objectives that align with the class visions you created.

Defining a Class Vision and Objectives from Scratch

In some instances, the instructor will not have the context clues to guide them as they work to define their class vision and objectives. For example, they could be offering a community class at a local park on Saturday mornings, which gives them the freedom to create a unique experience.

When the opportunities seem endless, it can be overwhelming to define the details of the class. In these instances, remember that the class vision and objectives are defined by identifying the desired outcomes for the class. To define the class vision and objectives, the instructor will consider the following:

- Class location and environment
- Who plans to attend
- The audience's goals
- Their own preferences, strengths, and passions

After speaking with community members interested in the class, the instructor might learn that most people have the desire to feel stronger but also hope to reduce some stress. This may inspire an instructor who is particularly passionate about mindfulness to offer a class that begins with strength-building exercises and ends with guided meditation. Likewise, this could inspire an instructor who is passionate about yoga to offer a power vinyasa flow.

Lesson 2: Class Environment

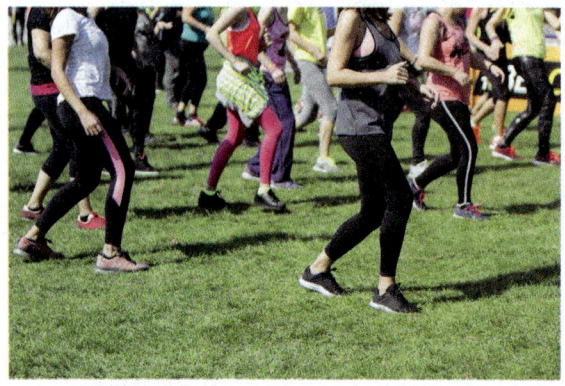
© Ivan Smuk/Shutterstock

Class Environment and Other Considerations

Details about the environment in which the class will take place are also going to influence the decisions the instructor makes as they determine the class vision and objectives and as they plan other logistics. Before designing the class, it is important to know the answers to the questions discussed in this section.

Who Are the Class Participants?

Sometimes, all the class participants will be of similar work capacity or conditioning level; other times, class participants will be a mix of fitness levels, abilities, and expectations. For example, although children in two groups are of similar ages, the fitness level and athletic ability of a group of 8- to 12-year-olds at a standard summer camp will be different from the fitness level and athletic ability of a group of 8- to 12-year-olds at a basketball camp. The standard summer camp instructor will appeal to a wider range of abilities by using movements requiring reduced complexity compared to the specific and demanding movements used by the basketball camp coach. Similarly, teaching a cycling class at a retirement community where all of the participants are 55 and older and may have similar needs is different from teaching a cycling class at a commercial health club with a membership diverse in age and fitness level. The instructor may have to prepare a larger variety of challenge options and modifications to meet the needs of their class at a commercial facility.

What Space Will the Class Take Place In?

The size of the space, the flooring, the safe maximum capacity, and other unique factors influence the decisions the instructor makes as they design a class. Whether a class takes place in a pool, in a studio, at a park, or virtually, each environment creates unique challenges and considerations. For example, an instructor may incorporate gliders into their weekly Core Strength and Stability class that takes place in a studio. Because gliders are designed to slide across a smooth surface like a wooden studio floor, the same class and equipment would not be suitable in a grassy area at a local park. Similarly, if the instructor were to offer the same class virtually, all participants following along from home may not have a surface suitable for gliders. When it comes to the size of the space, larger spaces like gymnasiums and large fields or parks are conducive to activities such as running sprints, which would not be as viable of an option in smaller spaces like a studio.

What Equipment Is Required and Available?

Each facility has a unique selection of equipment, which will influence the workouts the instructor crafts. Additionally, participants need to know if they are responsible for bringing anything with them, such as a yoga mat. Although the instructor needs to know what equipment they will have access to (e.g., medicine ball slams cannot be part of a workout in a facility without medicine balls), it is also crucial to know how much equipment is available. If a facility does not have multiple sets of the same-weight dumbbells, a circuit workout would be a better experience for participants to reduce the likelihood of using dumbbells that are too light or too heavy. It is also important that

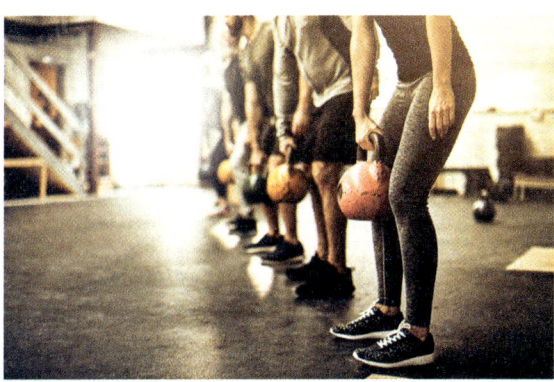

© Ground Picture/Shutterstock

an instructor knows which tools are at their disposal to avoid using equipment for unintended purposes (e.g., using a dumbbell for kettlebell swings) or redesigning the class at the last minute. This is especially important when an instructor is new to a facility. An instructor's ability to adjust and recover from unexpected changes will improve with experience, but knowing what equipment is available ahead of time, along with creating a backup plan for any variables they suspect could change, can prevent these stressful situations from happening in the first place.

How Will Participants Be Arranged?

Different arrangements are better suited for different class types (**Figure 8.3**). Instructors will think through certain characteristics of the class experience to determine which arrangement will work best: staggered, rows, circuits, or a circle. The staggered arrangement works well in a class where the participants closely follow the movements of the instructor, such as yoga, dance cardio, cycling, and some strength or interval training formats. In certain spots, participants may struggle to see the instructor's demonstrations, which the instructor can help overcome by regularly changing their position at the front of the room. The row arrangement works well in similar class types, but especially when participants are using large pieces of equipment, such as aerobics steps or barbells. Having participants in rows means that the instructor cannot see each individual from the front of the room, but it allows them to move through the room easily and safely in order to coach participants individually. The circuit arrangement is specific to the circuit workout format. Circuit training classes are a unique experience because each participant is performing a different exercise. These classes require thoughtful preparation by the instructor to ensure that participants can both perform their different exercises and move from one station to the next safely. The circle arrangement is a great way to create an interactive team environment. For this reason, an instructor may not have participants in a circle for an entire class but may start or end class by having the participants do an activity in a circle.

Participant Arrangement

STAGGERED ARRANGEMENT

Instructor

Allows the instructor to teach from the front of the room while being able to view all participants. This may create some obstructed views of demonstrations. It is important to ensure adequate space to be attentive through the various lines.

ROW ARRANGEMENT

Instructor

Allows instructors to move through the room to coach participants using large equipment. This may have some space limitations, and individuals at the ends may feel excluded. It is important to remember to visit those on the ends and ensure adequate space.

CIRCUIT ARRANGEMENT

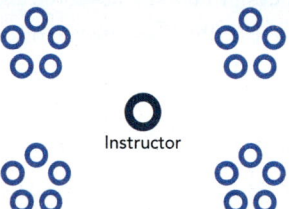
Instructor

Allows the instructor to move from station to station, coaching specific to the exercise at each one. This arrangement can create space and equipment constraints and may reduce the quality of feedback if multiple exercises are being performed simultaneously.

CIRCLE ARRANGEMENT

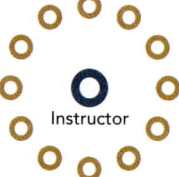
Instructor

Allows circular jogging, as well as forward and backward movement toward the center of the room. This arrangement requires an instructor's back to be turned to participants at times, which can complicate explanations and demonstrations. Instructors may have difficulty navigating among participants.

FIGURE 8.3 Participant Arrangement

How Long Will the Class Be?

If the instructor is leading a class at a facility, usually the facility will determine the class length that works best for their schedule and the members they are serving. Whether the instructor chooses the class length or not, it is important that all five components of the class (the intro, movement prep, body of the workout, transition, and outro) all fit within the allotted time (**Figure 8.4**). Participants expect the class to end at the scheduled time so that it does not interfere with their day. Classes at facilities need to start and end on time so that they do not interfere with the groups scheduled to use the space afterward.

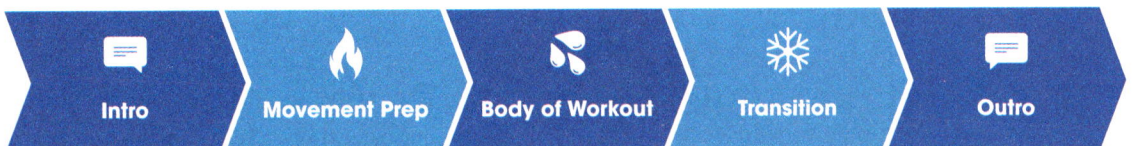

FIGURE 8.4 Five Components of a Group Fitness Class in the Order They Are Delivered

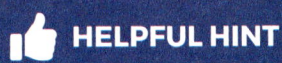 **HELPFUL HINT**

Is the class virtual? If so, is it live or on-demand? It is important to know the environment most participants are following along in. Factors such as carpeted floors and limited space to move around should be considered. For example, if the class is on-demand, specific references to the day of the week, weather, or season could lose their relevance to participants who follow along at a later date.

Lesson 3: Class Design Components

The Five Components of Class Design

Each component of class design, when properly planned, will help to create a positive, cohesive class experience for participants. The body of the workout is, so to speak, the star of the show, but the other four components play crucial supporting roles. Although they may not even realize it, a well-planned intro, movement prep, transition, and outro will strongly influence the participants' perception of their experience. This is why taking the time to set intentions and plan for each component is critical to both the participants' and the instructor's success.

The Power of a Great Intro

The simplicity of the intro can be misleading. A well-crafted intro can be a powerful tool, not only setting the tone for the experience, but also setting the participants' expectations for the class. During the intro, the instructor can encourage and inspire the participants to let go of what is happening in their world outside of the class, invite them on board with the class vision and objective, and encourage them to fully immerse themselves in this shared experience. Participants who feel especially connected to the community of people in their class report both a higher subjective rating of effort and greater levels of enjoyment once the class is over than they would if they felt less connected (Graupensperger et al., 2019). Initiating that connection and

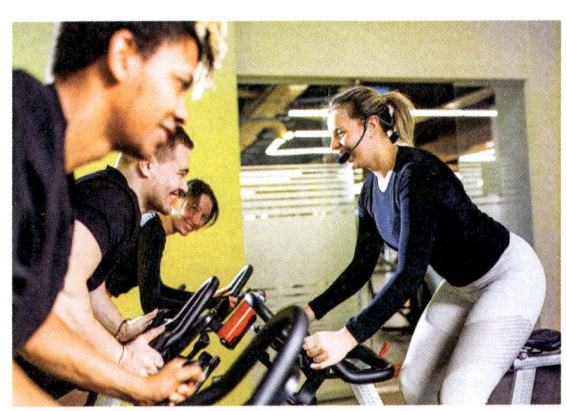

© Yurakrasil/Shutterstock

the shared purpose of the class vision and objectives during the intro can set the instructor and the participants up for success before the workout even begins.

In addition to creating a sense of community and shared purpose within the group, the intro is the instructor's opportunity to be clear about what is to come and to align the participants' expectations with the upcoming workout. This is why the intro is crafted after the instructor has written the body of the workout, movement prep, and transition. When the instructor communicates exactly what is about to come, new participants are able to adjust their expectations from what they predicted the class to be (based on descriptions or past experiences). This is also the time to communicate the vision and specific objectives of the class to everyone. The instructor's greatest challenge when crafting the class intro is keeping it brief. Participants arrive ready to dive in. Keeping the intro brief yet impactful can preserve that energy and anticipation.

Here is an example of a class intro: "Hey class! I'm Sarah, your instructor for this 45-minute strength workout. Today we're going to use a pair of dumbbells for overhead shoulder presses and a single, heavy dumbbell or kettlebell for goblet squats. If you haven't already, grab yours now, and please let me know if you'd like my help picking out your weights! Last class, we let loose and found our inner child while we targeted the muscles along our backside. Today we're going for a different vibe! We're going to unleash our inner beast as we tackle some challenging exercises that work multiple muscle groups at once! Of course, just like last week, I created the perfect playlist to set the mood. All right, let's get warmed up!"

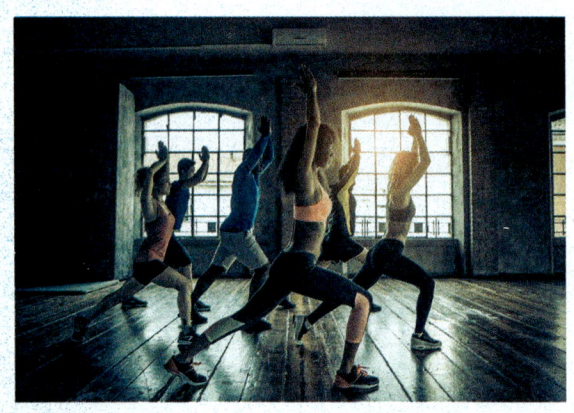

© Oneinchpunch/Shutterstock

Movement Prep: The Warm-Up

The movement prep is intended to prepare the participants, both physically and mentally, for the exercises they will perform in the body of the workout. Physically, the movement prep gradually generates heat in the participants' soft tissues and can reduce their risk of injury when higher-intensity movements are introduced (Scott et al., 2016). Also, introducing complex movement patterns at a lower intensity at the beginning of class can encourage successful technique when participants revisit those exercises at a higher intensity in the body of the workout. Mentally, movement prep serves as an extension of the class intro. It is an opportunity for the instructor to use language and demonstrate the energy that can get participants aligned with the class vision and objectives. For example, the energy level and tone of voice of a yoga instructor will likely be different from the energy level and tone of voice of a cycling instructor during the intro, movement prep, and the entirety of the class.

Building the Body of the Workout

Most of class time is spent in the body of the workout. Instructors will spend the majority of planning time on this section of the class. Because the four other components of the class are meant to support and complement the body of the workout, this section should be planned first. To build the body of the workout, the instructor will weave together the vision and objectives they have identified with their knowledge of proper technique and exercise physiology. What happens in the body of the workout will gradually lead participants from one stepping stone to the next until they have reached the desired outcome (**Figure 8.5**). It is a nuanced skill, which is why the next chapter is dedicated to planning this section of the workout.

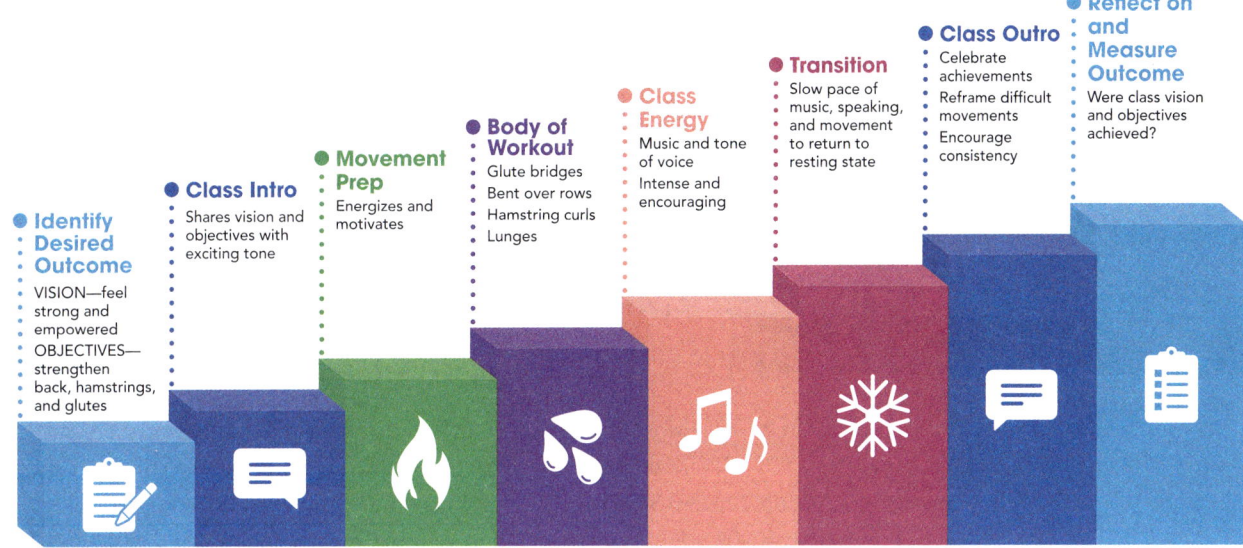

FIGURE 8.5 Class Vision and Objectives: Body of the Workout

Transition: The Cool Down

The transition is meant to cool down the participants' bodies and wrap up the class experience. Because the transition is a slower pace and lower intensity, this is a great time for the instructor to revisit the class vision and objectives, celebrate the ways in which the group met and exceeded those expectations, and offer encouragement about opportunities for progress in the future. For aerobic and high-intensity class formats, the instructor should aim to gradually reduce the participants' heart rates and guide their bodies back toward a resting state. Traditionally, this is accomplished with low-intensity movements and stretching. It is important to remember that transitions, particularly from supine to standing, should be gradual, otherwise participants could experience light-headedness, dizziness, or even fainting (Clark et al., 2018). Prioritizing stretches that address the muscles targeted during the body of the workout has long been recommended to improve muscle recovery and reduce delayed onset muscle soreness (DOMS), but the evidence neither supports nor contradicts these claims (Afonso et al., 2021). What is known, however, is that prioritizing joint mobility and range of motion can preserve people's independence and quality of life as they age (Ewing Garber et al., 2011).

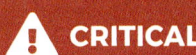 **CRITICAL**

Postural hypotension is when a person's systolic blood pressure falls by more than 20 mm Hg or their diastolic blood pressure falls by more than 10 mm Hg within 3 minutes of transitioning from lying down to standing up, causing light-headedness, dizziness, and potentially fainting (Ewing Garber et al., 2011). To limit the risk of these events, instructors should be mindful of both how frequently they transition from supine positions to standing positions, as well as how quickly they ask participants to make these transitions.

Outro

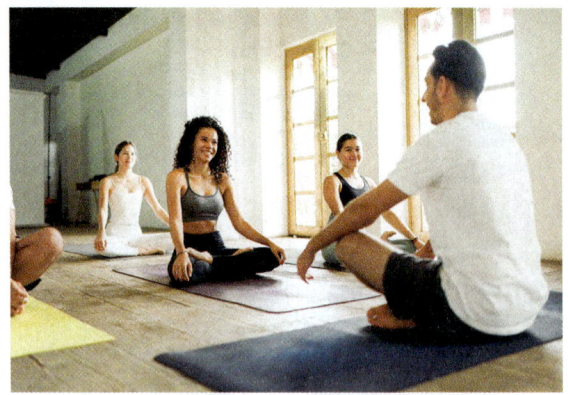

© Antoniodiaz/Shutterstock

As the class finishes, participants can be in a hurry, so it is best to keep the outro brief. The instructor could include any combination of the following in their outro:

- An invitation for participants with questions to speak with them before they leave
- Directions for cleaning and putting away their equipment
- A teaser of what's to come next class
- Promoting other classes they teach
- A quick plug for their social media channels

Most important, though, the outro is the participants' last moment of their experience with the instructor. This means that it is also the instructor's final opportunity to bring the class vision and objectives full circle and send participants on their way with a positive perception of their overall experience.

Planning Versus Delivering the Five Components of a Group Fitness Class

As briefly noted earlier, the five components were covered in the order they are *delivered* when instructing the class, but not the order they are *planned* when preparing for the class (**Figure 8.6**). This is because the movement prep and transition should be designed to complement the body of the workout, and the intro and outro should be relevant to the class experience as a whole. So, after determining the class type/format, the vision and objective, and the other logistics covered earlier, it is best to write the body of the workout first, followed by the movement prep and transition, and then finish with planning the intro and outro.

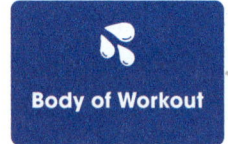   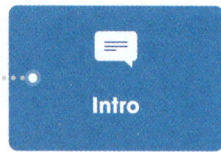 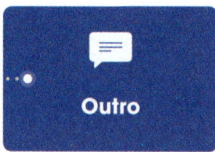

Body of Workout · · · **Movement Prep** · · · **Transition** · · · **Intro** · · · **Outro**

FIGURE 8.6 Five Components of a Group Fitness Class in the Order They Are Planned

Lesson 4: Class Flow

Flow

A class with excellent flow is delivered in a way that provides participants with a structured, organized, safe, and successful experience. The ability to lead a class that flows comes with practice and experience. New instructors will sharpen their skills as they repeatedly plan classes, teach them, and then reflect on their performance so that they can make necessary adjustments in the future.

Excellent instructors become great at what they do by consistently reflecting on their performance and adjusting details they noticed could have been prepared or done better. The moments that leave instructors feeling less than their best are not a failure if they are used to learn, grow, and improve future classes.

Structure

Although participants rely on and trust the instructor's expertise in crafting a safe and effective workout, it is important for them to feel as though there is a "method to the madness." Strategically planning similar exercises back-to-back can provide a sense of structure that creates a more efficient, enjoyable, and successful experience for the participants. When this is done well, it is so subtle that participants probably will not even notice. However, when it is not done well, participants may notice that the class feels a little rough. Consider the following examples of adjustments that can be made to create the subtle sense of structure that can ultimately improve class flow:

EXAMPLE 1

- **Good:** Glute bridges > bird dogs > Russian twists > plank hold (**Figure 8.7**)
- **Better:** Glute bridges > Russian twists > bird dogs > plank hold (**Figure 8.8**)

Why might this adjustment be better? The first option requires participants to start lying on their back, roll over so that they are kneeling on all fours, flip back over to a seated position, and then roll back over to a plank position. The second option leads participants from lying on their back, to sitting upright, to kneeling on all fours, and then to holding a plank, which makes for a smoother, gradual transition from one position to the next.

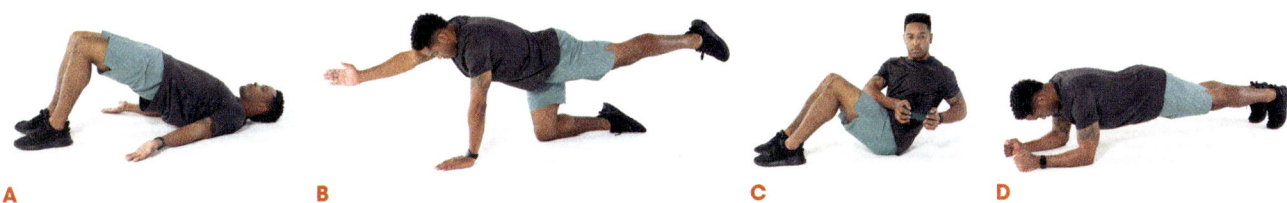

FIGURE 8.7 (A) Glute Bridge, (B) Bird Dog, (C) Russian Twists, (D) Plank Hold

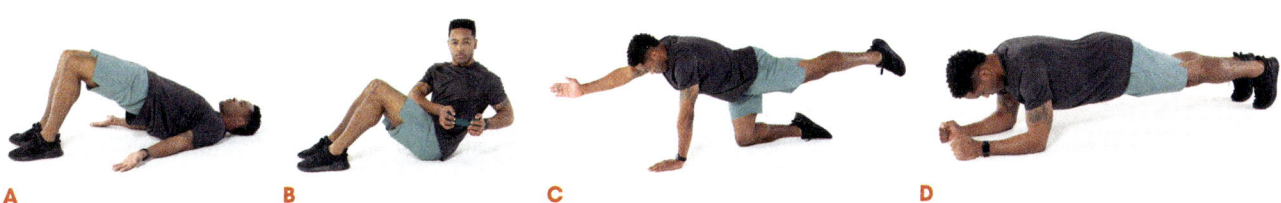

FIGURE 8.8 (A) Glute Bridge, (B) Russian Twists, (C) Bird Dog, (D) Plank Hold

EXAMPLE 2

- **Good:** Mini band kickbacks > dumbbell reverse lunges > mini band side steps > dumbbell squats (**Figure 8.9**)
- **Better:** Mini band kickbacks > mini band side steps > dumbbell reverse lunges > dumbbell squats (**Figure 8.10**)

Why might this adjustment be better? The first option requires participants to take the mini band off and put it back on every other exercise, which can slow down the pace of the class and frustrate participants who find the mini band difficult to get on and off. The second option requires half the number of transitions with the mini band, which keeps the class moving along and allows participants to move through the exercises with more ease.

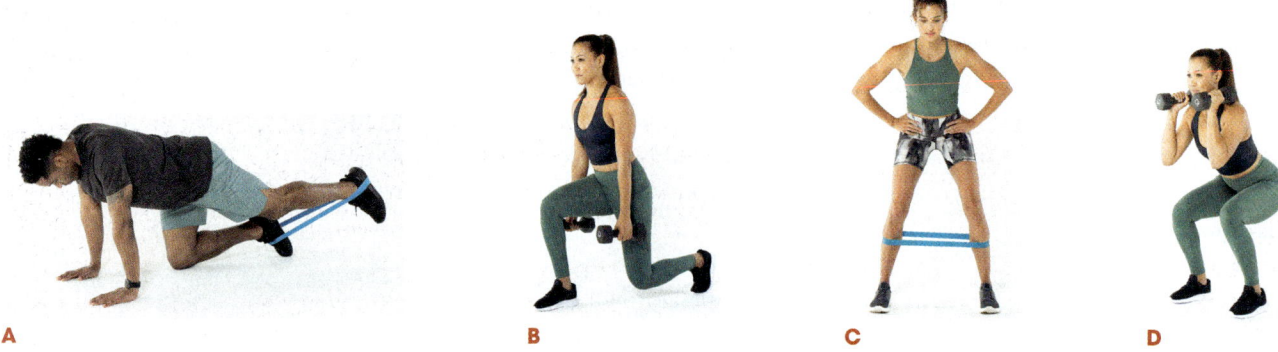

FIGURE 8.9 (A) Mini Band Kickbacks, (B) Dumbbell Reverse Lunges, (C) Mini Band Side Steps, (D) Dumbbell Squats

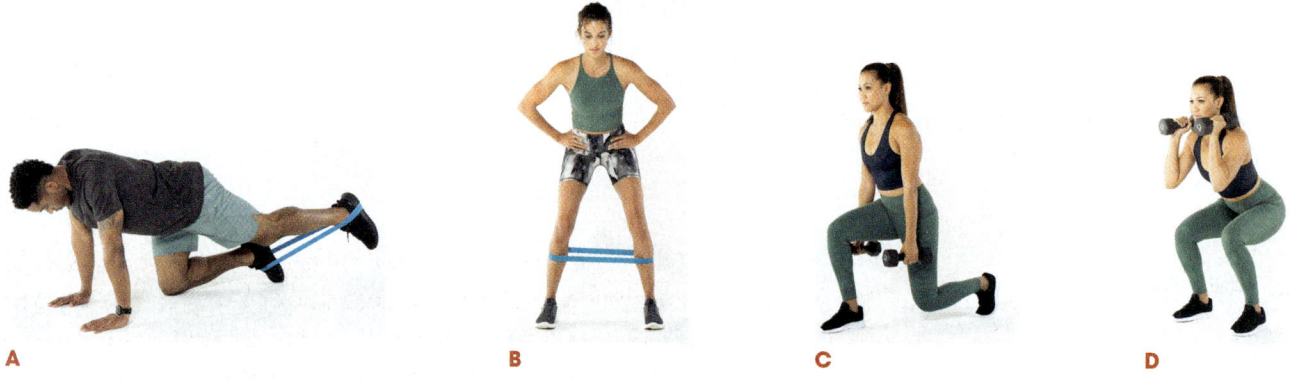

FIGURE 8.10 (A) Mini Band Kickbacks, (B) Mini Band Side Steps, (C) Dumbbell Reverse Lunges, (D) Dumbbell Squats

EQUIPMENT

Now, consider the equipment you will decide to use as an instructor for a specific class:

- **Good:** Using dumbbells, kettlebells, suspension straps, BOSU trainers, and resistance bands all within the same class
- **Better:** Taking a minimalistic approach and sticking with two to three of these equipment options

Why might this adjustment be better? Although the intention may be to create a class experience full of variety, asking participants to collect all those pieces of equipment can delay the start of class. In addition, having all that equipment in their space can create clutter that makes it difficult to move safely. It is also worth considering that using every tool available for each and every class can detract from the novelty for regular attendees. When it comes to equipment choices, variety from class to class will create a greater sense of structure than variety from exercise to exercise.

 INSTRUCTOR TIP

Keep it simple! As instructors gain experience, they gain an appreciation for simplicity. Although a series of exercises may seem ideal in theory, if they do not flow smoothly from one to the next in practice, the class experience will feel unstructured for participants.

Organization

An instructor cannot control all possibilities, but careful planning and minimizing of potential disruptions to class flow contributes to an instructor's confidence and, therefore, to their position as an authority in the group setting. Seemingly small details can make or break the participants' perception of control and organization. Although unpredictable moments happen to even the most seasoned instructors, having a mental (or written) checklist of things to confirm or address before class begins will often prevent the moments of disorganization that can interrupt its flow. The following are some specific examples of how instructors can improve the overall organization of their classes.

EXAMPLE 1
- **Good:** Grabbing a pair of backup batteries for the microphone pack in case it loses power mid-class
- **Better:** Replacing the batteries that are already in the mic pack with fully charged ones so that there is no disruption during class

EXAMPLE 2
- **Good:** Having music playing and greeting participants as they enter the space for class
- **Better:** Having music playing, greeting participants as they arrive, and communicating *all* of the equipment they will need for the class so that they do not have to search mid-workout

Safety

As they gain experience, instructors learn to think through variables such as participant arrangement, order of exercises, use of equipment, and how they will transition between work blocks to maximize safety. Being intentional about participant arrangement can prevent them from bumping into one another or tripping over each other's equipment. Mindfulness about the order of exercises can prevent participants from being distracted from proper form by having to keep up with transitions. Properly preparing the participants by communicating which pieces of equipment they will need during class and how to set them up safely can prevent accidents (e.g., plates sliding off a barbell because clamps were not used). Instructors should also not assume all participants understand proper equipment use. For example, it can be incredibly risky to have a whole class trying to balance on the flat side of a BOSU trainer. If one person falls, that can create a hazard for everyone else around them. Sacrificing safety for the sake of creativity may get a lot of likes on social media, but that will not automatically translate to a positive participant experience.

The instructor's thoughtfulness about structure and organization will directly affect participant safety. Recall the second example used previously for structure. Getting the mini band on and off can create a trip and fall hazard as participants fatigue and/or they feel rushed. Reflect on the second example used for organization. Participants scrambling to find the equipment they need mid-class can create a tripping hazard as they rush across the room when other participants' equipment is on the floor. It can also create the risk of an accident like a participant getting hit by a swinging kettlebell as they are rushing to get one for themselves. Although these kinds of incidents are rare, they demonstrate that disregard for class structure and organization will, at best, create a somewhat chaotic experience for participants and, at worst, put their safety at risk.

Success

The components of class flow just discussed—structure, organization, and safety—will influence a participant's perception of success and satisfaction with your class (Gilbert et al., 2017). In many group fitness formats, instructors want to challenge their participants. But keep in mind that although some challenges are empowering, (e.g., completing a set with a heavier weight than the last class), other challenges are downright discouraging (e.g., missing the first 10 seconds of an interval because the participant could not transition as quickly as the instructor). Reflect on the first example used for class structure and the two options for the order of four floor exercises. Some participants could keep up with the "good" option—which would require them to roll over to face the floor and then roll onto their back again more than once within the sequence—without an issue. However, certain fitness levels and body types may find it difficult and uncomfortable to roll back and forth for every single exercise. By opting for the "better" option, an instructor will not only improve the class flow but create a more inclusive experience for every participant in the class without sacrificing the challenge level.

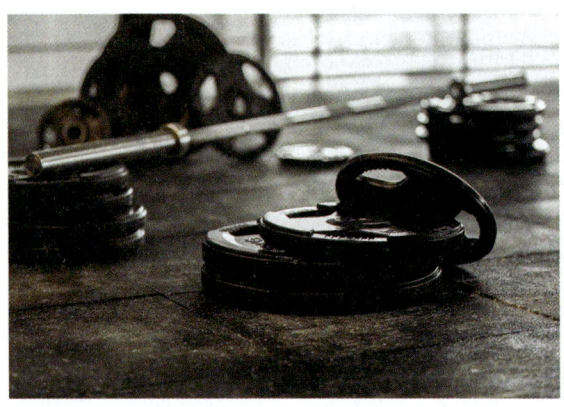
© Africa Studio/Shutterstock

SUMMARY

Creating a workout is similar to building a house. Although designing and decorating the interior of the house might be the most exciting part, the foundation and structure of the house must come first. The instructor lays the foundation of the workout by determining the class type/format, defining the class vision and objectives, and considering the environment in which classes takes place. They build the structure of the workout with the five components of a class by planning the body of the workout first, the movement prep and transition next, and the class intro and outro last. Structure, organization, and safety should not be underestimated in their influence on class flow and participant experience. Then, the instructor fills in the fun details by creating a play-by-play of what they will have the class do during each of those components.

REFERENCES

Afonso, J., Clemente, F. M., Nakamura, F. Y., Morouço, P., Sarmento, H., Inman, R. A., & Ramirez-Campillo, R. (2021). The effectiveness of post-exercise stretching in short-term and delayed recovery of strength, range of motion and delayed onset muscle soreness: A systematic review and meta-analysis of randomized controlled trials. *Frontiers in Physiology, 12*, 677581. https://doi.org/10.3389/fphys.2021.677581

Clark, C. E., Thomas, D., Warren, F. C., Llewellyn, D. J., Ferrucci, L., & Campbell, J. L. (2018). Detecting risk of postural hypotension (drop): Derivation and validation of a prediction score for primary care. *BMJ Open, 8*(4), e020740. https://doi.org/10.1136/bmjopen-2017-020740

Garber, C. E., Blissmer, B., Deschenes, M. R., Franklin, B. A., Lamonte, M. J., Lee, I. M., Nieman, D. C., Swain, D. P., & American College of Sports Medicine. (2011). American College of Sports Medicine position stand. Quantity and quality of exercise for developing and maintaining cardiorespiratory, musculoskeletal, and neuromotor fitness in apparently healthy adults: Guidance for prescribing exercise. *Medicine & Science in Sports & Exercise, 43*(7), 1334–1359. https://doi.org/10.1249/mss.0b013e318213fefb

Gilbert, M., Chaubet, P., Karelis, A., & Needham Dancause, K. (2017). Perceptions of group exercise courses and instructors among Quebec adults. *BMJ Open Sport & Exercise Medicine, 3*(1), e000278. https://doi.org/10.1136/bmjsem-2017-000278

Graupensperger, S., Gottschall, J. S., Benson, A. J., Eys, M., Hastings, B., & Evans, M. B. (2019). Perceptions of groupness during fitness classes positively predict recalled perceptions of exertion, enjoyment, and affective valence: An intensive longitudinal investigation. *Sport, Exercise, and Performance Psychology, 8*(3), 290–304. https://doi.org/10.1037/spy0000157

Scott, E. E. F., Hamilton, D. F., Wallace, R. J., Muir, A. Y., & Simpson, A. H. R. W. (2016). Increased risk of muscle tears below physiological temperature ranges. *Bone & Joint Research, 5*(2), 61–65. https://doi.org/10.1302/2046-3758.52.2000484

CHAPTER 9

BUILDING THE BODY OF YOUR WORKOUT

LEARNING OBJECTIVES

The intent of this chapter is to discuss how to select intensities, exercises, arrangements, and modifications for your class that will align with your class vision and enable you to meet your participants' needs.

After reading this content, students should be able to demonstrate the following objectives:

- **Identify** exercises for the body of the workout that are aligned with the class vision, objectives, and format.

- **Explain** proper exercise technique for a variety of exercises.

- **Identify** appropriate exercise modifications, including regressions and progressions.

Lesson 1: Intensity and Exercise Selection

Introduction

In order to write a safe, effective workout that fulfills the intentions of the written description, class vision, and objectives, the instructor must consider several essential components. These components include the physiological effects of exercise, the safety and effectiveness of the exercises chosen, and the way the movements flow together. In this chapter, you will examine how instructors take those factors into account when coaching participants through the exercises and their modifications to ensure that each participant ultimately achieves the desired class outcome.

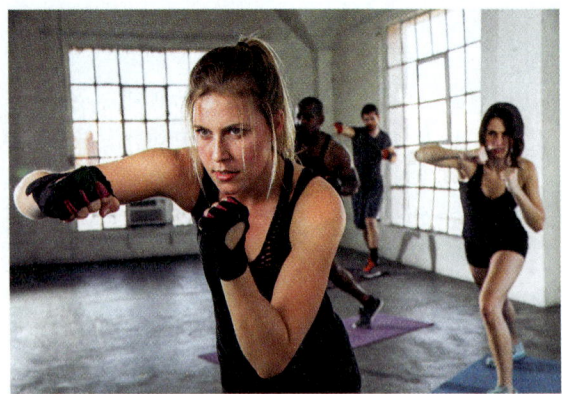

© El Nariz/Shutterstock

Determining Intensity and Building Work Blocks

The written description, class vision, and objectives are not the only factors that guide the instructor as they plan workouts; a basic understanding of bioenergetics helps instructors to choose and organize exercises in a way that creates an appropriate level of intensity for the class format they are preparing to teach. It is essential knowledge in crafting the right work and recovery periods. **BIOENERGETICS** is the study of how the body produces, stores, and uses the energy it needs for all functions of living (Neufer, 2018). Although instructors do not need to educate class participants about the complexities of bioenergetics, they should understand how they affect work capacity, output, and fatigue. A basic understanding of bioenergetics helps instructors with several aspects of planning and instructing their classes, including the following:

- Understanding how individual exercises integrate into work blocks for specific conditioning goals
- Effectively explaining how intensity and effort should feel to participants throughout the workout
- Knowing the ultimate physiological outcome of the workout they designed

A yoga class has a different feeling than an indoor cycling class, a muscular strength and endurance class, or a boxing class. One reason these unique formats feel so different is because they trigger different responses in the body because of the different energy demands. The following information will review previously discussed bioenergetics concepts and provide insight into how instructors write safe, effective workouts with the appropriate level of challenge for their class format.

> **BIOENERGETICS**
>
> The study of the three energy systems, also referred to as metabolic pathways, that produce adenosine triphosphate (ATP).

Bioenergetics

Recall that adenosine triphosphate (ATP) is produced via three different energy systems (two anaerobic, one aerobic). Exercise intensity, duration, and the availability of sufficient oxygen determine which system the body relies on most in a particular moment. These separate systems are integrated, and each one is always contributing to the production of ATP (Neufer, 2018). How fatigued participants get and how much their muscles burn during a bout of work depends on the energy system their body uses most to get the job done. Each of the three energy systems has its benefits and limitations and will affect how exercises and workouts feel.

ANAEROBIC ENERGY SYSTEMS REVIEW

Recall that although the two anaerobic energy systems are quick to produce ATP, they are also quickly depleted. Allowing the body time to recover gives these systems the opportunity to replenish their stores and support multiple bouts of high-intensity activity, but the amount of recovery time needed is dependent on the demands of the task and the fitness level of the person performing it (Monks et al., 2017).

The anaerobic ATP-PC energy system is the star of the show when the body performs movements with maximum effort, such as jumping as high as possible, deadlifting a one repetition maximum, or completing a short, all-out sprint (Baker et al., 2010). A benefit of this system is how quickly it can produce ATP, but its limitation is how little it can produce because it is depleted in a matter of seconds. Depending on how much phosphocreatine remains once depleted, the body will require anywhere from less than 5 minutes to as much as 15 minutes of recovery to replenish the amount of phosphocreatine to 100%, which would allow for another bout of work at maximum effort (Baker et al., 2010). Even when this energy system is depleted, though, the body can continue to work at a lower intensity while relying mostly on the other energy systems.

 HELPFUL HINT

The phosphagen system is associated with movements that require power and maximum effort, such as the long jump, Olympic lifting, or sprinting a 100-meter race. In a group fitness class, this system fuels bouts of work done with 100% effort, such as a 10- to 15-second sprint in an indoor cycling class or a burst of fast-paced, repetitive squat jumps in a high-intensity interval training (HIIT) class.

Also referred to as fast glycolysis, the glycolytic energy system produces ATP by metabolizing carbohydrates that are available in the blood (glucose) and in liver and muscle tissue storage (glycogen) when sufficient oxygen is not present. This energy system is the star of the show when the body performs high-intensity bouts of work for 2–3 minutes, such as a long sprint or completing multiple reps of a heavy strength exercise (Baker et al., 2010).

 HELPFUL HINT

Anaerobic glycolysis is associated with high-intensity, short-duration bouts of work such as sprinting a 400-meter race. In a group fitness class, this system fuels 2- to 3-minute bouts of work done at an intense effort level, such as completing a set of 20 heavy kettlebell swings in a strength and conditioning class or running fast-paced laps around a gym or track in a boot camp class.

AEROBIC ENERGY SYSTEM REVIEW

The aerobic energy system requires the presence of ample oxygen in order to produce ATP. A limitation of this energy system is that it is slow to produce ATP, which is why it is relied on primarily during a state of rest and for long-duration and low- to moderate-intensity activities. A benefit of this system, though, is that it eventually produces a large amount of ATP, which will support sustained effort (Bonora et al., 2012).

The aerobic energy system is associated with low- to moderate-intensity, long-duration bouts of work like walking, running, or cycling for several miles. In a group fitness class, this system will kick into gear when the anaerobic energy systems are depleted, allowing participants to continue moving but with less intensity. Recovery intervals are often performed in this system. This system is also the primary source of energy for mind–body classes such as yoga.

🤖 **GETTING TECHNICAL**

The Process of Aerobically Creating Energy

Stage 1: Aerobic Glycolysis

Also referred to as slow glycolysis, this is the first of the three stages in the aerobic energy system. Although this process starts out exactly the same as anaerobic glycolysis, the presence of sufficient oxygen results in a different outcome that will not only produce ATP, but create byproducts that will be used for ATP production in later stages of the aerobic energy system. **PYRUVATE** is the byproduct from metabolizing glucose changes into **ACETYL COENZYME A**, which will move along to the second stage of the aerobic energy system, the Krebs cycle (Bonora et al., 2012).

Stage 2: Krebs Cycle

The Krebs Cycle (aka the citric acid cycle) is the second stage in the aerobic energy system. It metabolizes acetyl coenzyme A generated from glucose, amino acids, and fatty acids to produce ATP and byproducts containing hydrogen ions that will be used in the final stage of the aerobic energy system, the electron transport chain (Bonora et al., 2012).

Stage 3: Electron Transport Chain

The electron transport chain is the third and final stage of the aerobic energy system. During this stage, the hydrogen generated by the Krebs cycle goes through a series of complex chemical reactions that ultimately produce a significant amount of ATP and the byproducts of water and carbon dioxide (Bonora et al., 2012). The process of producing energy in the cells aerobically is often termed cellular respiration because oxygen goes in and carbon dioxide goes out.

PYRUVATE

A byproduct formed during glycolysis, the metabolic process that breaks down glucose and produces adenosine triphosphate (ATP).

ACETYL COENZYME A

A byproduct formed from metabolism of glucose, fatty acids, and amino acids that is used for the production of adenosine triphosphate (ATP).

Using the Principles of Bioenergetics to Write Safe and Effective Workouts

An instructor's knowledge of bioenergetics should not only inform which exercises they ask participants to do and for how long they ask participants to do them, it should also inform how often and how long they will have participants rest and recover. For example, bioenergetics tells us that the ATP-PC system can only support a maximum effort for a matter of seconds and that anaerobic glycolysis can only support high-intensity efforts up to a few minutes, and then the body will need ample recovery before it can repeat those effort levels again (Baker et al., 2010). Knowing this, an indoor cycling instructor will be mindful of both how long they ask participants to sprint for, and how soon after they will ask participants to sprint again.

 INSTRUCTOR TIP

When designing a class template, building work blocks is not only about choosing the types of exercises that will make up the workout, it is also about choosing when and how long to rest.

Designing the right **CLASS TEMPLATE** allows instructors to write safe and effective workouts in terms of bioenergetics as well as with consideration of logistics such as the class environment, vision, and objectives. To design a template, the instructor will use the known length of the class to determine how long the body of the workout will be. Next, they will determine how many work blocks will make up the body of the workout and how long each block will last. For choreographed class formats, often the length of a work block is determined by the length of the song(s) that the movement is choreographed to. Then, the instructor will refer back to their knowledge of bioenergetics, the class environment, who the participants are, and the class vision and objectives to answer questions such as the following:

CLASS TEMPLATE

The outline of a group fitness class format that divides the class into blocks of work and provides guidance for the instructor as they choose which movements and exercises to fill in as they write the workout.

- Is it best to count repetitions (i.e., reps) or time intervals?
- Will I cycle through the exercises in a circuit, or complete all sets of an exercise before moving onto the next exercise?
- Should there be rest after every exercise?
- How many rounds of each block of work will be performed? And how long should the recovery be between those rounds?
- According to the written description and potential class vision and objectives, what kinds of movements and exercises should make up each block? What order should they happen in?

The relevant questions will vary depending on the type of class the instructor is preparing to teach, and it is likely that their answers will change as they gain experience leading the class. For these reasons, it is important for instructors to reflect on what worked well and what should be improved on after each class, and then edit the class template and exercise choices accordingly. Once the instructor designs a class template they feel confident about, preparing for future classes is as simple as plugging different exercises into the template. **Figure 9.1** presents a sample template of a total-body strength interval training class.

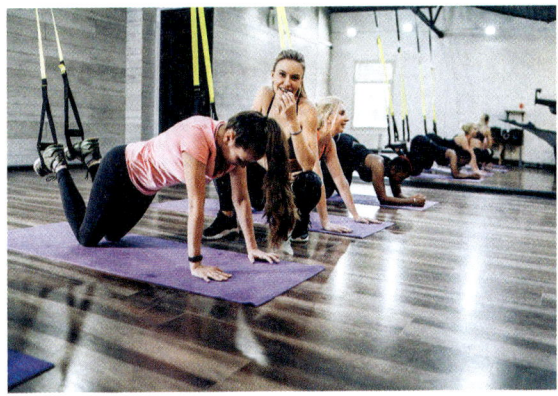

© GaudiLab/Shutterstock

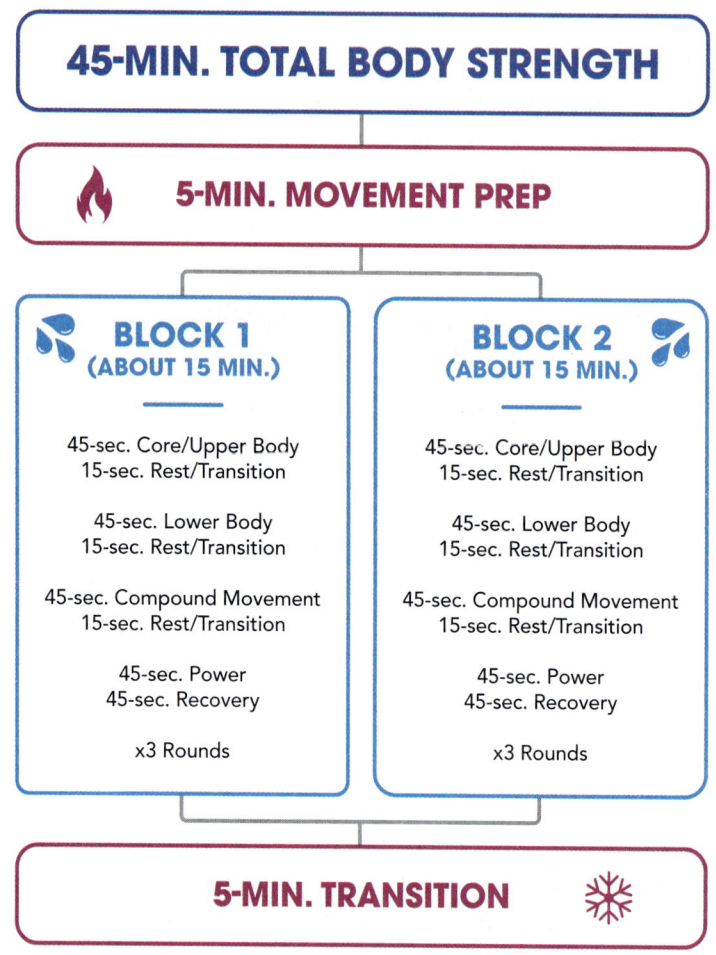

FIGURE 9.1 Sample Total-Body Strength Class Template

INSTRUCTOR TIP

When designing a class template, it is important to leave time for explanations, demonstrations, and transitions. In the sample total-body strength template provided in Figure 9.1, each block is noted to last approximately 15 minutes, but the programmed intervals add up to 13.5 minutes of work. This leaves 1.5 minutes for the instructor to explain and demonstrate the exercises before asking the participants to perform them.

Selecting Exercises

Once the class template is designed, each time a new workout is desired, the instructor will decide which movements and exercises are appropriate to plug into the template. The chosen movements and exercises should align with the class vision and objectives, fulfill the purpose that is specified in the template, and be safe and effective for participants. The following sections will reference the sample template for total-body strength provided in Figure 9.1.

Choosing Exercises That Align with the Class Vision and Objectives

Say the instructor's vision for their total-body strength class is to emphasize teamwork; this would give them the opportunity to incorporate some interactive exercises. In addition, knowing the broad objective of total-body strength building, the instructor has decided to narrow that down to a couple of specific objectives: to improve coordination and joint stability. With this in mind, when choosing the first exercise of the first block of work (core and/or upper body), the instructor could have participants partner up, hold a plank, and give each other high-fives as they try to hold a strong, steady plank. Simply having participants perform bent over dumbbell rows would absolutely fulfill the purpose of a core and/or upper body exercise, but the partner plank high-fives is an exercise that aligns with the class vision to emphasize teamwork, along with the class objectives to improve coordination and joint stability.

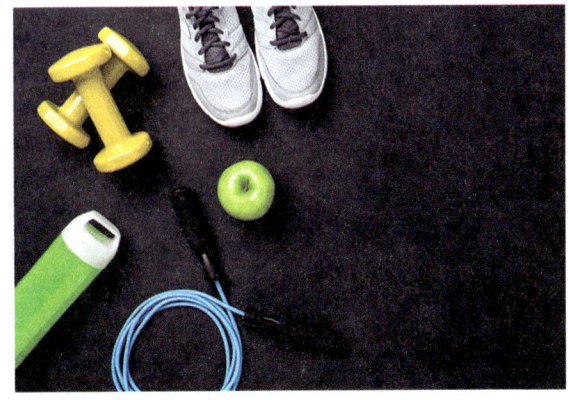

© Zerbor/Shutterstock

Choosing Exercises That Align with the Purpose Specified in the Template

As shown in the total-body strength template (Figure 9.1), sometimes the purpose is to target a specific muscle group or area of the body (e.g., upper or lower body), whereas other times the purpose is to use a specific approach to movement (e.g., compound movement or power). Choosing exercises that target a specific muscle group or area of the body can be fairly straightforward. The instructor is not going to use squats or lunges for the core/upper body interval, for example. Choosing exercises that use a specific approach to movement can be a little trickier. When deciding which movement or exercise they will use for the power interval, the instructor will consider explosive, plyometric options such as kettlebell swings and squat jumps. Before committing to complex exercises like these, however, the instructor will answer the AFAA 5 Questions to ensure that they are safe and appropriate for the class participants.

Using the AFAA 5 Questions™ When Selecting Exercises

Instructors should filter exercise selection decisions through the AFAA 5 Questions with the fitness level and ability of their class participants in mind (**Figure 9.2**).

The instructor not only answers these questions about each individual exercise, but they also consider how the answers to these questions may change depending on what comes before and after each exercise. For example, if the total-body strength instructor chooses goblet squats for the lower body interval, along with squats to an overhead shoulder press for the compound movement interval, they are asking the class participants to perform squats for two back-to-back intervals. This will affect the answers to Questions 2 and 4: "Are you doing it effectively?" and "Can you maintain proper alignment and form for the duration of the exercise?" After reflecting on the fitness level and ability of the class participants, if the instructor decides they can answer "Yes" to both, they may choose to move forward with those exercise choices. If the instructor answers "No" to those questions, they will change one or both exercises.

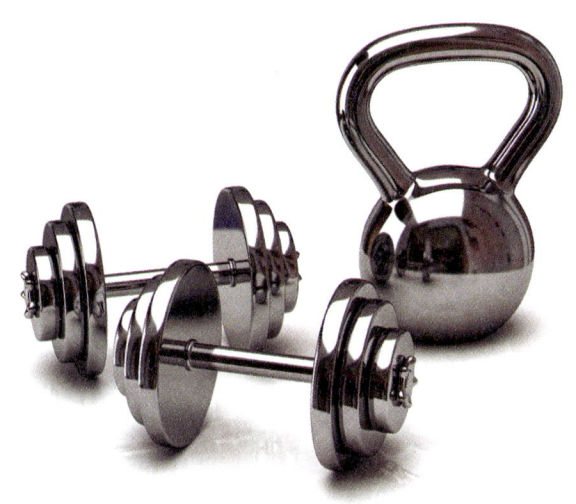

© Valdis torms/Shutterstock

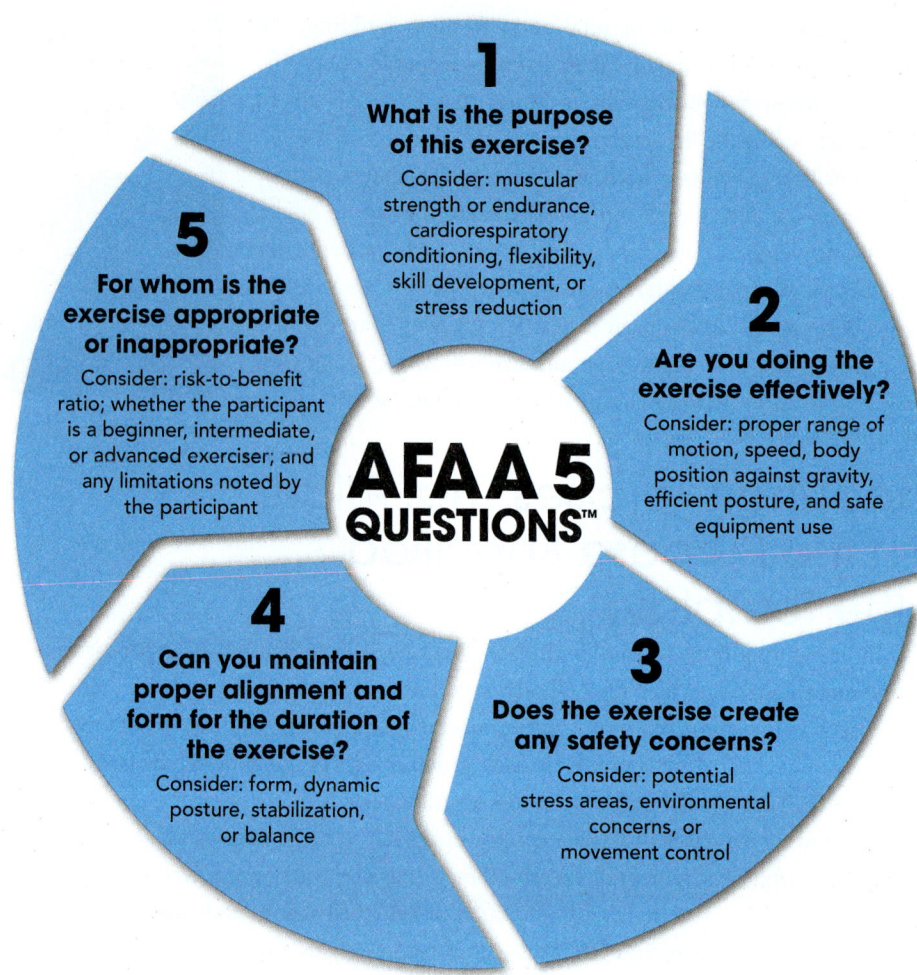

1 What is the purpose of this exercise? Consider: muscular strength or endurance, cardiorespiratory conditioning, flexibility, skill development, or stress reduction

2 Are you doing the exercise effectively? Consider: proper range of motion, speed, body position against gravity, efficient posture, and safe equipment use

3 Does the exercise create any safety concerns? Consider: potential stress areas, environmental concerns, or movement control

4 Can you maintain proper alignment and form for the duration of the exercise? Consider: form, dynamic posture, stabilization, or balance

5 For whom is the exercise appropriate or inappropriate? Consider: risk-to-benefit ratio; whether the participant is a beginner, intermediate, or advanced exerciser; and any limitations noted by the participant

AFAA 5 QUESTIONS™

FIGURE 9.2 The AFAA Five Questions™

Choosing Appropriate Equipment

Equipment availability is another factor that focuses an instructor's options as they choose exercises for classes. It is important to be intentional when deciding what equipment to incorporate into a class. A facility may have plenty of dumbbells, kettlebells, medicine balls, step benches, and resistance bands available, but it is likely the instructor will not use every option every class. One reason is that too many pieces of equipment can create clutter and become a tripping and safety hazard. Another reason is that it gives the instructor the ability to keep things fresh and interesting for regular class participants by switching up the equipment they use on a regular basis. In fact, as the instructor decides what their class vision and objectives will be, they can also decide which pieces of equipment inspire the kind of movements and exercises that best align with those intentions.

The instructor should also consider whether a piece of equipment is a safe and appropriate tool for the class participants and how the equipment will work within the participant's space. For example, suspension systems could create a safety hazard for a crowded class where participants are tightly packed in because they require a larger personal bubble to complete. Likewise, suspension systems need to be anchored to something. Thus, an instructor who teaches an outdoor class that takes place in an open field would not use that piece of equipment.

EQUIPMENT CLASSIFICATIONS

In **Table 9.1**, exercise equipment is classified into four categories: resistance, base of support, assistance, and flexibility/recovery. In some cases, a piece of equipment is essential in order to perform an exercise (e.g., step-ups cannot be performed without a base of support to step up onto). In other cases, a piece of equipment allows participants to get more out of a movement or exercise they are doing (e.g., many people get a far better supine hamstring stretch with the extra leverage of a yoga strap). When choosing equipment, the purpose of each tool should align with the desired outcome for the exercise, block of work, or the workout as a whole.

TABLE 9.1 Equipment Classifications

Equipment Type	Equipment Purpose	Examples
Resistance	These tools are used to trigger muscle contraction with the intention of improving muscular strength and performance.	Dumbbells Resistance bands Barbells and plates Medicine balls
Base of support	These tools are used for exercises that cannot be performed simply standing upright or lying on the ground.	Step bench Stability ball Indoor cycling bike Gliders
Assistance	These tools are used to provide support and stability so that movements and poses can be done more safely and effectively.	Mats Yoga block Barre
Flexibility/recovery	These tools are used to create more leverage when stretching and/or to support self-myofascial techniques.	Yoga strap Foam roller Trigger point balls

Lesson 2: Creating the Desired Outcome

Creating the Desired Outcome Through Exercise Selection and Instruction

A variety of group fitness class formats are available, and with so many of those formats being fusions of multiple exercise techniques, instructors must develop a range of coaching strategies and skills. The following sections explore the unique priorities, challenges, and intersections of coaching muscular strength and endurance, cardiorespiratory conditioning, and mind–body exercise techniques.

Muscular Strength and Endurance Formats

When selecting exercises for a muscular strength and endurance format, the instructor should consider exercises relevant to the desired outcome and think through how they either disrupt or contribute to class flow. If the class description tells participants they are going to target their lower body, the instructor probably will not incorporate exercises such as push-ups or tricep kickbacks. The instructor should also be mindful about how many different pieces of equipment the workout will require. If the instructor decides they want to use step benches for step-ups, depending on how much space is available, they may decide against incorporating stability ball hamstring curls into the same workout to avoid cluttering the space with too many large pieces of equipment.

Coaching participants through muscular strength and endurance exercises requires clear, concise direction to get participants moving with proper form, followed by individual coaching and feedback to keep participants safe and help them get the most out of each exercise. When teaching these exercises, it is common for instructors to perform the first few repetitions of an exercise along with the class participants, and then make their way around to individual participants to coach them through adjustments to their form or modifications of the movement. A unique challenge when coaching muscular strength and endurance exercises is educating participants about how the body gets stronger and empowering them to use a resistance that is truly challenging for them. The instructor should help the participants to understand that they should be challenged and not hurrying through a set or struggling.

 INSTRUCTOR TIP

A common question asked by many new participants is "What weight should I start with?" A simple way to determine the right load is using the concept of repetitions in reserve (RIR). One way to think of RIR is to ask, "How many more repetitions could I complete with good form at this weight?" If the answer is too high, then the weight is not challenging enough to yield desired results. If it is too low, then not enough resources will be "left in the tank" for subsequent sets. This will still take a little practice, but it will become an easy, intuitive way to select weights that provide just the right amount of challenge.

In general, strength endurance adaptations carry an RIR range of 0–2, particularly for single-joint exercises. If an RIR of 0 is desired, it is recommended to use that only in the last set of the exercise. Multi-joint movements may use an RIR of 2–4 to reduce undue fatigue. Movements for the purpose of power development use an RIR of 4 to allow the participant to maintain explosiveness throughout performance (Helms et al., 2016).

Instructing Cardiorespiratory Conditioning Formats

Coaching participants through cardiorespiratory conditioning exercises requires the instructor to set clear expectations that get participants moving safely and at the appropriate intensity, followed by plenty of encouragement to keep them motivated and engaged. Certain modalities for cardiorespiratory conditioning, such as indoor cycling, running, and rowing, have repetitive movement patterns. Although the instructor will regularly revisit safety and proper form, the repetitive nature of these exercise techniques often allows instructors more time to motivate and inspire their participants. Other approaches to cardiorespiratory conditioning, such as dancing, boxing, and the use of athletic drills, have greater movement variety, and the necessity to communicate changes in movement patterns will be the greatest priority. A unique challenge for instructors coaching participants through these formats is educating them about how to move with the appropriate intensity while creating minimal impact and stress on the joints.

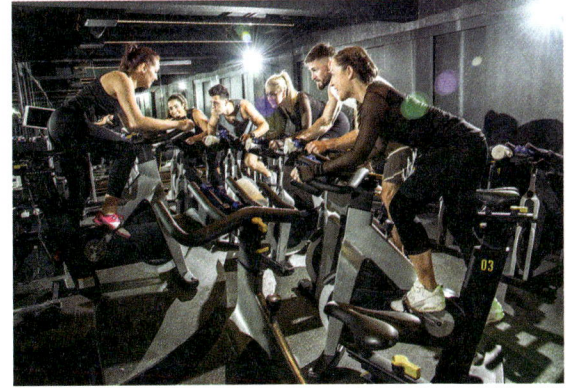

© Bojan Milinkov/Shutterstock

Instructing Mind–Body Formats

Coaching participants through mind–body exercises and movement flows requires coaching and cues that help participants become in tune with their bodies, usually in a way that inspires both physical and mental stress relief using structured challenge as a foundational tool. These formats often focus on mobility, flexibility, and breathing techniques. A unique challenge when coaching mind–body exercise techniques is encouraging participants to embrace what is probably a slower pace and lower intensity than they move through life with.

Regardless of the specific exercise technique, instructors are always coaching and encouraging participants to move safely and effectively. The following sections provide some insight into how instructors coach participants, both as a group and individually, to ensure they have a safe, effective class experience.

INSTRUCTING PARTICIPANTS TO ACHIEVE PROPER FORM AND INTENSITY

Group Fitness Instructors have the challenge and responsibility to reference their knowledge of anatomy, physiology, and biomechanics and then only communicate what is absolutely essential in order for participants to achieve the desired outcome. **Table 9.2** explores sound bites instructors often use when they are leading a class and what those sound bites mean in more technical terms. Although the "What Is Meant" and "What Is Being Fixed/Prevented" columns are probably too complex to explain while teaching, it is important that instructors know what outcome they are looking for so they can make sure they are getting their message across to the participants. Take some time to look the table over and see how instructors take their textbook knowledge and apply it in action.

OFFERING PROGRESSIONS, REGRESSIONS, AND MODIFICATIONS

Instructors can give class participants the opportunity to customize their experience by offering options and alternatives. They can also help participants feel more successful when they are unable to perform an exercise the instructor has planned by coaching them through modifications. These modifications and alternatives are vital to ensuring that each participant works at the right level of intensity with **PROGRESSIONS** or **REGRESSIONS**. It is the instructor's responsibility to observe each participant individually to determine whether it is appropriate to make an exercise more or less challenging or if the exercise itself should be modified.

PROGRESSION

A modification that increases the difficulty of an exercise or movement combination.

REGRESSION

A modification that decreases the difficulty or demand of an exercise or movement combination.

TABLE 9.2 Common Cues Instructors Use to Help Participants Move Safely and Effectively

What Is Said	What Is Meant	What Is Being Fixed/Prevented
"Check your posture." "Hinge your hips." "Keep your chest up." "Take an athletic stance."	Keep your spine neutral by shifting your pelvis back while leaning your trunk forward and bending your knees during a hip-hinging motion.	Rounding upper back (kyphosis) (**Figure 9.3**) Arching lower back (lordosis) (**Figure 9.4**) Chin jutting forward (**Figure 9.5**) Loading joints instead of muscles
"Engage your core." "Make sure you have a straight spine/**NEUTRAL SPINE**." "Keep your neck long." "Put your shoulder blades in your back pockets."	Support and stabilize your spine, hips, and shoulders by contracting the muscles that surround them.	Rounding upper back Arching lower back Tension in neck and shoulders Rib cage flaring out (**Figure 9.6**)
"We want to feel almost breathless." "We shouldn't be able to hold a conversation." "Push your pace."	This exercise/block of work is supposed to be challenging and even feel uncomfortable.	Going through the motions Not achieving the desired outcome of improved muscular and/or cardiorespiratory fitness
"Push through your heels." "Push the floor away from you."	Imbalances in weight distribution through the feet can lead to poor alignment and improper form.	Foot pronation/supination (**Figure 9.7**) Tension in ankles/knees/hips/back Loading joints instead of muscles
"Wrap around the bar with a strong grip."	Hold the handle firmly with the thumb on one side and the other four fingers on the other side.	Accidentally dropping equipment Tension in hands/wrists/elbows Not gripping with every finger (**Figure 9.8**)
"Deep breaths." "Exhale as you pull/stand/lift." "In through the nose, out through the mouth."	Ensures breath control during cardiorespiratory conditioning activities. Inhale through the nose to fill the lungs and expand the diaphragm on the eccentric portion of strength movements. Exhale through the mouth on the concentric portion of strength movements. Use breath to reduce tension when stretching.	Holding breath Dizziness Spike in blood pressure
"Land softly." "Strong stance."	When landing from a jump, keep knees soft and hips hinged to reduce impact on ankles, knees, hips, and back. Keep joints properly aligned on impact.	Foot pronation Valgus knee (**Figure 9.9**) Stress/strain in ankles, knees, hips, or back

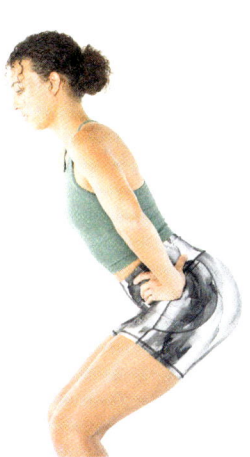

FIGURE 9.3 Rounding Upper Back

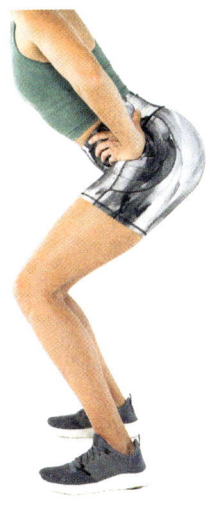

FIGURE 9.4 Arching Lower Back

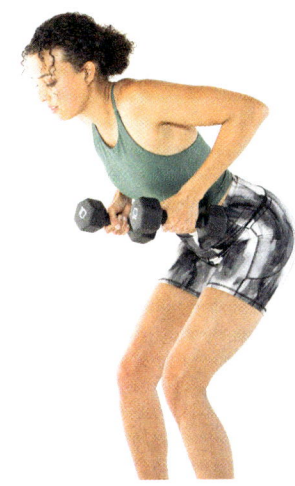

FIGURE 9.5 Chin Jutting Forward

NEUTRAL SPINE

Ideal alignment of the spine's curves to allow for safety, structural support, proper distribution of forces, and optimal muscular activation.

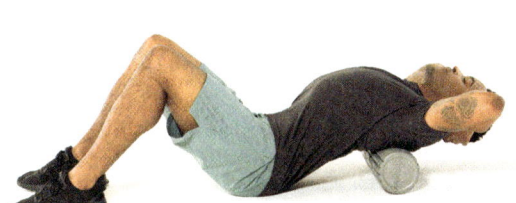

FIGURE 9.6 Rib Cage Flaring Out

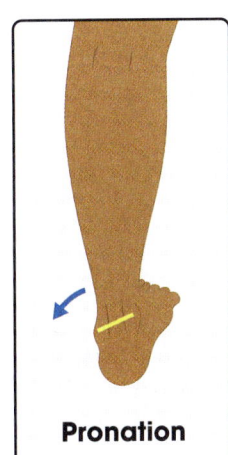
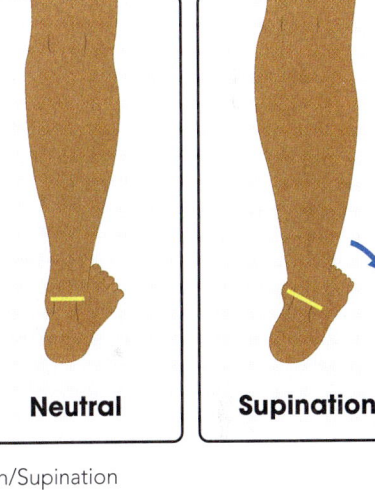

Pronation **Neutral** **Supination**

FIGURE 9.7 Foot Pronation/Supination

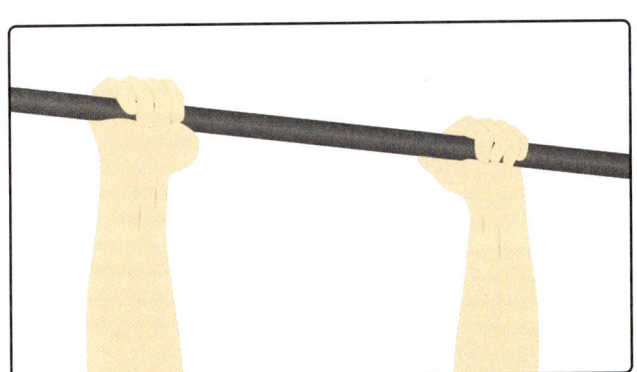

FIGURE 9.8 Not Gripping with Every Finger

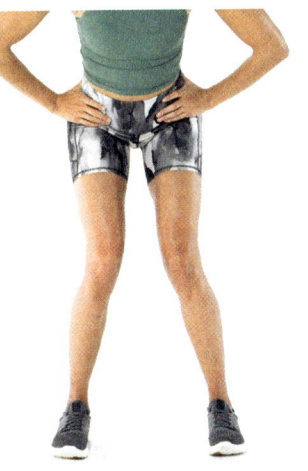

FIGURE 9.9 Knee Valgus

The progressions presented in **Table 9.3** are a great option for regular class participants who move with great form and would like to challenge themselves. The regressions are a great option for participants who would benefit from slowing down and/or practicing keeping their body aligned and moving with great form. If a participant has a limitation or injury preventing them from performing an exercise properly or comfortably, then the exercise itself should be modified. Modifications can be used to progress or regress an exercise. However, note that in most cases instructors offer modifications to regress movements that are either uncomfortable or inappropriate for a class participant. This can be done by adjusting the exercise so that it requires less coordination and/or stabilization or by having the participant perform a different movement that is more appropriate but trains similar muscle groups and patterns.

TABLE 9.3 Progressions and Regressions of Exercises and Movements

Progression	Regression
Increase range of motion (ROM) within safe technique.	Decrease ROM.
Speed up/slow down pace/tempo.	Speed up/slow down pace/tempo.
Add resistance.	Decrease resistance.
Increase number of reps per set.	Decrease number of reps per set.
Longer work interval/shorter rest interval.	Shorter work interval/longer rest interval.
Decrease points of contact.	Increase points of contact.
Mobile.	Stationary.
Decrease base of support.	Increase base of support.
Remove stability/challenge balance.	Add stability/do not challenge balance.
Increase movement complexity (e.g., add rotation to a lunge).	Reduce movement complexity.

INSTRUCTOR TIP

Although shortening the rest interval can be a simple way to make an exercise or workout more challenging, it is important for the instructor to revisit the principles of bioenergetics and decide whether that is the appropriate way to challenge their participants. After intense bouts of work that deplete the anaerobic energy systems, shortening the rest interval could mean sacrificing the opportunity for those energy systems to replenish. In this case, instructors should consider other strategies for progressing the workout to ensure that the workout is ultimately effective and not challenging simply because it is draining.

MODIFYING COMPOUND MOVEMENTS

Compound movements require coordination, which could be difficult for some participants. What is great about compound movements, though, is that they provide multiple modification options to participants. For example, if the instructor has the class doing dumbbell squats with an overhead shoulder press, they can coach a participant with sensitive knees to only do the overhead shoulder press. Likewise, they can coach a participant with a shoulder injury to only do the squats. Similarly, with renegade rows (holding a plank while performing alternating single-arm dumbbell rows), the instructor can coach participants with sensitive wrists to do a plank hold on their forearms if their priority is to target their abdominals or perform bent over rows if their priority is to strengthen their back. These adjustments can be made for new participants who are in the process of building foundational strength or for anyone who struggles with coordination. Encouraging these participants to focus on mastering a single movement pattern can prevent them from feeling frustrated and discouraged and reduce their risk of injury.

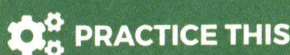 **PRACTICE THIS**

It is important to offer modifications in a way that helps participants feel successful. Think about how you would coach participants through a modification.

MODIFYING AND PROGRESSING TO IMPROVE BALANCE AND STABILITY

Challenging participants' balance and stability is a great way to provide a challenge to those who are looking for it, but it can be incredibly difficult and frustrating for those who struggle with maintaining balance and stability. A great way to empower participants who struggle with this is to provide them with a tool that will allow them to perform the movement or hold the pose with better stability. For example, if a yoga instructor has the class holding a dancer pose, they can coach a participant who is struggling to keep their balance to move close to a wall and do the pose facing the wall. This way, if they feel unstable, they can place their front hand against the wall to regain their balance without falling out of the pose.

Challenging participants' balance and stability can also be a great strategy for progressing exercises and helping participants to develop functional movement skills that will serve them in their daily life, especially as they age (Thomas et al., 2019). The progressions shown in **Figures 9.10** and **9.11**) require balance and stability.

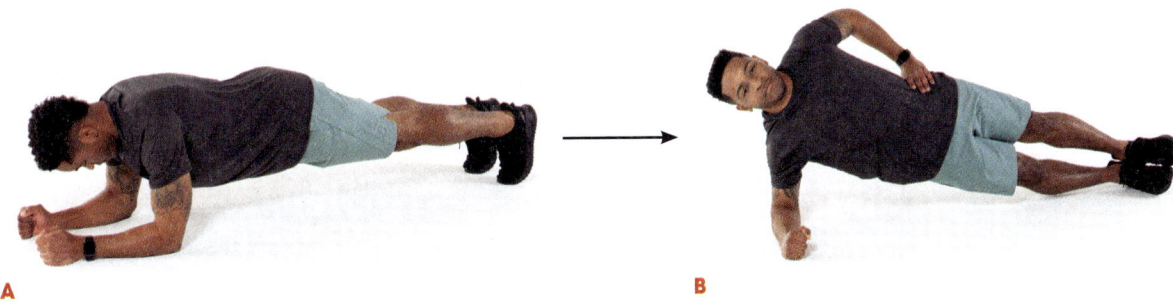

A   B

FIGURE 9.10 Progressing a Plank to Improve Balance and Stability: (A) Standard Plank Hold, (B) Side Plank

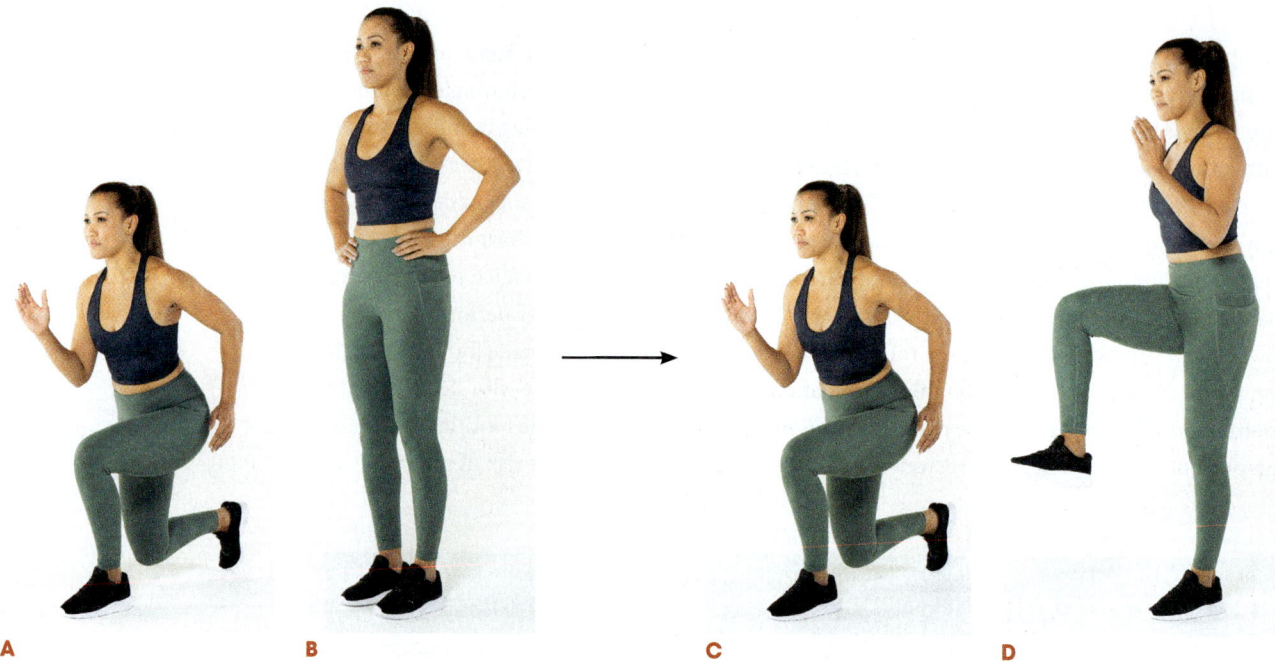

FIGURE 9.11 Progressing Reverse Lunges to Improve Balance and Stability: (A) Reverse Lunge (B) to Step Together, (C) Reverse Lunge (D) to Knee Drive

A   B   C   D

MODIFYING TO ADDRESS LIMITATIONS AND INJURIES

When a participant has an injury or limitation, certain movements and exercises will not be appropriate. In these situations, the instructor will provide alternatives that are more comfortable and will not further irritate the issue. Sometimes it will not be quickly apparent what the best modification is. When necessary, it can be helpful to prepare for these situations by making notes of alternatives, particularly for exercises that often prompt requests for modifications or alternatives. For example, an instructor who plans to include mountain climbers in a workout might anticipate that some of their regular participants will ask for an alternative because doing a plank on their hands irritates their wrists. Sometimes, though, providing modifications and alternatives will require instructors to improvise because every body and every situation is unique. In this case, it is helpful to reflect on Question 1 of the AFAA 5 Questions: "What's the purpose of this exercise?" With that purpose in mind, the instructor can choose a movement that fulfills the same purpose without putting the participant at risk of further injury.

Lesson 3: Flow Considerations

Considerations for Flow

As instructors plan workouts, their priority is not only to create fantastic workouts, but also to prepare an excellent class experience. This requires instructors to think through the decisions they make to ensure the workout is not only great on paper, but also great in practice.

Writing Safe, Effective Workouts That Flow

Writing an effective workout *and* a class that flows requires some creativity and compromise. Applying the principles of bioenergetics while also considering class flow is a great example of how skilled instructors create effective fitness experiences. For example, an instructor planning a high-intensity interval training class knows that the anaerobic energy systems could take several minutes of recovery to replenish, but they also know that having participants stand around for several minutes at a time can dramatically disrupt the flow of a class. To keep the class flowing after a high-intensity bout of work, the instructor may provide a short interval of complete rest (e.g., water break) followed by a low- to moderate-intensity movement or exercise that will still allow the anaerobic energy systems to replenish before the next bout of high-intensity work. For example, after an interval of mountain climbers, a HIIT instructor could have participants perform a slow, controlled exercise such as alternating bird dogs, which would keep the class moving and flowing while also giving the anaerobic energy systems the opportunity to replenish.

Flow Between Exercises

Timing the transition between exercises is a skill instructors refine as they gain experience. Providing too little time can be discouraging for participants who feel like they cannot keep up, and providing too much time can be frustrating for participants who feel like they are losing momentum or want more challenge. For these reasons, the instructor should consider any adjustments that need to be made after participants finish one exercise and before they begin the next:

- Are we changing positions? (Lying on back to facing the floor, seated to standing, etc.)
- Are we putting down/picking up/switching out equipment?
- Will we need time to recover in order to perform the next exercise safely and effectively?

If any of these adjustments need to be made, it is important for the instructor to provide enough time for them to happen. When participants keep up with the pace and demands of the class, they feel far more successful and satisfied with their class experience (Gilbert et al., 2017).

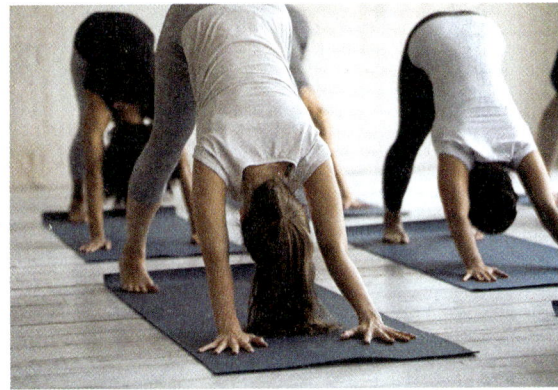

© Fizkes/Shutterstock

Here is an example of cueing a transition between exercises in a muscular strength and conditioning class: "Wrapping up in 3 … 2 … 1. Take 15! Next, we'll pick up both our dumbbells and hold them by our sides for alternating reverse lunges (*instructor demonstrates three to four reps*). We've got 5 seconds until we start; so get ready! 3 … 2 … Let's work!"

Flow Between Work Blocks

Timing the transition between work blocks is another skill instructors refine as they gain experience. Leaving enough time for the adjustments listed previously is still relevant when transitioning between work blocks, but the instructor's greatest priority between work blocks is to set clear expectations and provide concise instructions. The instructor should provide enough information for participants to understand what they are about to do without spending so much time on explanations where energy and enthusiasm decline.

The instruction between work blocks can also give participants a sense of structure and organization, especially for classes that are a fusion of multiple exercise techniques. In classes that are strictly one exercise technique, the different work blocks usually have a similar focus and feel. In classes that fuse together multiple exercise techniques, the different work blocks can have unique objectives and dramatically shift the energy of the class. For example, in a class that combines blocks of cardiorespiratory conditioning with blocks of muscular strength and endurance exercises, the instructor will have to guide participants through a shift in both the approach to movement and the intention of the exercises. Through communicating the intention and purpose of the class in its entirety, and communicating how each separate block of work contributes to achieving that intention and purpose, the instructor provides a sense of continuity and structure, no matter how different each work block may be.

Here is an example of cueing a transition between blocks of work in a fusion cardiorespiratory conditioning and muscular strength and conditioning class: "And rest! Awesome job, team! That's a wrap on the cardio portion of class; so use this 60 seconds of rest to take some slow, deep breaths and feel free to sip some water while I show you what's coming next! In the next block of work, we're going to move some weight around; so it's important that we slow down, control our movements, and really feel our muscles work. We're going to begin with lateral shoulder raises. You'll hold your lightest set of dumbbells, sweep them to the side and up until they're shoulder height, then control them back down again (*instructor performs three to four reps*). After that, we'll have a quick break to set those dumbbells down and pick up our heavier set for squats (*instructor performs three to four reps*). We'll alternate between those two exercises for three rounds. You have 25 more seconds of rest; so keep bringing that heart rate down and I'll count you down when it's time to start!"

⚙ PRACTICE THIS

When preparing to teach a class, the instructor may find it beneficial to plan and practice their transitions between exercises and blocks of work to ensure that the class flows smoothly. The goal is to provide participants with all the essential information they need to get moving without talking for so long that it disrupts the momentum of the class. Using a class you are going to or would like to teach in the future, practice leading participants through transitions between exercises as well as transitions between blocks of work.

SUMMARY

Writing the body of the workout requires the instructor to juggle a number of factors to ensure that they follow through on the intentions they have set with the class vision and objectives. Instructors should think through the demands they are putting on the body's energy systems to make sure the class is the appropriate level of intensity. In addition, they should consider the exercise techniques they are coaching participants through and how those exercises flow together to make sure the class experience has the intended outcome and overall feeling.

REFERENCES

Baker, J. S., McCormick, M. C., & Robergs, R. A. (2010). Interaction among skeletal muscle metabolic energy systems during intense exercise. *Journal of Nutrition and Metabolism, 2010*, 905612. https://doi.org/10.1155/2010/905612

Bonora, M., Patergnani, S., Rimessi, A., De Marchi, E., Suski, J. M., Bononi, A., Giorgi, C., Marchi, S., Missiroli, S., Poletti, F., Wieckowski, M. R., & Pinton, P. (2012). ATP synthesis and storage. *Purinergic Signalling, 8*(3), 343–357. https://doi.org/10.1007/s11302-012-9305-8

Gilbert, M., Chaubet, P., Karelis, A., & Needham Dancause, K. (2017). Perceptions of group exercise courses and instructors among Quebec adults. *BMJ Open Sport & Exercise Medicine, 3*(1), e000278. https://doi.org/10.1136/bmjsem-2017-000278

Helms, E. R., Cronin, J., Storey, A., & Zourdos, M. C. (2016). Application of the repetitions in reserve-based rating of perceived exertion scale for resistance training. *Strength and Conditioning Journal, 38*(4), 42–49. https://doi.org/10.1519/SSC.0000000000000218

Monks, M. R., Compton, C. T., Yetman, J. D., Power, K. E., & Button, D. C. (2017). Repeated sprint ability but not neuromuscular fatigue is dependent on short versus long duration recovery time between sprints in healthy males. *Journal of Science and Medicine in Sport, 20*(6), 600–605. https://doi.org/10.1016/j.jsams.2016.10.008

Neufer, P. D. (2018). The bioenergetics of exercise. *Cold Spring Harbor Perspectives in Medicine, 8*(5), a029678. https://doi.org/10.1101/cshperspect.a029678

Thomas, E., Battaglia, G., Patti, A., Brusa, J., Leonardi, V., Palma, A., & Bellafiore, M. (2019). Physical activity programs for balance and fall prevention in elderly: A systematic review. *Medicine, 98*(27), e16218. https://doi.org/10.1097/md.0000000000016218

CHAPTER 10

OTHER VITAL COMPONENTS OF YOUR WORKOUT

LEARNING OBJECTIVES

The intent of this chapter is to show how the body of a workout is used to inform your selection of the other workout components to align with your class vision and objectives and support your participants' expectations and success.

After reading this content, students should be able to demonstrate the following objectives:

- **Identify** exercises for movement prep and transition that are aligned with the class vision, objectives, format, and body of the workout.

- **Explain** proper technique and intensity for movement prep and transition exercises.

- **Identify** appropriate exercise modifications, including regressions and progressions.

- **Identify** the characteristics of effective intros and outros.

- **Evaluate** all components of a workout as a cohesive class.

Lesson 1: Planning Movement Prep and Transitions

Introduction

A well-planned class begins with a thoughtful vision and clear objectives that will guide the instructor as they create an effective body of the workout, but the preparation does not end there. Four other components of the class must be planned to create a complete experience: movement prep, transition, intro, and outro. Because the intro and outro both reference the entire class experience, the instructor creates the movement prep and transition first. Once those components are prepared, the instructor will know exactly what information is essential to communicate in the intro and outro and devise the best transitions between each component. By preparing each component in that specific order, instructors create a cohesive experience that flows from beginning to end. Once an instructor has mapped out the five components for a workout, they can use a more detailed workout template (see Appendix) to plan for the equipment, music, and environment to bring everything together.

Planning the Movement Prep and Transition

Once the instructor knows what exercises and movement patterns the participants will need to execute and recover from in the body of the workout, they can plan the appropriate movement prep (warm-up) and transition (cool down). The purpose of the movement prep is to increase blood flow and generate heat in soft tissues to prime the participants' bodies for the movements they will perform in the body of the workout. The purpose of the transition is to guide the body back to a pre-workout resting state, often while gently moving and stretching the muscles and joints that were primarily used.

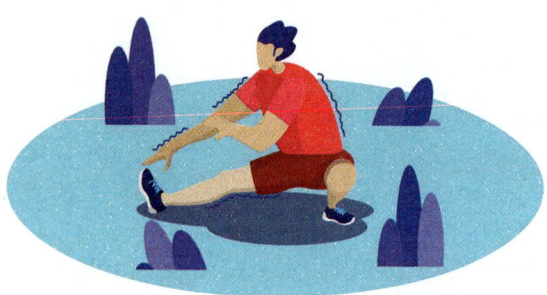

© Perzeus/Shutterstock

Effective Movement Prep Technique and Exercises

A well-planned movement prep block should not be treated as an afterthought, because it can translate to a positive initiation of the class experience and even improve participants' performance during the body of the workout. During the movement prep, the instructor will continue their efforts to set the stage for the class experience, something they began to do in the intro. Note that the term *warm-up* does not fully capture the nuance of this class component; the music the instructor plays, the tone of voice they use, and the things they say can all prompt the appropriate energy and inspire an ideal mindset for the class ahead. With those details in mind, the instructor chooses movements that adequately prepare the heart, muscles, joints, connective tissues, and nervous system for the demands of the rest of the workout. It is important to distinguish that although movement prep has the power to improve performance during the body of the workout, movement prep that results in fatigue can diminish performance (Fradkin et al., 2010). In class formats that emphasize intensity, it can benefit instructors to educate their class participants about this. Most people want to achieve the best results possible and instinctually believe that the harder they push themselves, the better the outcome, which simply is not true during the movement prep.

👍 **HELPFUL HINT**

Compare the body of the workout to baking cookies. It is best practice to preheat the oven and wait until it has reached the ideal temperature before putting raw cookie dough into the oven to bake. The movement prep of a workout is equivalent to letting the oven preheat before putting cookie dough in the oven. Properly preparing for the body of the workout can ultimately improve performance and outcome (Fradkin et al., 2010).

The class type and length influence which movements are used and how long the movement prep lasts. The movement prep for a cycling class is generally done on the bike, pedaling against light resistance. The movement prep for mind–body classes can look and feel similar to the body of the workout because these formats are low-impact and low-intensity, which are qualities of an effective movement prep. The movement prep for a strength class format usually includes movements and exercises that prepare the muscles that will be targeted in the body of the workout. High-intensity and high-impact class types, such as high-intensity interval training (HIIT) or cardio kickboxing, can require more time spent preparing the body in order to reduce stress and strain on the participants' joints and soft tissues. It is important for the instructor to be mindful of both the amount of time spent on movement prep and how to adequately prepare the body for the workout ahead.

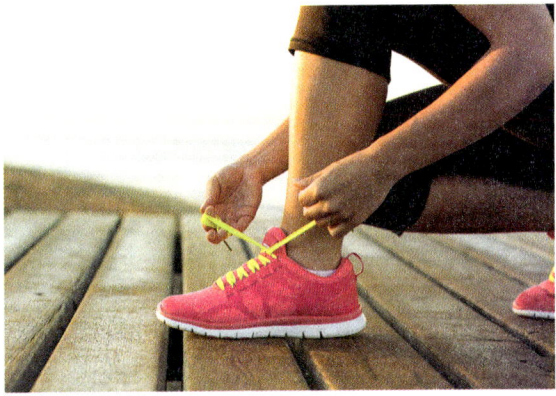

© Halfpoint/Shutterstock.com

FLEXIBILITY TRAINING

Flexibility plays an important role in physical performance and quality of life. During a workout, a participant's lack of flexibility can inhibit their movement patterns, creating stress and strain on the body, and potentially leading to injury. Flexibility is not only important during exercise, though. A person's ability to bend over and tie their shoes or slide into the driver's seat of a vehicle is dependent on the ability of their muscles and joints to move freely. This is why prioritizing flexibility is important, especially as we age.

When the average person thinks about flexibility, they think of static stretching, which is just one tool that can improve range of motion and flexibility, but it is not the only tool (Afonso et al., 2021). Instructors can educate their participants on the variety of tools and strategies that can be used to improve flexibility, including strength training, dynamic stretching, and soft tissue techniques such as foam rolling.

STATIC STRETCHING BEFORE A WORKOUT

In leading participants through an effective movement prep block, Group Fitness Instructors will use various stretching techniques to enhance participants' flexibility and joint **RANGE OF MOTION (ROM)**. Both static and dynamic stretching exercises provide similar increases in joint ROM (Beedle & Mann, 2007). Note that some confusion exists around static stretching, given that research has demonstrated that it can reduce power production and strength for 10 minutes or even up to an hour following completion of the stretching (Fowles et al., 2000; Power et al., 2004). However, this assumes that no other dynamic movements are being performed after the static stretch and that the participant proceeds directly into the workout. If static stretching is done for no longer than 60 seconds per muscle group and is part of a larger movement prep sequence that finishes with dynamic and workout-specific activities, performance impairments are not a concern (Behm, 2018; Behm et al., 2016; Behm & Chaouachi, 2011; Kay & Blazevich, 2012). Movement prep can improve performance during a workout when it is specifically tailored to the activity in the body of the workout (Fradkin et al., 2010). The key takeaway for movement prep is this: to prepare to move with any intensity, specific movements that do not lead to excessive fatigue should be an instructor's primary method of delivery. The four qualities of movement prep that are both efficient and effective are shown in **Figure 10.1**.

RANGE OF MOTION (ROM)

The amount of motion available at a specific joint.

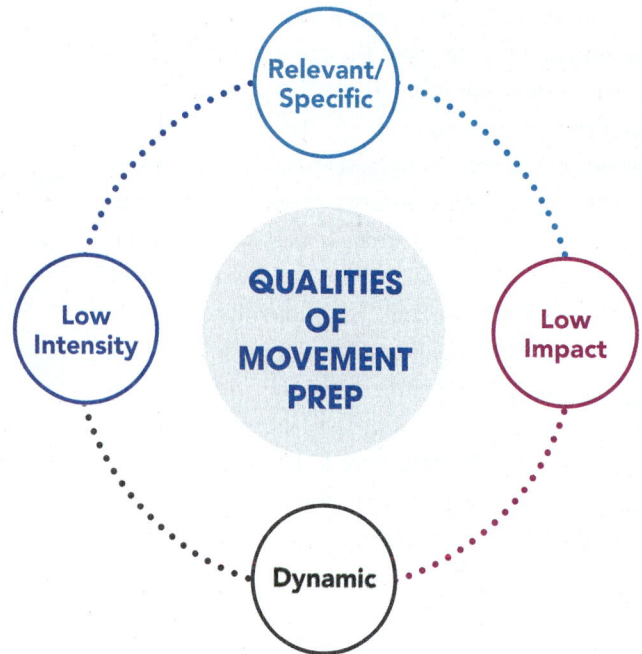

FIGURE 10.1 Qualities of Movement Prep

LOW-INTENSITY AND LOW-IMPACT MOVEMENTS

In every class type, but especially for formats with high-intensity or high-impact efforts, the movement prep progressively escalates intensity to prepare participants for the mental and physical demands in the body of the workout. Because the goal is to prime the body without fatiguing it, the intensity of the movement prep generally will not exceed that of a brisk walk or light jog, and it should focus on the same muscle groups and similar movement patterns as the upcoming workout. In addition, to minimize stress on participants' joints, the movements and exercises incorporated into the movement prep are low impact. To ensure that the movement prep is both low intensity and low impact, instructors may stick to movements that are slower paced, use bodyweight/minimal resistance, and avoid activities such as running or jumping. Dynamic stretching is a great low-intensity, low-impact tool for efficiently and effectively warming up soft tissue and can potentially "optimize the subsequent muscle performance" (Opplert & Babault, 2019).

👍 **HELPFUL HINT**

When choosing movements for the movement prep, it is important to stick to options that minimize stress on the participants' joints, muscles, and connective tissues when they are not adequately warmed up. Although an exercise such as jumping jacks may be a lower intensity than some of the exercises participants will perform in the body of the workout, jumping jacks are not a low-impact movement, and when they are done too early, they can create undue stress on the ankles, knees, hips, and back.

DYNAMIC STRETCHING

Dynamic stretching actively moves muscles and joints through their available and pain-free range of motion. This can look and feel a lot like exercising in a slow, controlled manner, which is why it is common for the terms *dynamic stretching* and *dynamic movements* to be used interchangeably. This kind of movement increases blood flow and generates heat, which is why it is such a great tool when preparing participants' bodies for higher-intensity and/or higher-impact efforts. Remember, the instructor's task is to guide participants toward finding a pace and effort level that efficiently and effectively prepares their muscles, joints, and connective tissues without creating too much fatigue.

Table 10.1 and Figures 10.2 through 10.12 provide some examples of dynamic stretches and movements an instructor might incorporate into the movement prep.

> ⚠️ **CRITICAL**
>
> Dynamic stretching before exercise can improve muscular contraction and performance during exercise (Opplert & Babault, 2019).

TABLE 10.1 Dynamic Stretches and Movements

Dynamic Stretch/Movement	Category	Why It Is Effective for Movement Prep
 **FIGURE 10.2** Glute Bridges	Supine	Increase blood flow to core and glutes. Warm up soft tissues around the pelvis with minimal stress on hips and back (with proper form).
FIGURE 10.3 Superman	Prone	Increase blood flow to back and glutes. Warm up soft tissues around spine with minimal stress on neck and scapula (with proper form).
FIGURE 10.4 Bird Dogs	Prone	Move hips and shoulder joints while using the core to maintain balance and control. Promote kinesthetic awareness, coordination, and good posture.
FIGURE 10.5 Plank	Prone	Work the core, increase blood flow, and generate heat throughout the entire body.

(continues)

TABLE 10.1 Dynamic Stretches and Movements (*continued*)

Dynamic Stretch/Movement	Category	Why It Is Effective for Movement Prep
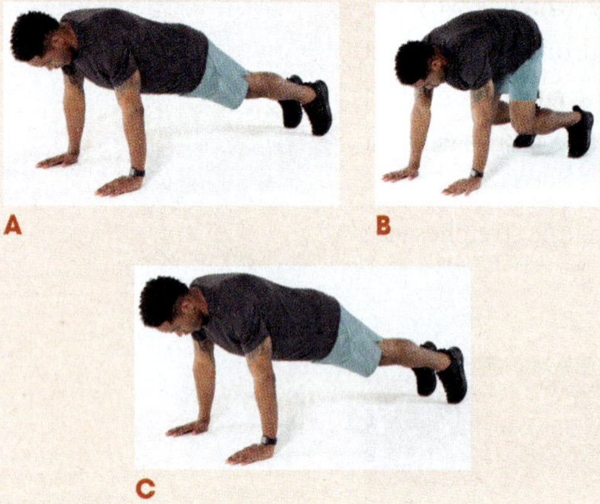 **FIGURE 10.6** Inch Worms	Prone	Warm up soft tissues surrounding wrists and shoulder joints. Promote shoulder stability. Actively lengthen hamstrings and calves.
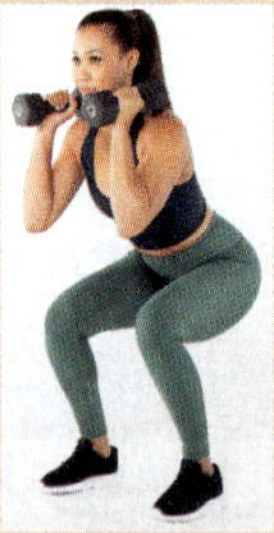 **FIGURE 10.7** Squats	Squatting	Warm up muscles and other soft tissues surrounding ankles, knees, hips, and spine. Promote kinesthetic awareness and good posture.
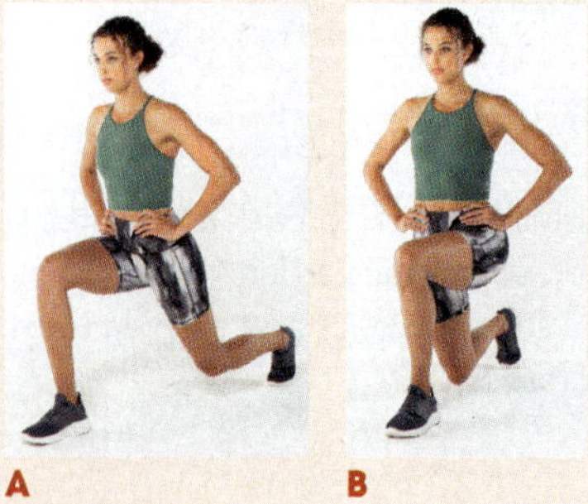 **FIGURE 10.8** Walking Lunges	Squatting	Warm up muscles and other soft tissues surrounding ankles, knees, hips, and spine. Promote kinesthetic awareness, coordination, and balance.
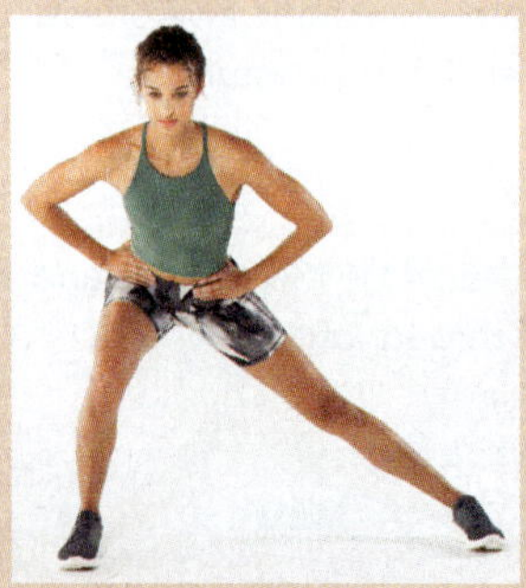 **FIGURE 10.9** Lateral Lunges	Squatting	Warm up muscles and other soft tissues surrounding ankles, knees, hips, and spine. Actively lengthen adductors (inner thigh).

Dynamic Stretch/Movement	Category	Why It Is Effective for Movement Prep
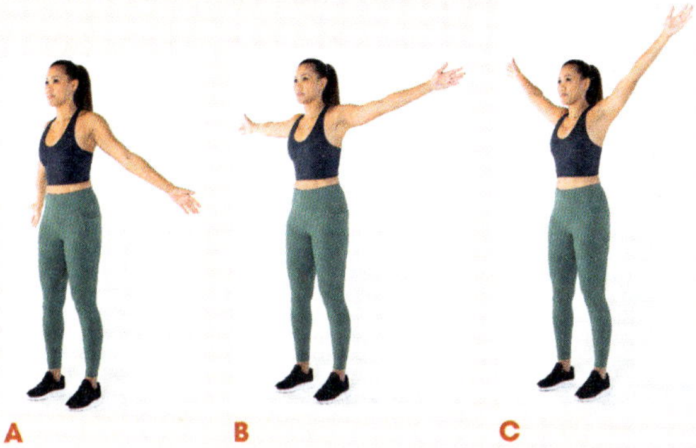 A B C **FIGURE 10.10** Shoulder Rotations/Arm Circles	Rotational	Prepare shoulder joints for range of motion that may be neglected in daily activities.
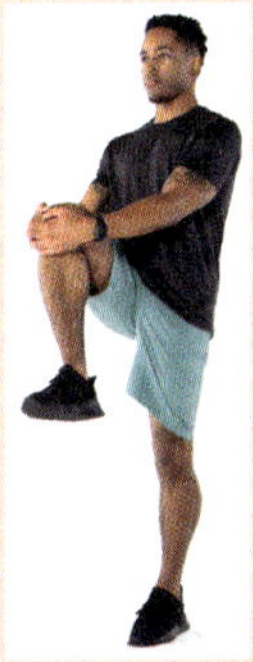 **FIGURE 10.11** High Knee	Hip hinging	Prepare hips for range of motion that may be neglected in daily activities.
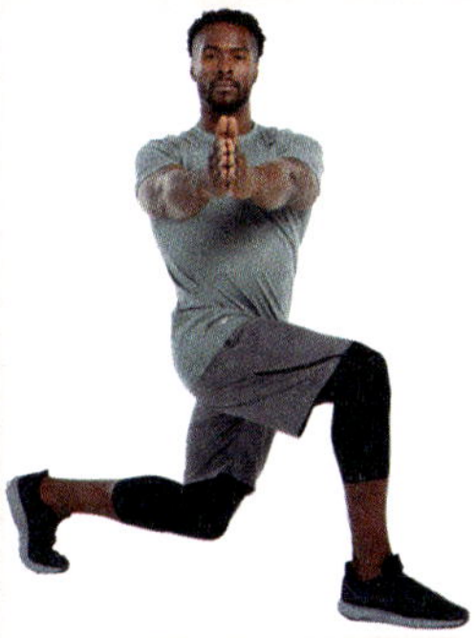 **FIGURE 10.12** Lunge with Rotation	Rotational	Prepare spine and hips for range of motion that may be neglected in daily activities.

RELEVANT AND SPECIFIC MOVEMENT PATTERNS

To adequately prepare participants for the workout ahead, the instructor can prioritize warming up the muscle groups and introducing the movement patterns used in the body of workout. For example, if push-ups are an exercise in the body of the workout, the instructor can use the movement prep to adequately warm up the shoulder joint, pectorals, and triceps with dynamic movements such as inch worms and arm circles. Because a push-up is a moving plank, the instructor may also incorporate a plank hold into the movement prep, which gives them the opportunity to coach participants into a strong plank position and help them understand proper form. By doing this, when it comes time for the push-ups later in class, the instructor can reference the plank hold they did at the beginning to help participants understand what the proper form for a push-up looks and feels like.

Similarly, if the body of the workout has a high volume of squats and lunges, the instructor may choose to do movements such as glute bridges and bird dogs during the movement prep to ensure that the joints and muscles in the participants' legs, hips, and spine are prepared for the workout ahead. If they plan to do the lunges with heavy weights or do squat jumps during the body of the workout, the instructor may also incorporate dynamic squats and lunges into the movement prep, which gives them the opportunity to coach participants through the proper breathing technique, posture, landing technique, and form. This way, when the instructor introduces the heavy lunges and squat jumps later in class, the participants have already begun to master these movement patterns.

INSTRUCTOR TIP

The movement prep and transition are also a great opportunity to address common postural imbalances and muscular tension participants may live with because of a sedentary lifestyle, especially with so many people working jobs that require them to sit at a desk for extended periods of time. If the instructor identifies a common need within the group, they may decide that it is appropriate and relevant to address these issues in the movement prep and transition, even if it is not specific to the workout they planned.

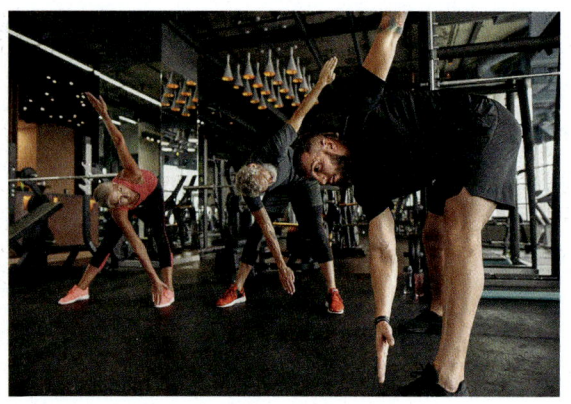

© BAZA Production/Shutterstock

INSTRUCTING MOVEMENT PREP

To ensure that the movement prep effectively prepares the participants for the body of the workout, the instructor can coach and cue participants in ways that encourage energetic yet gentle movements and proper form while speaking in a tone that prepares and excites them for what comes next. The instructor might notice some participants attacking the movement prep with an intensity that is best saved for later in the workout. In these situations, the instructor could take the opportunity to educate participants about the purpose of a warm-up and provide them with tools to monitor their intensity to ensure effort is at an appropriate level. The instructor could also count out the tempo of the movement or connect it to slow, deep breaths in order to guide participants back to an appropriate pace and effort level. Because the movement prep is generally slower paced, it is also a great opportunity for the instructor to coach participants through breathing techniques, posture, alignment, and form. This does not just benefit participants during the movement prep, it will continue to benefit them through the remainder of the workout. As the movement prep builds in intensity, if appropriate, the music and the instructor's speech patterns may also build in intensity.

MOVEMENT PREP PROGRESSIONS AND REGRESSIONS

Completing the movement prep successfully can kick off each attendee's class experience on a positive note. Because the purpose of the movement prep is to prepare the body for the physical challenges that are planned in the body of the workout, it is not the most appropriate time to challenge participants with progressions. That said, although the movement prep is generally low intensity and low impact, instructors still need to be mindful about the fitness level and ability of their class participants and, when necessary, provide alternatives that help them feel confident and successful. For participants who have trouble getting down on the floor, the instructor may choose to plan alternative movements that will not require them to kneel, sit, or lay down. For participants who struggle to keep their balance, the instructor may proactively give them the option to stand next to a wall or barre before beginning certain movements. Sometimes, though, the instructor will notice that a participant is having a difficult time with a movement for which they did not plan any alternatives or modifications. This will require the instructor to improvise before offering a regression or modification.

For example, say that a class is performing inch worms during the movement prep sequence. Most participants are comfortably and safely performing them, but the instructor notices two people who are struggling. The first person informs the instructor that the movement hurts their wrists. As a modification, the instructor suggests that they hold a forearm plank and alternate reaching each arm straight forward. The second person lacks flexibility in their hamstrings, preventing them from safely walking their hands all the way back to their feet. The instructor suggests that instead of inch worms, they alternate between a plank and a downward dog. Both of these modifications allow these participants to continue engaging their core in the plank position while warming up their shoulder joints. Providing regressions and modifications can require quick thinking and creativity, but as long as the instructor keeps the purpose of the original movement in mind they cannot make a wrong decision. The ultimate goal is to create an inclusive and positive experience for each participant.

Movements and Techniques for an Effective Transition

The purpose of the transition is to guide the body back to a resting state, often while gently moving and stretching the muscles and joints that were primarily used during the body of the workout. Now that the body is warmed up, the instructor may choose to incorporate any combination of static stretches and dynamic movements. The transition shares three of the same qualities as the movement prep: low intensity, low impact, and relevant/specific (**Figure 10.13**).

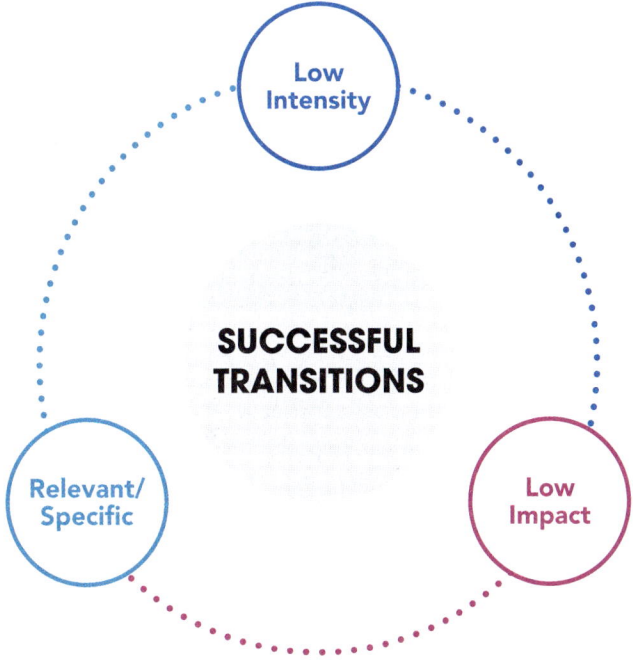

FIGURE 10.13 Transition Qualities

LOW-INTENSITY, LOW-IMPACT, AND RELEVANT/SPECIFIC MOVEMENTS AND STRETCHES

Similar to the movement prep, to ensure that the transition is both low intensity and low impact, instructors generally stick to movements that are slower paced, use bodyweight/minimal resistance, avoid activities such as running or jumping, and aim not to fatigue the participants any further. Instructors can also incorporate movements and stretches that target the joints and muscle groups that were especially taxed and fatigued during the body of workout. For example, if plenty of lunges were performed in the body of the workout, the instructor may choose to incorporate dynamic movements of the hip joints, along with some static stretches for the gluteals, quadriceps, hamstrings, and adductors.

INSTRUCTING THE TRANSITION

Instructing the transition is usually a combination of coaching and cueing participants through gentle movements and stretches that will help return their body to a resting state and celebrating things the group did well and accomplished during the workout. Being mindful of the fatigue class participants may feel during this time, instructors often focus on providing cues that help participants slow their breath while maintaining great posture and alignment. Instructors might notice that some participants move forcefully into their stretches, which gives them the opportunity to inspire participants to connect their movements and workouts to their ultimate goals. If participants wish to reduce stress and tension in their body, the instructor can remind them that aggressively forcing their body into stretches will not reduce stress and tension as effectively as easing and breathing into them.

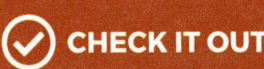

CHECK IT OUT

In some class spaces, instructors have access to tools that allow them to manipulate the class environment in ways that help them to achieve the desired outcome for each class component, such as altering the lighting in a space. During the transition, in addition to speaking in a lower or slower tone and playing music with a slower tempo, the instructor might dim the lights or close the shades to make the space darker and encourage the participants to relax.

Lesson 2: Planning Intros and Outros

Planning the Intro and Outro

The intro is the first impression of the class experience, and the outro is the last impression of the class experience. Although both play an important role in the class experience, participants usually want to make the most of their time in class. This is why it is in the instructor's best interest to keep both brief yet impactful.

Anatomy of an Intro

Every class format is meant to have a unique energy throughout the experience and create a unique outcome at the end. The vibe and outcome of a yoga class is usually far different than that of a cardio dance class. Instructors set the tone for the experience and initiate the participants' journey toward the intended outcome by speaking with the appropriate tone of voice for the class ahead. Other details, such as what music is playing in the background and the lighting of the class space (if that is something the instructor can control), also affect the participants' experience and perception of the class. This also applies to when participants enter the class space and have their first interaction with the instructor.

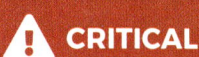

CRITICAL

A great intro does two things:

1. Sets the tone for the experience.
2. Sets the participants' expectations for what is to come.

A participant's experience begins the moment they enter the class space, and there are ways instructors can create a specific vibe and initiate a positive experience before the class officially begins (**Figure 10.14**). Once it is the scheduled start time, the instructor will address the whole class in the intro (**Figure 10.15**).

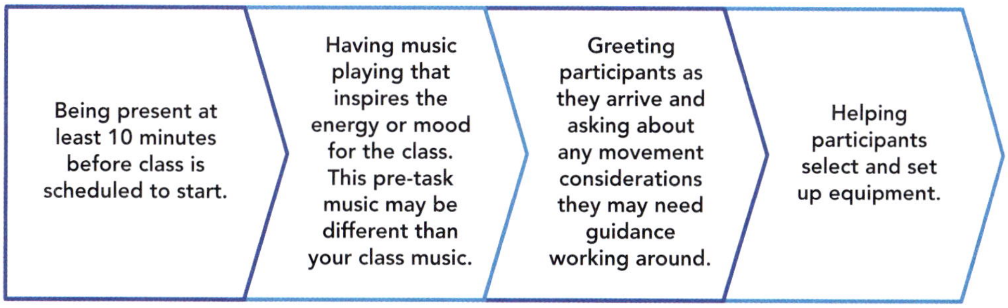

| Being present at least 10 minutes before class is scheduled to start. | Having music playing that inspires the energy or mood for the class. This pre-task music may be different than your class music. | Greeting participants as they arrive and asking about any movement considerations they may need guidance working around. | Helping participants select and set up equipment. |

FIGURE 10.14 Before Class Starts

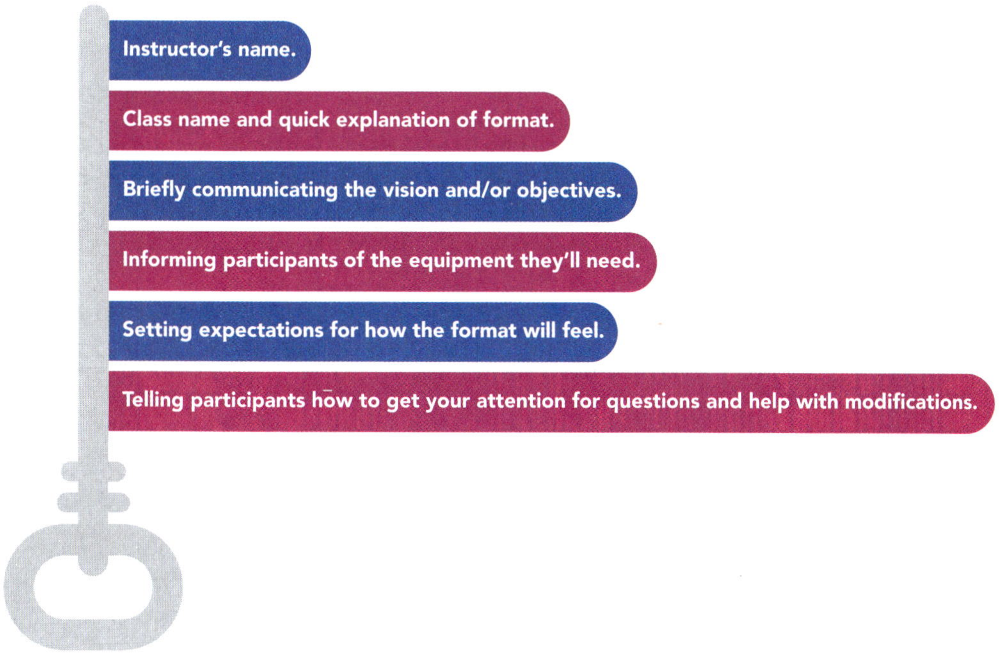

- Instructor's name.
- Class name and quick explanation of format.
- Briefly communicating the vision and/or objectives.
- Informing participants of the equipment they'll need.
- Setting expectations for how the format will feel.
- Telling participants how to get your attention for questions and help with modifications.

FIGURE 10.15 Keys to a Successful Intro

INTRO EXAMPLES

Table 10.2 provides some example intros.

TABLE 10.2 Intro Examples

Class Type	Sample Intro
Mat Pilates	"Hi everyone! Welcome to Mat Pilates. I'm [name], and I'll be guiding you through this 45-minute, total-body workout. In case I didn't catch you on your way in, we're going to be using a Pilates ring. So, if you haven't yet, you can grab one now! Today we're going to focus on releasing unnecessary tension as we prioritize movements that strengthen our core and rotate our joints. We're going to take our time building up the intensity, but, by the end, the burn is going to have us sweating! If we ever get to a movement that's not appropriate for your body, just give me a wave and I'll come give you a modification. Before we dive into the workout, we'll spend about 10 minutes warming up. Let me show you what that's going to look like!"
Cardio dance	"Hey dance crew! Welcome to Cardio Hip Hop. I'm [name], and by the end of this 30-minute class I'm determined to help you find your inner diva! Today, we're going to start with songs that are a slower pace and build our way up until we're going all out! We're definitely going to get our heart pumping for the majority of the class, but we'll finish with a slow routine to bring our heart rate back down before we wrap up. Because the routines are choreographed, it may take me a few extra seconds to get to you if you need a modification, but as soon as I get the class into the groove, I'll come help you. Singing along isn't mandatory, but it's highly encouraged. Having fun, though, that's mandatory! Who's ready to move their body to the music and have a blast?!"
Indoor cycling	"Good morning! Thank you all for getting out of bed early enough to join me for today's 60-minute ride! I'm [name]. Today we're going to focus on maintaining excellent posture, especially when we push through the challenging hills and sprints we'll get to later in class. We'll kick off our ride together soon, but until then get your bike set up and start pedaling with light resistance. I'm going to finish helping a couple more people set up their bike. Just give me a wave if you'd like me to help you find your ideal set up too!"
Total-body strength	"Hey squad! I'm [name] and I'm so pumped that you're here for Total-Body Strength! This is a 45-minute class, and because it's the end of the week, I've put together a playlist of awesome throwbacks that are guaranteed to boost our mood! Those of you who were here earlier this week already prioritized pushing and knee dominant movements; so, today, we're going to focus on pulling and hip dominant movements. Before we get started, let's make sure that we have all the equipment we need: a kettlebell for swings, one dumbbell for single arm rows, and a pair of dumbbells for deadlifts. Please let me know if you'd like my help as you pick your weights! Our warm-up and first block of work will both be entirely bodyweight, then we'll put the kettlebells and dumbbells to good use after that. If you decide you need a different weight than the ones you grabbed already, please let me know. I'm happy to grab what you need and bring it to you! And if we ever get to a movement that doesn't work for you today, just wave me over and I'll give you a modification. Let's get started! Get ready to get sweaty!"

CRAFTING YOUR INTRO

To practice crafting an intro, choose a class format you know you will be teaching or aspire to teach one day and create an intro that sets both the tone and the expectations for the class participants. If you find it helpful, you can use the Class Intro Template provided in the Appendix and fill in the blanks.

Anatomy of an Outro

As the class ends, instructors have the opportunity to leave participants with a positive perception of their experience by doing the items outlined in **Figure 10.16**.

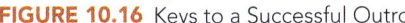

Celebrating things the group did well.

Congratulating participants for achieving the class vision and objectives.

Recapping what was just accomplished and why it benefits the participants.

Reframing things participants may have struggled with in a positive way.

FIGURE 10.16 Keys to a Successful Outro

This time is also an opportunity for instructors to do the following:

- Invite participants to approach them with questions or concerns after class.
- Provide directions about how to clean up their space and equipment.
- Share teasers of what the next class will be like.
- Promote other classes taught at that facility.
- Plug their social media channels (if appropriate).

OUTRO EXAMPLES

Table 10.3 lists example outros that complement the example intros provided in Table 10.2.

TABLE 10.3 Outro Examples

Class Type	Sample Outro
Mat Pilates	"Fantastic work today, everyone! I was thrilled to see you so focused on engaging your core without tensing up your neck and shoulders. Even when our muscles burned so much that we started shaking, you all kept your core solid! That kind of determination will have you walking taller and feeling stronger. So keep it up! Please wipe down your mat and Pilates ring before you put them away. There's another class starting in here shortly. So, if you have any questions for me, please find me in the lobby. If you'd like to join me for another class this week, you can catch me on Thursday at 6:30 p.m. Have a great night!"

(continues)

TABLE 10.3 Outro Examples (*continued*)

Class Type	Sample Outro
Cardio dance	"What a fierce group this dance crew is! You all brought the heat! Props to every single one of you for contributing to the incredible energy that filled the room today. We certainly got our hearts pumping, which is great for our heart health, but we don't want to forget the amazing impact that letting loose and having fun can have on our mental health. So, let's make a date to do it again next week, same time, same place! I'm working on a fun, new routine I plan to debut then, too. If you have song requests for future classes or any questions or concerns for me, don't hesitate to come chat before you head out. See you all soon!"
Indoor cycling	"That was an amazing ride, team! I could tell you loved the songs during that long climb because you were all in the zone! I noticed a lot of us got pretty gassed during the last few sprints; so, I want to reassure everyone that sprints are all about finding and pushing our body's limits. If you hit your limit today that doesn't mean you're out of shape, it means you found your body's limit. So, well done! It got pretty steamy in here too; so, we should all be sure to drink plenty of water. I'm here again tomorrow morning for a 30-minute express ride at 7:00 a.m. and you can see my entire schedule of classes here in my Instagram bio. My handle is [handle]. Please use the sanitizing wipes in the bins on the walls to wipe down your bike before you leave. Way to kick off your day doing something great for yourself! Take care!"
Total-body strength	"You all absolutely crushed this workout! Today's exercises targeted our posterior chain, which can address issues with our posture or tension in our body that can happen if we spend most of our day sitting. I know those kettlebell swings are a complex exercise. They take plenty of practice to master; so, I plan to hang around in here for an extra 5 to 10 minutes to work with any of you who would like some more pointers. If you don't have the time today, let's try to connect before or after class in the future! Next week's class, we'll target the same muscle groups, but I'm going to put a fun twist on some of the exercises we did today. Please sanitize the equipment you used before putting it back where you found it. Again my name is [name], thank you for joining me tonight! See you next week!"

CRAFTING YOUR OUTRO

Using the same class format you chose for your practice intro, create an outro that provides class participants with specific directions on how to leave the space, celebrates what they accomplished, and ends the experience on a positive note. If you find it helpful, you can use the template in the Appendix and fill in the blanks.

Lesson 3: Finalizing the Workout Plan

Putting Your Class Template and Workout Together

Because the class experience is prepared in a different order than it is delivered, once each individual component of the class is planned, the instructor pieces them together in the proper order (**Figure 10.17**).

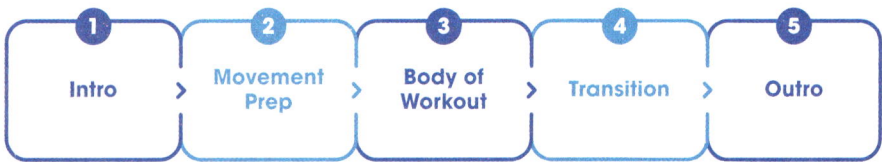

FIGURE 10.17 Workout Component Order

To ensure the class experience flows, the instructor will think through the transitions between each individual class component. A class experience that flows can give participants a sense of structure, organization, safety, and success. With these goals in mind, the instructor decides how much time they will leave between each class component and what needs to happen to prepare for what comes next. In some cases, it is simply leaving enough time to demonstrate the next exercises. In other cases, as in the following examples, there are more details to finalize. You can use the workout template provided in the Appendix to write down and plan any of these extra details.

- **Example 1:** Imagine teaching a fusion class format that alternates between blocks of rowing and blocks of strength training done standing next to the rowing machine (aka as an *erg* or *ergometer*). Because class participants are using ergs directly next to one another, if one participant steps off the right side, and the other participant steps off the left side, they are both going to end up in the same space for the strength training blocks. By telling participants which side of their erg to step off from during strength training blocks, the instructor proactively keeps the class flowing and organized.

- **Example 2:** Imagine teaching a fusion class format that is 40 minutes of cycling followed by 20 minutes of yoga. If the instructor leads participants through exactly 40 minutes of cycling, by the time the class transitions to their yoga mats, there may be 15 minutes or less to dedicate to yoga. In an effort to keep the 40:20 ratio participants expect, the instructor can strategically shave off a little time from each portion of the class to create enough time to transition. There is also the decision about when to have participants set up their space for yoga. The instructor could have participants set it up at the beginning of class, or they could decide to have participants set it up as they transition from the cycling portion of class. The second option could take up more time in the middle of the class, but the instructor may decide that is the best course of action because that may allow more time for participants' heart rates to decrease before they get on the floor for yoga.

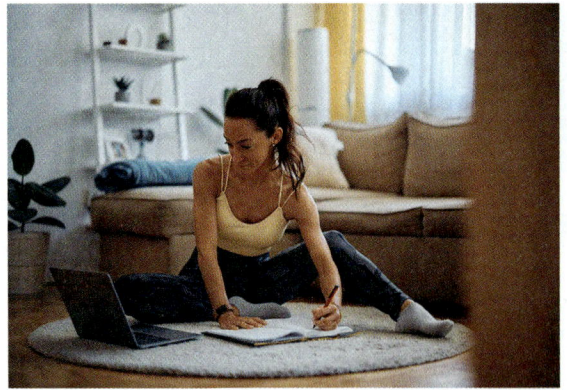

© Drazen Zigic/Shutterstock

Creating Multiple Class Experiences from a Single Workout

Although writing a workout from scratch may take a lot of time and thought, a single workout, or certain parts of it, can be altered and reworked to create multiple unique class experiences. For example, when planning a new workout, if the instructor wants to dedicate a block of work toward strengthening the core, they could take a core strength block from a previous workout they have created for that same format and plug it into the new workout. For the instructor, this can create a more efficient preparation process for each individual class they teach. When done strategically, it can improve the results for regular class participants and keep things fresh and engaging for them no matter how long they have been attending.

CLASS PREPARATION THAT BOOSTS PARTICIPANTS' POTENTIAL FOR RESULTS

PROGRESSIVE OVERLOAD

Gradually increasing the demand of an exercise or workout over time in order to make small, consistent improvements in a person's overall fitness.

Personal trainers apply the principle of **PROGRESSIVE OVERLOAD** to programs they write for their clients. Group Fitness Instructors can leverage this principle in order to boost their regular class participants' potential to gain results. Progressive overload is the practice of gradually increasing the demand of an exercise or workout over time in order to make small, consistent improvements in a person's overall fitness (American College of Sports Medicine, 2009). This approach can also reduce the risk of injury by ensuring adjustments do not increase the workload so dramatically that it creates excessive stress or strain on the participant's body. Participants will need to attend class consistently in order to reap the benefits of progressive overload, and instructors can use this to their advantage! Educating participants about why it is beneficial to repeat exercises and workouts can inspire and motivate them to keep coming back.

The following variables can be gradually altered over time to increase the demand of an exercise or workout:

- Increase range of motion (without loss of technique).
- Alter pace/tempo (speed up or slow down).
- Increase resistance/load.

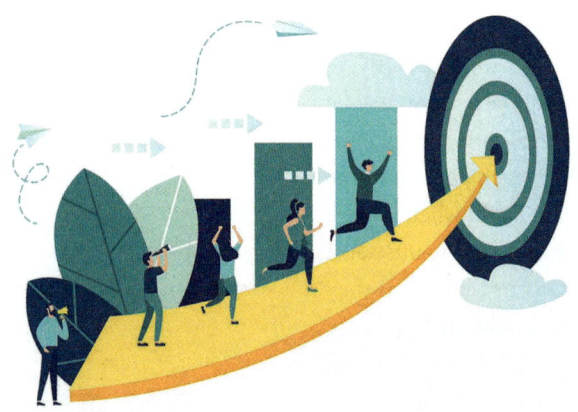

© Viktoria Kurpas/Shutterstock

- Progress exercise/movement complexity.
- Increase repetitions per set or round.
- Increase sets or rounds per workout.
- Lengthen work time.
- Shorten rest time.
- Reduce stability/challenge balance.

Figure 10.18 provides examples of applying progressive overload to create multiple class experiences from a single workout. In both examples, each class was developed from the same original workout, which was gradually altered over the course of several classes.

In this example, an interval training circuit, the instructor created five different class experiences from the same workout. With each class they taught, the instructor either lengthened the work

	Class 1	Class 2	Class 3	Class 4	Class 5
Work Interval	30 sec	40 sec	40 sec	50 sec	50 sec
Rest Interval	30 sec	30 sec	20 sec	20 sec	15 sec
Progression		↑ work interval	↓ rest interval	↑ work interval	↓ rest interval

FIGURE 10.18 Interval Training Circuits: Work Time and Rest Time

interval or shortened the rest interval to progress the challenge level. As the work interval lengthens, participants will likely complete more repetitions of each exercise, which can build strength and endurance (American College of Sports Medicine, 2009). As the rest interval shortens, participants will have less time to recover between exercises, which can improve conditioning (American College of Sports Medicine, 2009).

In **Figure 10.19**, progressing a single exercise within a workout, the instructor created three different experiences from the same foundational exercise. With each class they taught, the instructor added another element to the exercise. In doing so, participants progressed from isometrically challenging their hamstrings and gluteals while strengthening their back with bent over rows, to dynamically engaging their hamstrings and gluteals by adding the deadlift, and ultimately challenging their balance with a single-leg deadlift. In both examples, the instructor created new variations of the same workout to make the experience feel fresh and new to regular participants while also gifting them the benefits of progressive programming.

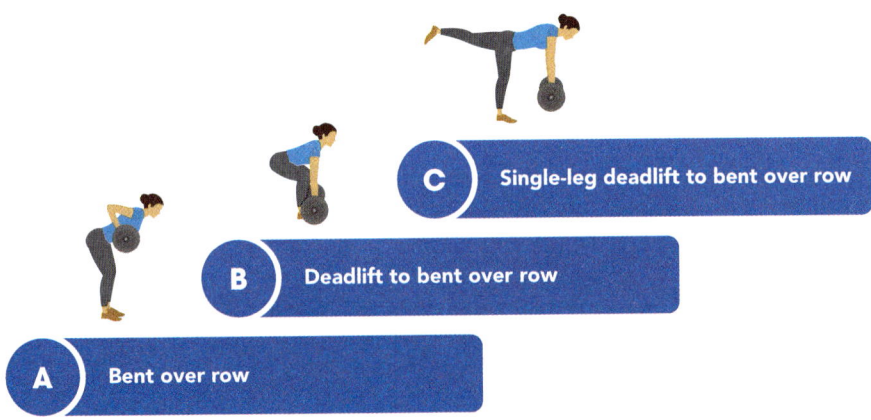

C Single-leg deadlift to bent over row

B Deadlift to bent over row

A Bent over row

FIGURE 10.19 Progressing a Movement

ADDITIONAL STRATEGIES FOR CREATING A VARIETY OF CLASS EXPERIENCES

Another great way to create multiple class experiences without writing an entirely new workout for each class is to mix and match elements of different workouts (**Figure 10.20**). Referencing the sample Total-Body Strength class template, an instructor could pair Block 1 from one workout with Block 1 from another workout to create a body of the workout the class has never done before. The same strategy can be used with the movement prep and transition, as well as with individual exercises and movements within a block of work.

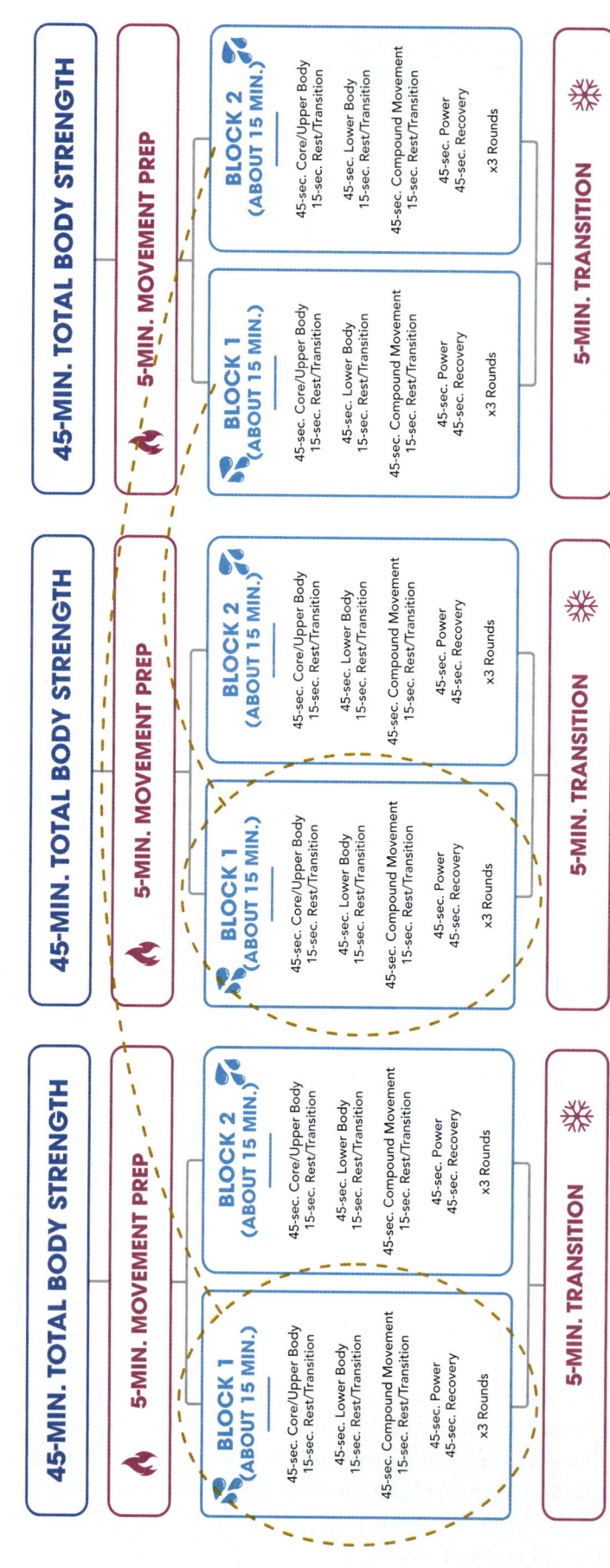

FIGURE 10.20 Mixing and Matching Elements of Different Workouts to Create New Workouts

As instructors develop relationships with class participants, they will learn about each person's unique priorities and goals. When a participant shares a particular desire or goal, in addition to writing effective workouts and programs, instructors can help set them up for success by educating them about SMART goals. SMART is an acronym that stands for specific, measurable, attainable, relevant, and time-based. Defining all five of these components can help participants to set clear, achievable goals (White et al., 2020):

Specific: A clear outcome is identified and defined.

Measurable: Progress toward that outcome can be tracked.

Attainable: The goal is achievable by the end date they have decided on and the workload of pursuing it is appropriate for their current life demands/ routine.

Relevant: The goal is appropriate for their body and current health status.

Time-based: A realistic end date or deadline is identified in order to prepare a clear game plan.

SUMMARY

Once the instructor writes the body of the workout, they plan the movement prep, then the transition, followed by the intro and outro. Once all five components of the class are prepared, the instructor organizes them in the proper order and plans how they will transition between each component as they teach the class. Although the body of the workout is the star of the show, by properly preparing the other class components and prioritizing class flow, the instructor can improve the participants' perception and overall experience of the class.

REFERENCES

Afonso, J., Olivares-Jabalera, J., & Andrade, R. (2021). Time to move from mandatory stretching? We need to differentiate "Can I?" from "Do I have to?" *Frontiers in Physiology, 12*, 714166. https://doi.org/10.3389/fphys.2021.714166

American College of Sports Medicine. (2009). American College of Sports Medicine position stand. Progression models in resistance training for healthy adults. *Medicine & Science in Sports & Exercise, 41*(3), 687–708. https://doi.org/10.1249/MSS.0b013e3181915670

Beedle, B. B., & Mann, C. L. (2007). A comparison of two warm-ups on joint range of motion. *Journal of Strength & Conditioning Research, 21*(3), 776–779. https://doi.org/10.1519/r-19415.1

Behm, D. G. (2018). *The science and physiology of flexibility and stretching: Implications and applications in sport performance and health.* Routledge. http://doi.org/10.4324/9781315110745

Behm, D. G., Blazevich, A. J., Kay, A. D., & McHugh, M. (2016). Acute effects of muscle stretching on physical performance, range of motion, and injury incidence in healthy active individuals: A systematic review. *Applied Physiology, Nutrition, and Metabolism, 41*(1), 1–11. https://doi.org/10.1139/apnm-2015-0235

Behm, D. G., & Chaouachi, A. (2011). A review of the acute effects of static and dynamic stretching on performance. *European Journal of Applied Physiology, 111*(11), 2633–2651. https://doi.org/10.1007/s00421-011-1879-2

Fowles, J. R., Sale, D. G., & MacDougall, J. D. (2000). Reduced strength after passive stretch of the human plantar flexors. *Journal of Applied Physiology, 89*(3), 1179–1188. https://doi.org/10.1152/jappl.2000.89.3.1179

Fradkin, A. J., Zazryn, T. R., & Smoliga, J. M. (2010). Effects of warming-up on physical performance: A systematic review with meta-analysis. *Journal of Strength & Conditioning Research, 24*(1), 140–148. https://doi.org/10.1519/jsc.0b013e3181c643a0

Kay, A. D., & Blazevich, A. J. (2012). Effect of acute static stretch on maximal muscle performance: A systematic review. *Medicine & Science in Sports & Exercise, 44*(1), 154–164. https://doi.org/10.1249/MSS.0b013e318225cb27

Opplert, J., & Babault, N. (2019). Acute effects of dynamic stretching on mechanical properties result from both muscle-tendon stretching and muscle warm-up. *Journal of Sports Science & Medicine, 18*(2), 351–358.

Power, K., Behm, D. G., Cahill, F., Carroll, M., & Young, W. (2004). An acute bout of static stretching: Effects on force and jumping performance. *Medicine & Science in Sports & Exercise, 36*(8), 1389–1396. https://doi.org/10.1249/01.mss.0000135775.51937.53

White, N. D., Bautista, V., Lenz, T., & Cosimano, A. (2020). Using the SMART-EST goals in lifestyle medicine prescription. *American Journal of Lifestyle Medicine, 14*(3), 271–273. https://doi.org/10.1177/1559827620905775

CHAPTER 11

MUSIC

LEARNING OBJECTIVES

The intent of this chapter is to describe the connection between music and movement, explain the various components of music, and outline the various sources of music and the legalities associated with each. Most important, the chapter details how you can align music with your class vision and objectives so that you can meet your participants' needs.

After reading this content, students should be able to demonstrate the following objectives:

- **Explain** the connection between music and movement.

- **Differentiate** between synchronous and asynchronous uses of movement in group fitness.

- **Explain** music concepts such as BPM, phrases, and music mapping.

- **Identify** considerations (such as genres, styles, and demographics) that might inform music selection for a group fitness class.

- **Discuss** various sources for music and related licensing or rights requirements.

- **Explain** methods for aligning music selections to class components or work blocks.

Lesson 1: Music and Movement

Introduction

Music transports us to wonderful places. Places we have been, and places we want to go. Music can send us back in time to high school, to college, or the night we fell in love for the first time. It reminds us of that crazy road trip, our honeymoon, when our baby was born, and when that same baby graduated high school. Music connects us to our memories and to each other. It provides relaxation, inspiration, and motivation. Without a doubt, music has the power to move us emotionally. But it does not stop there. Anyone who has ever felt the uncontrollable urge to nod their head, tap their toe, or jump up and dance when the right song plays can attest that music

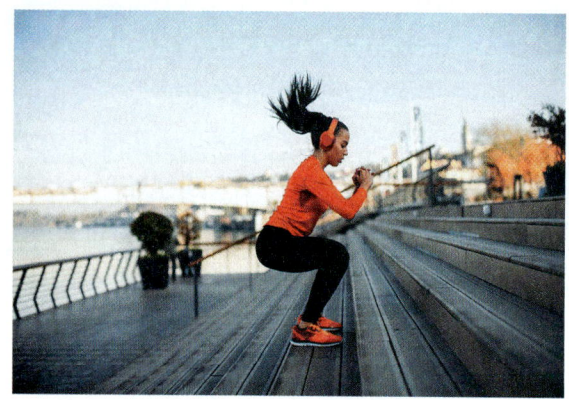

© BGStock72/Shutterstock

also moves us physically. Research has found that moving to music can be one of the most important factors in keeping people engaged, motivated, and committed to an exercise program (Terry et al., 2020). Therefore, regardless of format or style, when it comes to group fitness, there is magic in music.

The Connection Between Music and Movement

Understanding and maximizing the role of music in group fitness is one of the most important skills an instructor can learn. It is no secret that exercise is difficult for many individuals. Some of the most frequently cited barriers to regular exercise include lack of motivation, boredom, fear of being uncomfortable, and the absence of social support (Biddle et al., 2021; Herazo-Beltrán et al., 2017). Fortunately, group fitness, specifically when performed with music, provides one of the most effective solutions for overcoming those barriers. When movement is combined with music, it can have powerful and far-reaching effects on exercise enjoyment, adherence, and effectiveness.

Rationale for Using Music for Movement

To observe how innately wired humans are to respond to music, one need only watch how a baby reacts when upbeat music begins to play, smiling and bobbing their head to the beat. The

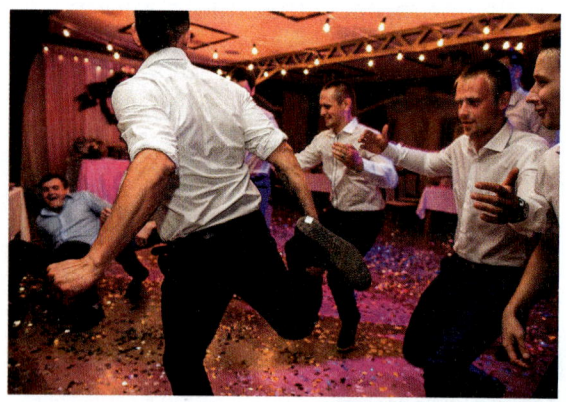

© Wedding and lifestyle/Shutterstock

same kind of reaction can be witnessed at a wedding reception when people of all ages rise to their feet and dance to a familiar song. Of course, it can also be observed when, without thinking about it, you find yourself tapping your feet or moving your hands to a catchy beat.

As human beings, music can affect both our emotional state and our physiology. An up-tempo song can elevate our heart rate, whereas a slower song can lower it. Music can boost our mood or calm us down (Levitin, 2006). It can agitate us, and it can put us to sleep. It can also (as observed by the need to tap our feet to that catchy song) incite the urge to move. Given the growing body of research on music, movement, and the brain, it is no surprise that music is inextricably linked with movement in nearly all forms of group fitness. Through intentional music selection and utilization, Group Fitness Instructors can influence not only the energy and mood states of participants but also their intensity and performance potential (Terry et al., 2020).

THE MAGIC OF GROUP FITNESS IS THE MUSIC

Performing group fitness to music became increasingly popular in the 1980s when, inspired by fitness leaders such as Jane Fonda, people discovered how enjoyable it was to "exercise in sync with a musical beat" (Karageorghis, 2017). Today, for many individuals, group fitness is synonymous with exercising to music and is one of the most important reasons a participant will choose to attend one class in favor of another (Wininger & Pargman, 2003).

However, it is not just the music that attracts participants to group fitness; it is the joy of moving to it with others. Throughout human history, moving together to music has been a social glue, bringing people together on a deeply connected level. Consider that if music is affecting our own brains and physiological responses, it is also affecting those of others around us. When we are moving together and experiencing those responses simultaneously, it can foster relationships, forge social bonds, and strengthen the sense of community (Karageorghis, 2017). For many group fitness participants, that sense of belonging may be the greatest reason they remain committed to an exercise program.

MUSIC MAKES YOU FEEL GOOD

In addition to the considerable social benefits of exercising to music within a group, there are numerous physiological and psychological benefits as well. Not only does music make exercise more enjoyable, it can also make it more effective. Studies indicate that exercising to music can distract people from pain, elevate mood, and increase performance (Jabr, 2013). The mental diversion music provides as a function of distraction, or **DISSOCIATION**, has been shown to improve endurance by as much as 15% and to decrease the perception of exertion by up to 10% at lower to moderate intensities (**Figure 11.1**) (Karageorghis, 2017). At higher-intensity ranges, although there is a notable switch to **ASSOCIATION** (more intense focus on what is happening physically), music can still have a positive effect on the way individuals interpret fatigue (Patania et al., 2020; Terry et al., 2020).

DISSOCIATION

The act of mentally separating or disconnecting from a physical task and focusing on other external elements, such as sounds or visual input.

ASSOCIATION

The act of focusing intently on internal feedback while performing a task, such as breath rate or muscle activity.

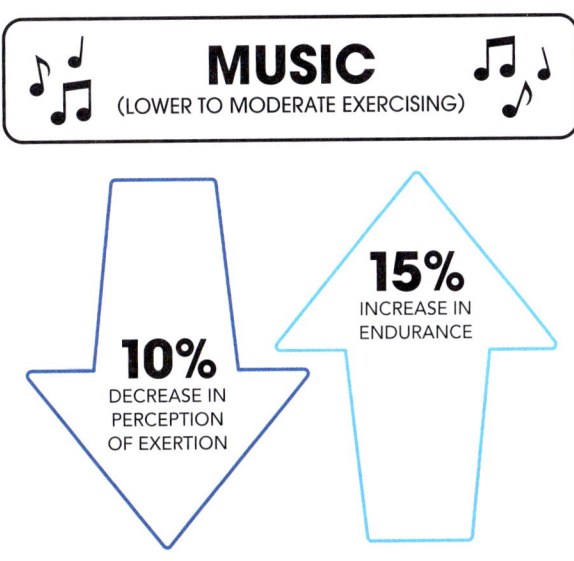

FIGURE 11.1 Music's Influence on Exertion and Endurance

Well-chosen music can also enable participants to work harder, longer, and with less physical discomfort across a range of intensities (Hutchinson et al., 2015). Additionally, some research has shown that when movement is performed perfectly in sync with music it "appears to promote feelings that verge on that of a spiritual experience" and that these feelings of "intense pleasure" are augmented when they are shared with others (Karageorghis, 2017). Although exercise and intense pleasure are not typically associated with each other, music can often be the element that brings them together. One only has to witness the joyful smiles, whoops, and cheers emanating from a dance fitness class to see that music can transform exercise from a dreaded chore to a joyful celebration.

Simply put, both exercise and music contribute to feelings of physical and emotional well-being. When they are effectively combined in the group fitness environment, they form the fundamental platform upon which group fitness exists. As a Group Fitness Instructor, whether

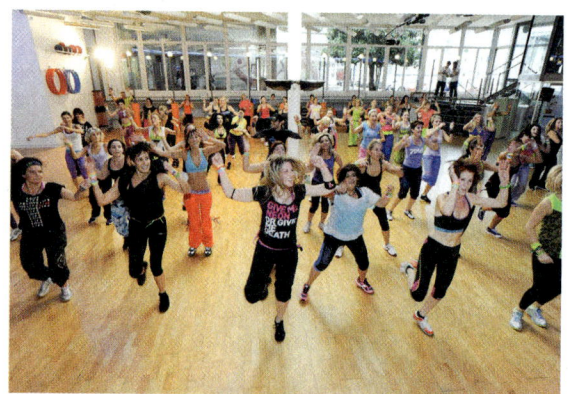
© Stefano Ember/Shutterstock

your format of choice involves movement choreographed perfectly to the beat or uses music in the background, it is imperative to recognize the relevance of music in group fitness and harness its power to create extraordinary experiences that participants enjoy and will return to.

Common Uses of Music in Group Fitness

Although music is used in almost all forms of group fitness, the role that it plays varies significantly by format. Broadly speaking, the role of music can be broken down into two categories: (1) formats where music is used to set the precise pace of movement or choreography (such as dance-based fitness or step aerobics) and (2) formats where the movements are self-paced and the music provides an energetic backdrop (such as circuit training or boot camp). Although both applications have significant benefits, as an instructor, it is important to know how and when to use them.

Synchronous Versus Asynchronous

Movement purposely done in time with music is considered **SYNCHRONOUS**, whereas movement that is performed with music in the background is considered **ASYNCHRONOUS** (**Table 11.1**). In synchronous activities, the music acts like a metronome, setting the pace and coordinating every movement to the beat. Group fitness formats commonly associated with (and frequently defined by) synchronous movement are dance-based formats, step aerobics, traditional hi/lo, cardio kickboxing, choreographed resistance training formats, barre formats, and aqua aerobics. Indoor cycling is also often performed synchronously, with the beat of the music setting the **PEDALING CADENCE** measured in **REVOLUTIONS PER MINUTE (RPM)**.

SYNCHRONOUS

When movement is purposely done in time with music.

ASYNCHRONOUS

An application of music where there is no conscious synchronization between the tempo or meter of the music and an individual's movement.

PEDALING CADENCE

Often used interchangeably with revolutions per minute (RPM) in reference to pedaling speed.

REVOLUTIONS PER MINUTE (RPM)

A measure of pedaling speed, or cadence.

🤖 GETTING TECHNICAL

Synchronous movement is very effective in group fitness for a variety of reasons. Not only does it keep the class together, making it easier to organize and control movement, some studies indicate it may improve movement quality by reducing kinetic chain inefficiencies (Karageorghis, 2017). For example, a study of stationary cycling indicated that "participants who cycled in time to music required 7 percent less oxygen to do the same work as cyclists who did not synchronize their movements with background music" (Bacon et al., 2012). According to research "a credible explanation for the observed effect is that the rhythmical elements of music enhance the biomechanical or neuromechanical efficiency of physical movements during exercise … resulting in slightly reduced energy cost for a given workload" (Terry et al., 2020, as cited in Bood et al., 2013). Although these effects may be small, they may still contribute to better performance, particularly when the movements are rhythmic and repetitive in nature (Terry et al., 2012). Besides the practical and performance-based benefits of moving in time with music, there is also the satisfying social benefit. It just feels good to move together.

TABLE 11.1 Synchronous Versus Asynchronous Formats in Group Fitness

Synchronous	Asynchronous
Dance based	Circuit training
Traditional aerobics (hi/lo)	High-intensity interval training (HIIT)
Step aerobics	Boot camp
Cardio kickboxing	Equipment-based boxing
Group resistance training	Time-based/self-paced strength training (e.g., EMOM)
Indoor cycling (some formats)	Indoor cycling (some formats)
Barre	Yoga (most styles)

Although there are significant and well-documented benefits to synchronous movement, it is not practical or possible in all scenarios. Moreover, much of the research on the positive benefits of music and exercise has been performed using asynchronous movement. Just because music is not always setting the pace does not mean its presence is less significant. When selected appropriately, it still can delay the onset of fatigue and improve the capacity for work, resulting in better endurance, power, strength, and productivity (Karageorghis, 2017). For this reason, class types that use music in the background still benefit tremendously from the use of a well-selected playlist. Formats that typically use music asynchronously include circuit-style workouts, boot camp classes, time-based strength formats, some types of indoor cycling, and most styles of yoga.

✓ CHECK IT OUT

Although the music selection during exercise is of great importance, the music playing prior to and after class should also be considered. Pre-task music, or the music played prior to the activity, can be very effective in either exciting participants or calming them down (Karageorghis, 2017). For example, playing up-tempo, high-energy music prior to a HIIT or cardio kickboxing class can get people pumped up and ready to "hit it hard." Conversely, playing down-tempo, calming music before a mindful yoga practice can help participants to relax and focus. For optimum benefits, instructors should be intentional about their music selection in every phase of the class experience.

WHEN TO USE EACH IN VARIOUS FORMATS

The choice to teach classes that use music synchronously or asynchronously is largely determined by the type of format and the class objective. Certain formats, such as dance fitness or step aerobics, use music very specifically to dictate the pace of movement. Not only does moving in time with the beat keep participants together at a safe, controlled pace, but it also enables the instructor to use features of the music to influence choreography and intensity. Conversely, some formats necessitate that the participants move at their own pace in order to maintain an appropriate range of motion and personal intensity level. Typically, these formats use time or rep counts as the element that keeps the group together while the music supports the desired energy. Common examples of each include the following:

CHOREOGRAPHED MOVEMENT

- Dance-based fitness: The instructor uses different parts of the song to dictate recognizable and repeated patterns of choreography (e.g., performing one move during the verse of the song, another during the chorus, and a third pattern during the bridge).
- Step aerobics: The choreography is structured to match the beat structure of the music, allowing participants to follow along in perfect synchrony with the instructor and each other. The instructor will build and break down movement patterns that correspond with the changes in the music, making it easy to follow and perform as a group.

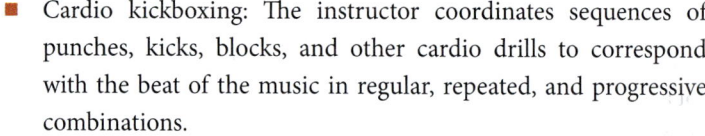

- Cardio kickboxing: The instructor coordinates sequences of punches, kicks, blocks, and other cardio drills to correspond with the beat of the music in regular, repeated, and progressive combinations.
- Group resistance: Participants use barbells or other types of resistance equipment to lift weights in time to the music. Although the weight chosen will vary by individual, each participant lifts the weights at the same speed and for the same number of repetitions.
- Indoor cycling: Many indoor cycling formats use the beat of the music to specifically determine RPM for the pedaling speed, or cadence. These classes may also include body position or intensity changes that precisely correspond with changes in the music.

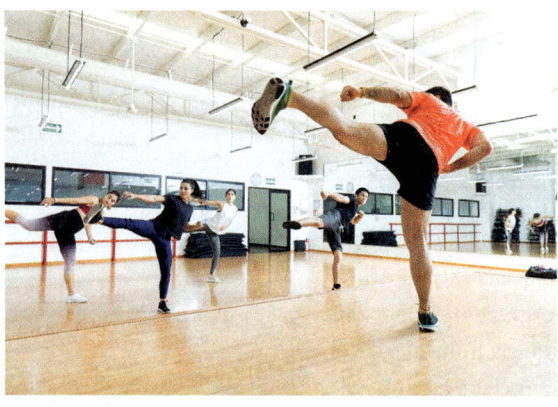

© Antoniodiaz/Shutterstock

NON-CHOREOGRAPHED MOVEMENT

- Circuit formats: Participants work at stations featuring cardio drills, resistance exercises, or both for a specified period of time before moving on to the next station or exercise. Due to the nature of these workouts, it is neither practical nor effective to perform them in time with the music.
- HIIT, boot camp, and equipment-based boxing: Similar to circuit-style workouts, HIIT, boot camp, and equipment-based boxing formats feature a variety of exercises that are best done at the participant's preferred pace in order to achieve the correct intensity.

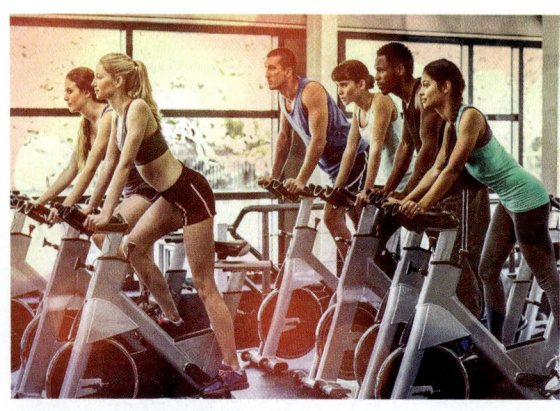

For example, when the goal is to perform a maximum number of repetitions in a given time period, it is important that each participant is able to work at their own level of challenge to achieve the desired benefits and maintain proper form.

- Indoor cycling: Although many indoor cycling formats use the beat of the music to set the cadence, in others, riders are encouraged to select their own optimal pedaling speed to achieve intensity goals dictated by power (watts), heart rate, or rating of perceived exertion. In this style, the music provides energy and motivation but does not dictate the pedaling speed.
- Flexibility: When training flexibility, music is often in the background to enable participants to achieve the optimal duration and range of motion for each exercise.

© Vectorfusionart/Shutterstock

Lesson 2: Music Structure and Alignment

Music Structure

Whether the class uses music to set the pace or simply the mood, selecting music with the right energy for the format is critical to the overall experience. To use music to its fullest capacity in the group fitness setting, it is important to have a basic understanding of the fundamental structure and features of music as well as how they influence class design, organization, and intensity.

Considering the role of energy in music selection, instructors must first understand the role of **BEAT** and **RHYTHM**. The beat is the regular, consistent pulse that sets the pace of music and anchors all the other elements together. This can be observed when the drummer of a band begins a song by tapping out the beat (often with a "one, two, three, four"), or the conductor of an orchestra waves a baton before the musicians start to play. These actions are performed to establish the speed at which a particular piece of music will be played. The speed of music is also called the **TEMPO** and, just like a heartbeat, is measured in **BEATS PER MINUTE (BPM)**.

⚙ PRACTICE THIS

Listen to a song and see if you can identify the beat. Tap your foot along with it in a regular pulse, then hum or sing the lyrics along with it. Notice how the length of the sounds of the words change, but the beat does not.

Studies on exercise and music indicate a strong relationship between music tempo and how individuals physically respond to it. Music with a faster BPM is typically considered to convey higher, more uplifting energy. Indeed, research shows that songs with faster tempos, specifically 120–140 BPM, are preferred for higher-intensity activities (Karageorghis, 2017; Terry et al., 2020). In addition to BPM, another critical element that influences the energy of the song is the rhythm; exercisers tend to respond best to music with strong rhythmic qualities (Karageorghis, 2017).

Although the terms *beat* and *rhythm* often are used interchangeably, they are not the same. The beat is the steady underlying pulse that remains constant throughout a piece of music. It is what you feel in your body and typically notice yourself tapping out when it is stimulating. The rhythm refers to the length of the sounds on top of the beat. Rhythm is what makes a song interesting and often is responsible for how energetic it feels. In group fitness, the most frequently utilized **TIME SIGNATURE** is 4/4 (common) time, which denotes that there are four beats in each measure of music (**Figure 11.2**). The regular pulse of "1, 2, 3, 4, 1, 2, 3, 4" provides an energetic, predictable pace at which to perform movements and, conveniently, is also the time signature used in most popular music. Musicians often compose songs in eight-bar (measure) segments that correspond with the verses and choruses, providing a built-in structure that can be used to build predictable movement patterns.

BEAT

The audible, metrical division that occurs within the foundational layer of music.

RHYTHM

A pattern of repeated movement or sound.

TEMPO

The speed of music, or how fast it is played; typically measured in beats per minute (BPM).

BEATS PER MINUTE (BPM)

A musical term that refers to measurement of the tempo (speed) of music.

TIME SIGNATURE

A convention in written music that denotes how many beats are contained in a measure.

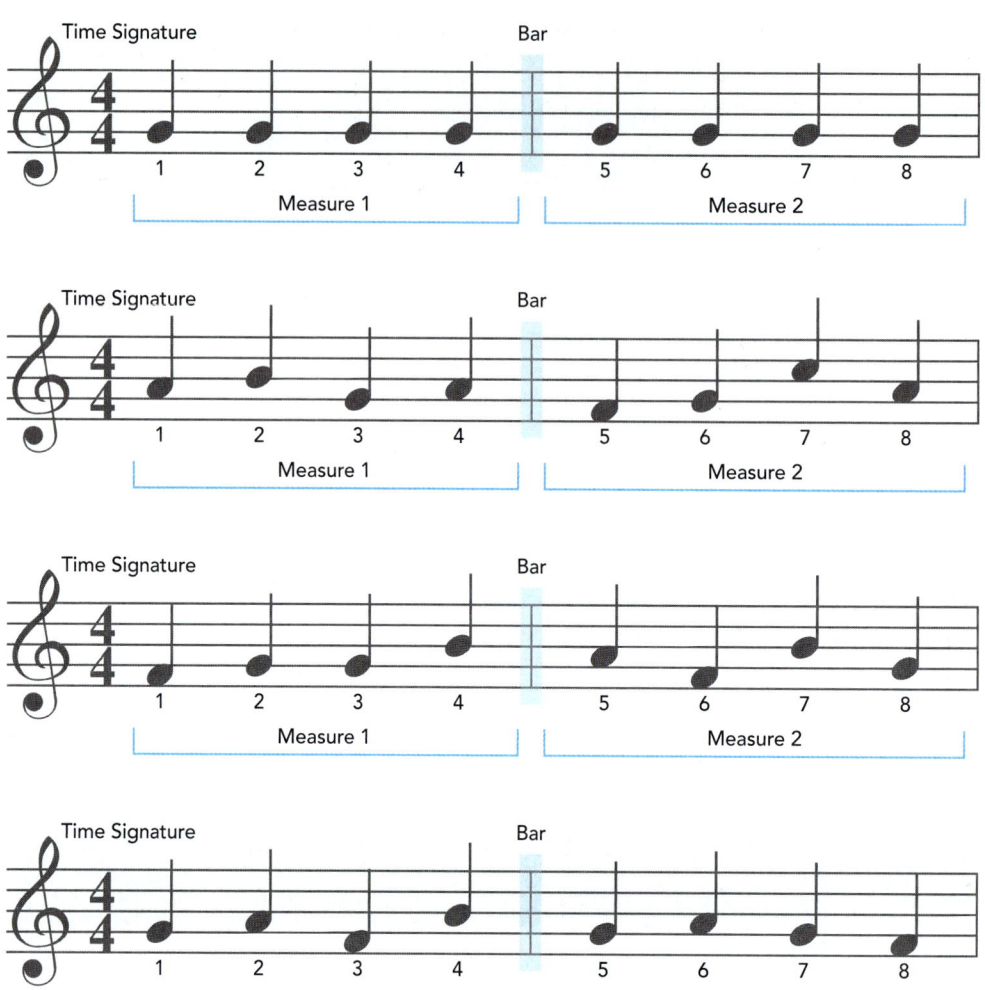

FIGURE 11.2 Music Time Signature

✓ **CHECK IT OUT**

Although 4/4 is the most often used time signature in group fitness, there are certainly other time signatures that feature interesting rhythms. You may recognize 3/4 time as that of the waltz, featuring three beats per measure rather than four (e.g., "raindrops on roses and whiskers on kittens" from "My Favorite Things" by Oscar Hammerstein II and Richard Rodgers), or **SYNCOPATED** rhythms, such as those found in salsa or dubstep (or the catchy rhythm in the song "Superstition" by Stevie Wonder). Although it can be more challenging to choreograph movements to some of these other rhythms, in certain formats they can provide diversion and interest (and they are heavily featured in Latin dance–based formats).

The Role of BPM

Research indicates that two of the most important qualities in setting the pace of movement are the tempo (speed) of the music and the **RHYTHM RESPONSE**, or how likely the song is to incite movement (Cadwell et al., 2007). When the music is driving, energetic, and uplifting, it has the potential to affect mood, elevate heart rate, and increase the speed of movement (Cadwell et al., 2007; Karageorghis, 2017). With that in mind, selecting music with the appropriate BPM is an essential element of class design. The right BPM varies by format, but it is especially critical in classes where the movements will be performed synchronously with the music. For choreographed formats that coordinate each movement to the beat, the BPM must not only support the desired intensity but also the participants' ability to execute safe and effective range of motion while moving to it. Additionally, a predictable and consistent music structure enables the instructor to design logical combinations and patterns that are easy to follow. Fortunately, this can be accomplished by choreographing movements to correspond with the regular pattern in music known as the **MUSICAL PHRASE**.

CHECK IT OUT

It is easier than ever to discover the BPM of any song. In the past, to determine the BPM of a song instructors had to use the tap method. This involved listening to a song with a stopwatch or a watch with a second hand and tapping the beat while watching an interval of time. For example, when listening to a song, if you tapped the beat 32 times in 15 seconds and multiplied by 4, it would confirm that the BPM is 128. Fortunately, today a variety of websites, apps, and music-mixing software can do this in an instant. Many apps or programs will quickly and easily sort an entire music library by BPM. Of course, another excellent option is to purchase formatted songs at your desired BPM from professional fitness music companies.

32-Count Phrases

One of the most essential and commonly utilized practices in group fitness is choreographing blocks of movement to align with 32-count phrases of music. In songs written in 4/4 time, there are four beats per measure; thus, eight measures of music will have 32 counts. This is known as a 32-count phrase.

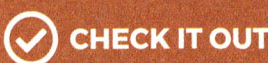 PRACTICE THIS

Search online (or in your favorite streaming service) for "32-Count Workout Music" and then listen to several tracks. See if you can identify the 32-count musical phrase by counting on the first strong beat as follows:

"**1**, 2, 3, 4, 5, 6, 7, 8"
"**2**, 2, 3, 4, 5, 6, 7, 8"
"**3**, 2, 3, 4, 5, 6, 7, 8"
"**4**, 2, 3, 4, 5, 6, 7, 8"

You will notice a distinctive shift in the music at the beginning of each 32-count phrase, typically with a change in the instrumentation or the fullness of the sound. Although this can be difficult to identify at first, with practice you will be able to identify when these shifts are coming, even without counting.

By choreographing movement to correspond with this predictable 32-count phrase, instructors can easily plan movement changes and cues that are telegraphed in the music, making them easier to teach and easier to follow. Consider the example of four simple moves performed to a 32-count phrase in **Figure 11.3**.

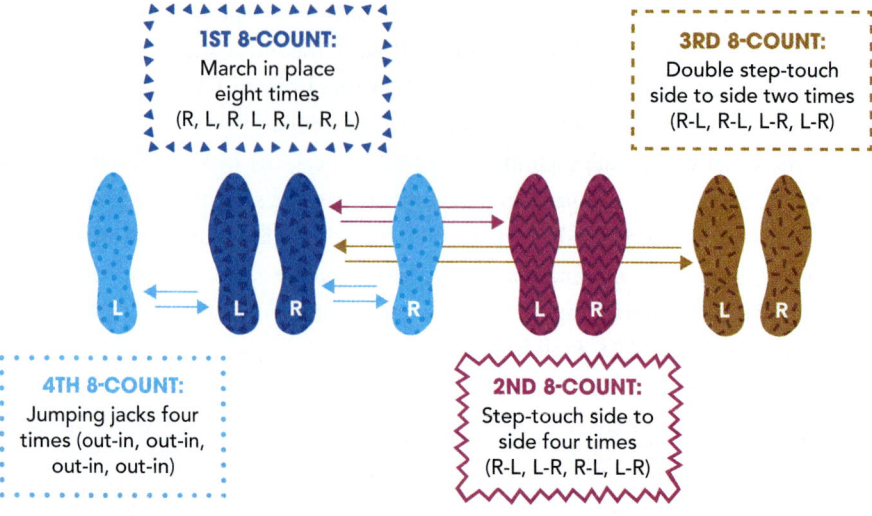

FIGURE 11.3 Steps in a 32-Count Phrase

Using the jumping jacks as a neutral movement (neither starting with the right or left leg), after the last jumping jack, the combination could be repeated starting with the left leg. If this combination were performed at 128 BPM, two times through each side would be equivalent to 1 minute of movement (i.e., 32 counts on the right, 32 counts on the left is 64 counts; performed twice it is 128 counts).

Although this is a simple example of basic movements, this same logic can be applied to a variety of formats, including dance fitness, cardio kickboxing, step aerobics, or group resistance. In group resistance, knowing the BPM and the duration of each phrase can be useful in determining how long to perform a specific movement. For example, if you want to do 1 minute of squats without looking at the clock, you could use 32-count music as follows:

- 8 reps at half time (down, down, up, up) = 30 seconds
- 16 reps at single time (down, up, down, up) = 30 seconds

Both examples illustrate how useful the structure of 32-count phrases in music can be when designing and delivering class formats that benefit from repetition of logical patterns.

⚙ PRACTICE THIS

Listen to a 128-BPM song and see if you can identify the 32-count phrase. Note that you can hear a change in the sound and often observe changes in the line patterns as you watch the song play. Listen to the song and notice that every 32 counts (count them in four groups of eight) something changes. Because this music is at 128 BPM, 32 counts takes 15 seconds. Once you have identified it, practice one of the patterns described in the examples. Then, try to make up your own 32-count movement pattern. Although this skill may seem challenging at first, it is invaluable as a Group Fitness Instructor.

Although not all formats utilize 32-count phrasing as a fundamental feature, those that rely on it heavily include the following:

- Dance-based fitness
- Step aerobics
- Cardio kickboxing
- Group resistance

If you are interested in teaching these formats, this is a particularly important skill to master. Fortunately, professional music-mixing services are available that specialize in producing music that features 32-count phrasing specifically for group fitness.

Music Anatomy

In addition to the role of the beat and rhythm in music, it is also useful for Group Fitness Instructors to understand the basic elements of popular song structure (especially those who want to choreograph movement song by song, such as in dance fitness). Although there are many ways of composing and structuring music, it is helpful to understand the musical form most often utilized in popular music (i.e., what is likely to be heard on the radio and used in group fitness). Most songs in this category are composed using common elements that frequently include an intro, verse, pre-chorus (or **BEAT DROP** in some styles), chorus, bridge, and outro (**Figure 11.4**; **Table 11.2**).

BEAT DROP

The dramatic release of progressive tension within a song. Typically occurs two to three times within a song.

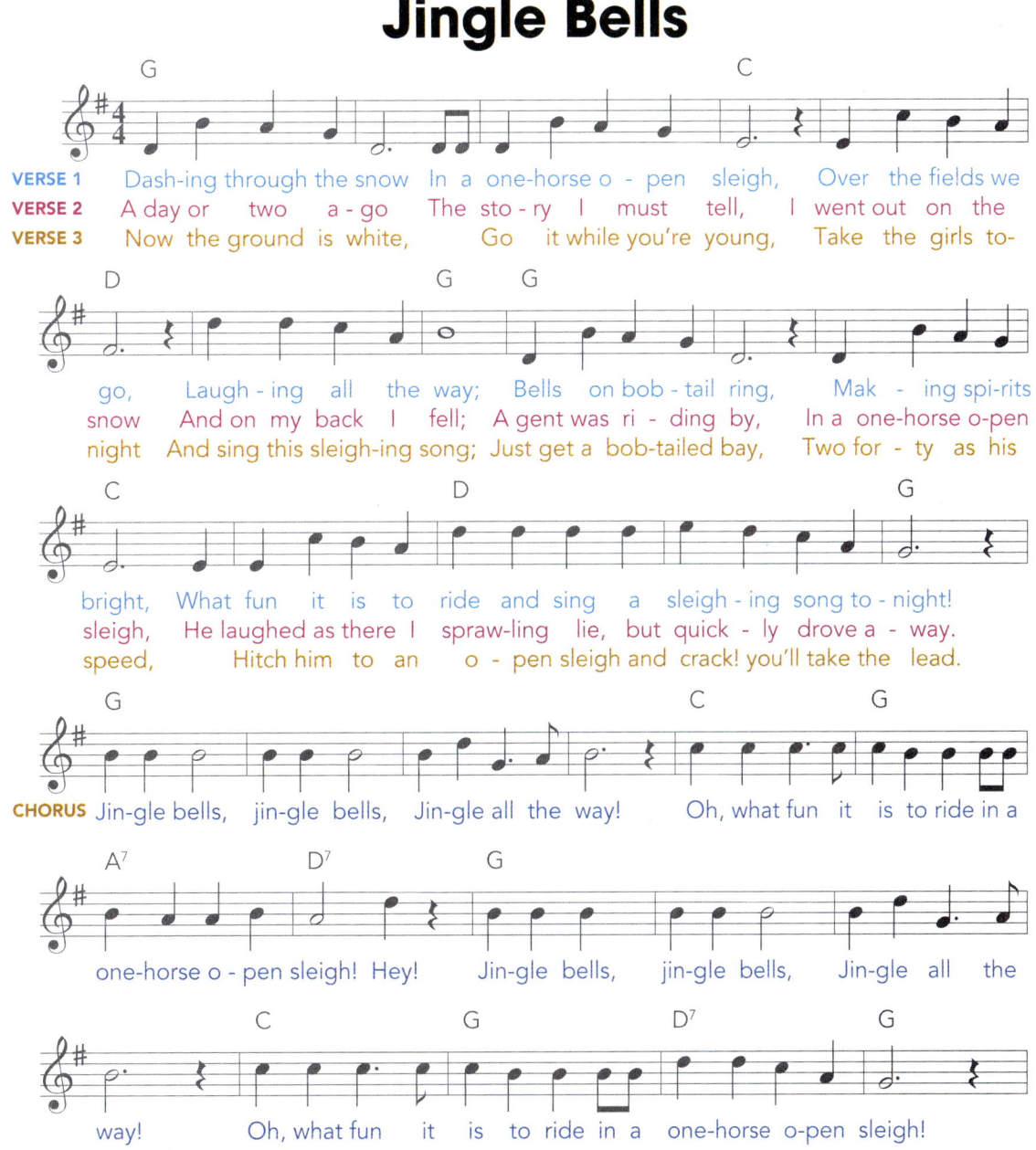

FIGURE 11.4 Verse Versus Chorus

TABLE 11.2 Common Musical Components

Component	Description
Intro	The intro to a song may be short or long, but its purpose is to set the initial tone of the song. If it has a strong beat, it can be particularly useful for establishing the pace at which the movement will be performed before it begins. Additionally, because it typically does not feature lyrics, it is a great time to provide brief instructions without competition from the lyrics in the verse.
Verse	The verse is the part of the song that relates a story, even if there are no words. Often, we remember the melody that accompanies the verse even when we do not know the words. The verse is typically repeated at least two times with an identical melody.
Pre-chorus	In some songs, between the verse and the chorus there is a transitional pre-chorus. The pre-chorus builds anticipation of the chorus that is about to come (or in some musical styles, the beat drop).
Chorus	The chorus is the repeated part of the song that is most recognizable. It often contains the words found in the title and is the "big moment" that all other parts of the song complement. Typically, it repeats three times. Instructors can use both the energy and consistency of the chorus to correspond with high points in choreography or intensity.
Bridge	The bridge is just like it sounds; it is a unique musical "bridge" between two sections of a song, often to the final chorus. The bridge typically sounds very distinct and, due to its frequently dramatic nature, can be used for a special purpose in the choreography.
Outro	Often, but not always, the song will have an outro that signals the song is coming to an end and the energy fades.

In songwriting, the primary components of the verse, chorus, and bridge often are notated as follows:

- A = Verse
- B = Chorus
- C = Bridge

Figure 11.5 shows how a typical pop or rock song might look with this notation.

Instructors can use the parts of a song to create more effective and engaging experiences for participants. Instructors in a dance fitness class might use the verse for one move or combo, the chorus for another, and the bridge for a third (**Figure 11.6**).

A	B	A	B	C	B
VERSE	CHORUS	VERSE	CHORUS	BRIDGE	CHORUS

FIGURE 11.5 Breakdown of a Song

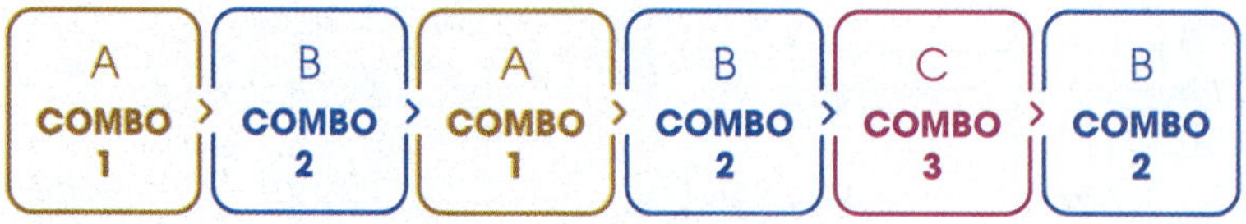

A	B	A	B	C	B
COMBO 1	COMBO 2	COMBO 1	COMBO 2	COMBO 3	COMBO 2

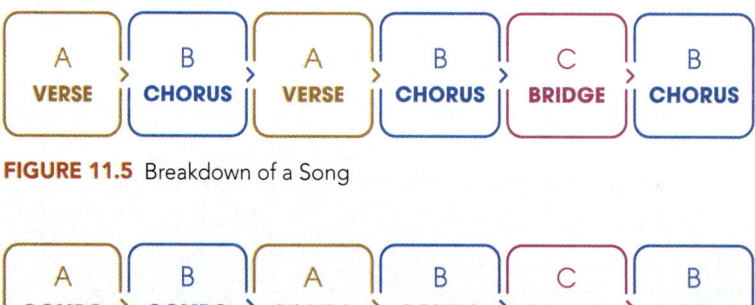

FIGURE 11.6 Breakdown of Exercises to Match a Song

In a group resistance class, the intro might be used to set up the exercise, the verse used for one move (e.g., lunges), and the chorus for a different but complementary movement (e.g., squats). In this example (**Figure 11.7**), the song structure could be used as follows:

- Verse 1: Right leg lunges
- Chorus 1: Squats
- Verse 2: Left leg lunges
- Chorus 2: Squats
- Bridge: Alternating lunges
- Chorus 3: Squats

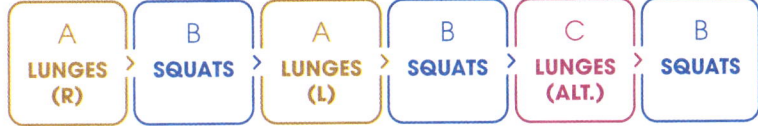

FIGURE 11.7 Example of Matching Exercises to a Song

Because each section of the song is typically the same length, it ensures that equal reps of each exercise are performed and that the changes in the movements match the changes in the music. Although it can take time to hone this skill, the ability to perfectly match movement to music is a quality shared by the most successful instructors.

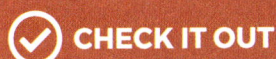

CHECK IT OUT

Examples of this common song form include "Happy" by Pharrell Williams and "Hot N Cold" by Katy Perry. Recognizing and utilizing each part of a song to correspond with the movements, intensity, or energy can be extremely useful in many group fitness formats.

Music Mapping

Knowing the features of the music and using them intentionally in class starts with **MUSIC MAPPING**. Often, what separates a novice from an expert instructor is their ability to coordinate their choreography, exercises, and drills with the musical features in the songs. Most songs have elements that, when used effectively, can greatly enhance the workout by connecting every movement to the energy shifts in the music. Doing this requires the instructor to not only be familiar with each feature, but also to be aware of how long it lasts.

There are a variety of methods to notate the music mapping process. Some instructors keep a spreadsheet, notebook, or index cards; others may use digital notations in the comments section of their playlist or a specialized app. The notation method is not important if it works for the instructor. What matters most is understanding and using the elements of the song individually or linked together to create interval sets, choreography blocks, or movement segments that align so perfectly with the music that it feels as if it was written to match, like the soundtrack of a movie.

This skill is of particular importance to formats such as dance fitness classes, indoor cycle, and group resistance classes and begins with knowing (and often notating) the relevant features of each song to be used. These include the song length, BPM, dramatic features and changes, and

MUSIC MAPPING

The process of identifying the basic elements of a song such as the intro, verse, chorus, and other notable features so that they may be applied in class design.

the length and number of repeated elements such as choruses or beat drops (**Table 11.3**). With that information and a little artistic flair, an instructor can deliver every element of their class with musical precision. The following example illustrates how a mapped song could be used for three perfectly timed 30-second intervals in an indoor cycle class; however, the same basic process could be used in a variety of formats.

TABLE 11.3 Song Mapping Example for Use in Indoor Cycle Versus Strength Training

Indoor Cycle	
Song name	"Feel So Close" by Calvin Harris
Length	3:45
BPM	128
Base pattern	65–75 RPM
Choruses/drops	30 sec. at 1:15, 2:15, 3:15
Use	3 × 30-second cadence pickups with music shifts
Strength Training	
Song name	"Feel So Close" by Calvin Harris
Length	3:45
BPM	128
Base pattern	2/2 biceps curl
Choruses/drops	1/1 at 1:15, 2:15, 3:15
Use	3 sets of biceps curls 2/2 during lyrics, 1/1 with shift (instrumental)

To map a song of your own, you must first identify a song with the right energy, length, and BPM for the desired class segment (**Figure 11.8**).

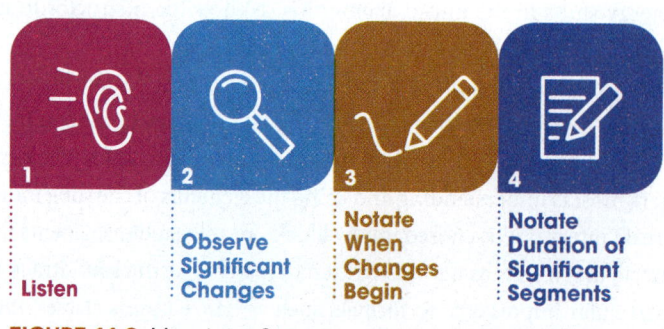

1 Listen
2 Observe Significant Changes
3 Notate When Changes Begin
4 Notate Duration of Significant Segments

FIGURE 11.8 Mapping a Song

Then, while listening to the song, watch the time counter on the device from which the song is playing and note the following:

- When the intro ends and the verse (or the main melody) of the song begins
  - This is usually indicated by additional fullness coming into the sound, the beat coming in, or the verse starting.
- The shift leading into a notable change (e.g., the chorus or beat drop)
  - After the verse or a rhythmic build, the next feature is typically a chorus or a beat drop, depending on the music genre. As your musical intuition improves, it will become easier to identify when this is about to happen.
- The time when the change begins (e.g., chorus or beat drop)
  - Watch the timer on your music player to see when this happens in the song. Fortunately, due to the mathematical nature of music, this will likely be a consistent interval of time. Although not always the case, a great many choruses or beat drops last 20–45 seconds. Typically, these elements repeat at least once, if not twice. Be sure to locate all of these changes as they are important for class design.
- The number of changes you want to use
  - Once each beat drop or chorus has been identified, note how many times it happened and how long it lasted.
- Any other interesting features observed
  - There might be a quiet point with powerful spoken words, a fun sound effect, a rhythm shift, or any number of other interesting elements might be incorporated; take note of those as well.

Now the song is ready to be paired with other mapped songs for use in your class.

Although the mapping process can be time consuming in the beginning, once your musical familiarity and intuition improve, you will be able to quickly navigate a song to determine the important features. If you want to be the best, this is an invaluable skill to master in certain formats. See **Figure 11.9** for a music mapping example.

 **INSTRUCTOR TIP**

Five Simple Steps to Mapping a Song

1. Note the length of the song.
2. Note the BPM of the song (especially if the pace of the movement will correspond to the beat of the music).
3. Note when the verse/melody begins as well as the beginning of each chorus.
4. Note the duration of each chorus or other repeated element (this is important if you are using it as a timed bout of work).
5. Note how many times the repeated element occurs (this enables you to inform participants of the number of upcoming bouts of intense work, or how many times through participants might perform an identical drill).

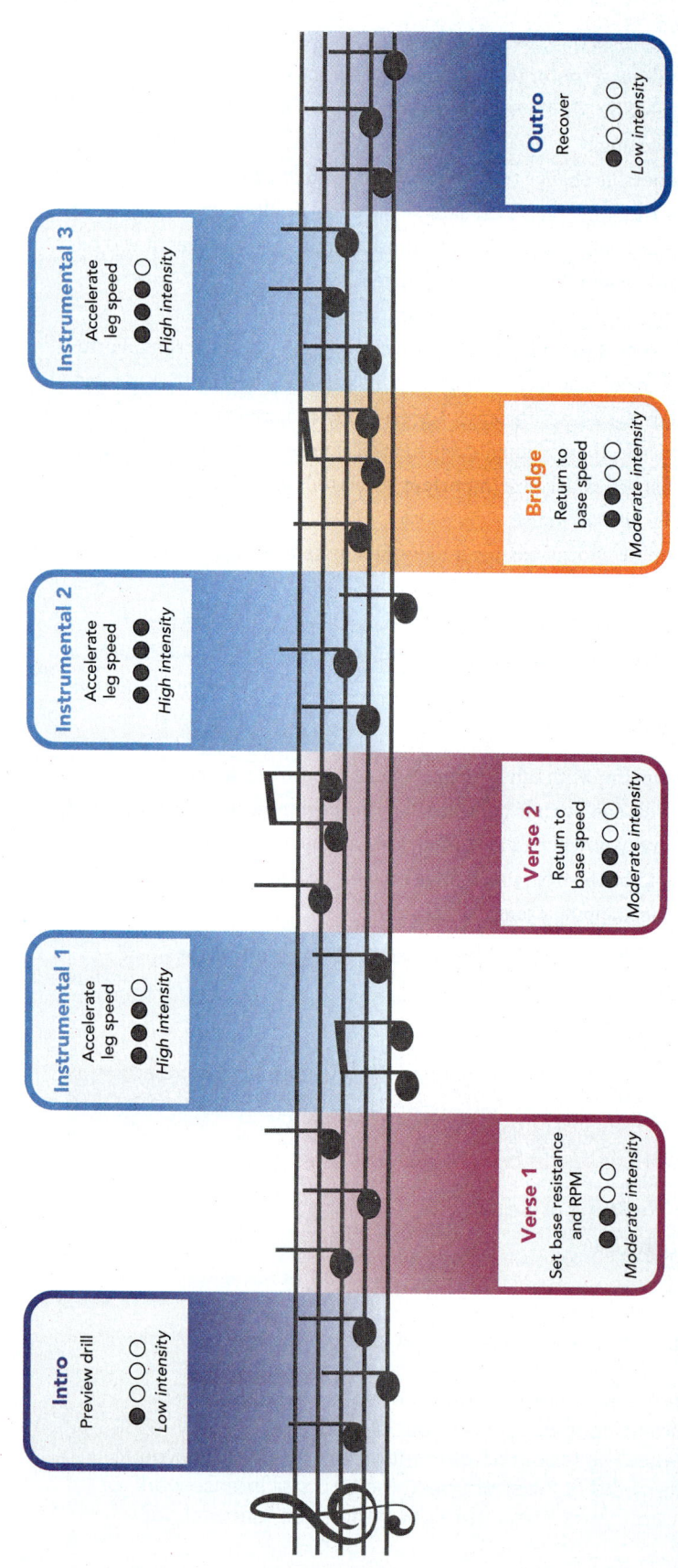

FIGURE 11.9 Music Mapping Example

Aligning Music to Class Description, Vision, and Objectives

To create an effective, motivating, and dynamic group fitness experience, music selections should be based on the context, vision, and objective of the class. Just like the soundtrack of a movie is composed to evoke specific emotions and feelings that align with the action onscreen, the music that accompanies a group fitness class should support the energy, intensity, and objectives of the format. Imagine the effect it would have in a scary movie if the accompanying music sounded like the theme for a circus? It would seem completely out of place and diminish whatever hard work the director did to create suspense and drama. In the same way, the most well-designed class could fall flat if the music selected to accompany it does not complement the energy and vibe.

Music Selection Considerations

When selecting music for a group fitness class, a number of important factors need to be considered:

- What is the class format?
- What is the intended class vibe?
- What are the demographics of the participants who will be attending?
- Is it dance based or athletic?
- Is it aggressive and powerful or lighthearted and fun?
- Is it mindful and relaxed or non-stop and intense?
- Are there segments with different energetic needs?
- Is it best suited to a diverse playlist with song-to-song structure or a continuous mix at the same BPM?

Although it may seem obvious, music in a boot camp, HIIT, or cardio kickboxing class should feel very different from what might be found in a step, dance, or barre class. Because music can have a priming effect (imagine a boxer walking toward the ring to an aggressive theme song or football players running onto the field to their team anthem), the right music selection can be extremely motivating and put participants into the appropriate mindset for the activity. Conversely, when the genre or style of music fails to match the energetic style of the workout, it can have the opposite effect. For example, a remix of "Eye of the Tiger" by Survivor might have the perfect energy to fire up a boot camp or kickboxing class but might not fit the mood of a lighthearted dance fitness workout. In that case, it might be more appropriate to play a remix of a current, popular radio hit or an uplifting classic such as "Don't Stop Me Now" by Queen.

⚙️ PRACTICE THIS

When listening to the radio or a favorite streaming service, notice the feelings certain songs evoke. Do they make you want to move? Do you feel energized or relaxed? Imagine the type of activities that seem intuitive for them. Make a note or use an app to remember the names of the songs and how you might use them in a workout.

Genres and Styles

Given the great variety of formats and workout styles, as well as the vast variety of music that exists, choosing music for group fitness classes can feel overwhelming at first. When starting out, it is advisable to consider choosing from genres that have proven consistently successful for many instructors in the most common class formats. These include electronic dance music (EDM), pop, rock (both classic and alternative), hip-hop, world music genres, and instrumental (ambient). However, because music genres are broad and ever evolving (and highly subject to individual interpretation and preference), it is unrealistic to suggest that one type of music is always better than another for a specific class type.

Although it is true that due to a variety of factors (e.g., tempo, rhythm, energy, lyrics, cultural significance, and popularity) certain genres or styles of music are generally better suited to some formats than others, ultimately, the instructor's personality and style play a significant role in determining what works best for them and their participants. An instructor's ability to sell their music should not be underestimated. However, just as important, instructors should avoid the pitfall of only playing music they personally enjoy or listen to themselves. When it comes to playing music in group fitness, it is not always about what you like but rather what works for the style of class and the participants who come.

 HELPFUL HINT

One effective tactic to expand your knowledge of music is to search trending songs in different genres on websites or streaming services and identify the most popular and current songs in categories that are less familiar to you. Although you might not love some of them at first, it is a great first step to identify what individuals who like these genres are listening to. Additionally, you can seek out professional fitness music providers and may find that they have ready-to-use music by category that perfectly aligns with the vision and objective of your class.

 CRITICAL

Explicit lyrics or subject matter are a common feature of many of today's musical genres. Instructors should be mindful when choosing which songs to include. Clean versions or radio edits of popular songs can often be obtained through professional fitness music services or other resources.

APPROPRIATE TEMPO (BPM) BY FORMAT

The pace, intensity, ability to achieve full range of motion, and other components of safety have a direct relationship to the tempo of the music. For that reason, it is important to understand and adhere to the established guidelines for safe and effective BPM ranges by format shown in **Table 11.4**.

TABLE 11.4 BPM Guidelines by Format

Format	BPM Range	Rationale for BPM Range
Resistance training	125–135	This BPM range supports safe and effective range of motion when using resistance equipment at appropriate loads and with a variety of eccentric/concentric tempo patterns (e.g., 1/1, 2/2, 3/1, and 1/3).
HIIT/Tabata	150–160	The high energy of this fast BPM supports the high intensity of HIIT workouts. However, participants should always be encouraged to go at their own pace if they cannot maintain proper form.
Boot camp	130–140	Because boot camp is typically taught asynchronously, this BPM range supports the high intensity without requiring participants to move in time with it.
Step	128–132	This BPM range supports safe and effective choreography. Stepping above this BPM can limit range of motion and lead to injury.
Barre, Pilates	124–128	This BPM is appropriate for the slightly slower pace and precise movements of these formats.
Kickboxing	140–150	Kickboxing is a high-energy, intense format that requires participants to aggressively punch and kick. However, as with all higher tempos, it is critical that participants move with proper form and range.
Aqua/water/seniors	122–128	Because of the nature of working out in the water and the resistance it provides, a slower BPM is necessary for optimal benefits.

Demographics

For many group fitness participants, music may be the first step to committing to exercise long enough to achieve results, regardless of the quality of the content (Wininger & Pargman, 2003). As anyone who has suffered through a class with poor music selection will attest, music can be the difference between a highly enjoyable experience and a decidedly unpleasant one. Moreover, research indicates that the benefits of exercising to music may be most significant in individuals who are new or returning to exercise, making it an extremely valuable tool to influence adherence for those populations (Terry et al., 2020). However, given the diverse musical preferences of individuals, planning music that appeals to an entire group can often be challenging to get right (Karageorghis, 2017). With so much at stake, careful consideration of participant demographics is another critical component of music selection.

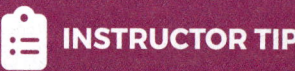
Social media is a very effective tool to let members know what is on the music list for your upcoming classes. Seeing which kinds of playlists generate the most buzz is a great way to get to know the participants' preferences. It may also be helpful to put out a poll that invites participants to share their favorite songs or artists.

Depending on variables that range from format, time of day, and geographical location to participant age, occupation, and gender, there are a dizzying number of factors that can influence participant preferences (Karageorghis, 2017). Given the futility of attempting to satisfy the unique musical taste of every individual in every class, instructors can work toward successful outcomes by employing the tactics in **Figure 11.10**. Instructors who actively observe and adapt to participants' responses to their music will quickly develop a loyal and consistent following (Karageorghis, 2017).

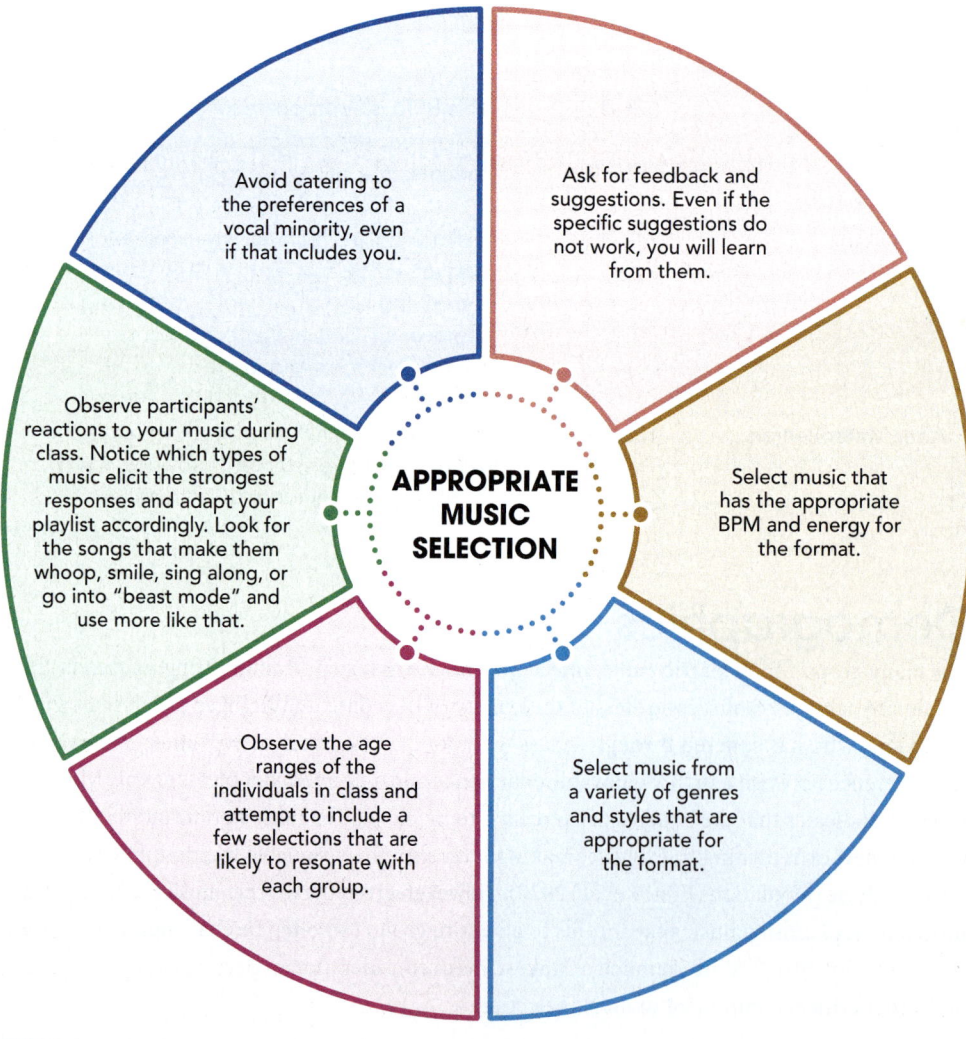

FIGURE 11.10 Appropriate Music Selection

The unique demographics of the facility and the time of day the class is offered can have a significant influence on the music that will be most effective during a particular class. The following points may be helpful in determining how to approach music selection depending on your location and class time:

- The average age of the participants and the location of the club or studio must be considered because the preferences of individuals who live and work in urban areas may be significantly different from those in the suburbs.
- Young working professionals will likely have very different tastes than a community of retirees. Getting to know them, trying to understand what they like, and then seeking out appropriate music will go a long way to ensuring success.
- Early morning exercisers tend to be very focused and may prefer more driving music to get them moving for the day.
- Mid-morning hours in many fitness centers often attract individuals who work from home or have flexible schedules. These participants tend to be more social and interested in having a good time than the early morning crowd. In those time periods, it might be wise to play plenty of fun, recognizable music that allows them to connect with other participants.
- Evening exercisers are likely coming to exercise after a long day at work. Play music that allows them to blow off some steam and decompress.

Lesson 3: Music Sources and Building Playlists

Music Sources

Digital music has reshaped the way we acquire and listen to music. With the growing number of streaming services and fitness-specific resources available today, it is easier than ever to keep music in classes fresh, motivating, and fun. However, when sourcing music for group fitness, instructors need to consider many factors. Does the music need to be a continuous mix at the same BPM, or will the class be more effective taught in a song-by-song format? Will participants be moving in time with the music (synchronously), or will it be in the background? What type of device will be used to play the music? How much time does the instructor have to devote to finding music? How much money are they willing to spend? And, critically, can the music be played legally in a public setting? With consideration of these factors and awareness of the available options, instructors can make informed choices that work best for the formats they teach, the facilities they teach in, and the budget they have.

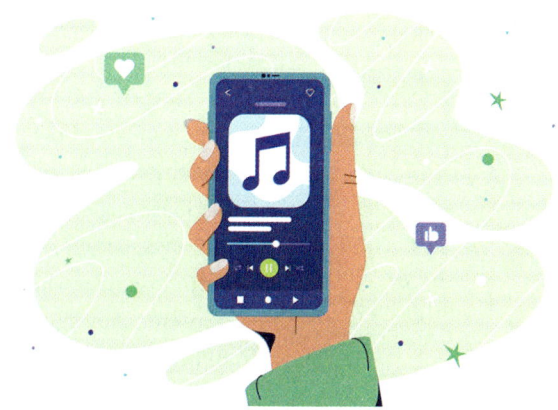

© Redgreystock/Shutterstock

Rights/Licensing Considerations

A responsible discussion of music resources in group fitness begins with some important legal considerations. To play music created and produced by original artists, it is imperative that instructors adhere to the laws surrounding the use of music in public places or performances. In the era of the Internet, music often is downloaded and used illegally, preventing artists, producers, and record companies from receiving the royalties to which they are entitled. For example, subscribing to a popular streaming service allows individuals to listen to the music in a private setting, but it does not include the licensing fees for playing the same music in a public setting (such as a group fitness class).

Instructors who wish to play music by original artists (even remixed versions) in class must first ensure that the facility or organization for which they work has paid the required licensing fees (IHRSA, 2022). Typically, these fees are paid to performance rights organizations (PROs) such as BMI and ASCAP. Although it is likely that most large commercial facilities have paid these fees, instructors should make a point to understand what music they can legally use. Moreover, instructors who teach independently must secure the appropriate licensing rights before using music in a class. Finally, because music licensing laws vary by country as well as by the intended use, instructors are advised to learn about the regulations specific to their personal situation and to act within the confines of the law. When in doubt, instructors are advised to only use music they have purchased (or streamed) from reputable, professional fitness music services or **ROYALTY-FREE** music they have purchased for this purpose. However, if instructors are operating within the legal parameters of their specific situation, there are additional resources available.

Non-Stop Mixes, Radio Edits, and Remixes

When planning music for your group fitness class, you will need to decide whether it is appropriate to use a **NON-STOP MIX** (often produced by a professional music service or DJ) or to create your own unique playlist that features individual songs you have selected. Non-stop mixes are compilations of songs mixed together, one after another, typically (but not always) at the same BPM. Formats commonly taught using non-stop mixes with consistent BPM are those that utilize 32-count phrases in their class design. These might include cardio kickboxing, step, and some resistance training formats. Continuous mixes also are effective in formats such as circuit training, boot camp, and HIIT where it is important that the energy of the music stays consistent throughout the class.

Conversely, formats that have a variety of BPMs and energy shifts to complement different class segments are often taught using playlists crafted by the instructor. Indoor cycling, yoga, and song-by-song dance formats are examples of formats commonly taught using instructor-created playlists. Both types of playlists can be very effective depending on the format and song choices.

Songs included in continuous mixes will almost always be remixed in order to meet the BPM requirements of the playlist as a whole, whereas songs included in individual playlists may feature the original, remixed, or radio edit versions. Each format has pros and cons. A **REMIX** of a familiar song can be an effective way to add an element of familiarity while still sounding fresh. However, because the BPM is often sped up in remixes, the altered version may not be appropriate in instances where the energy or slower BPM of the original song would better complement a specific movement. For example, if an indoor cycling instructor wanted to use a song at 100 BPM to be ridden at 100 RPM, a remixed version at 120 BPM would not be effective. Conversely, if an instructor loves a particular song but finds the **RADIO EDIT** version is too slow, too short, or overplayed, then a remixed version might be more effective for their desired use.

With so many options available, instructors can be extremely creative and specific with their music choices (if they have the time and resources). They can also find great success by using music sourced from professional fitness music companies who have already done the work to select songs and create playlists appropriate for many styles and formats.

Professional Fitness Music and Royalty-Free Options

A variety of fitness-specific companies offer cover versions of popular songs or royalty-free music that can either be purchased individually by song or as part of a monthly service. Monthly services are a great resource because it means the instructor does not need to purchase a trendy song they may only use a few times. With most services, instructors can easily drag and drop the songs they like in the order they choose into their audio device and play them at the BPM they desire.

Professional fitness music is a great option for many formats because it features covers of popular songs mixed exclusively for use in a group fitness setting. These remixed versions of hit songs are typically formatted to optimize the driving beats that support synchronous movement. Additionally, they offer a fresh take on songs that have been overplayed, making them feel simultaneously recognizable yet updated. Critically, music purchased from professional resources is legal and keeps instructors from violating laws related to the public performance of licensed music. The only downside to this option is that because these songs are covers (i.e., they are not the original artist versions), they do not always work as well in formats that rely heavily on emotional connection to music.

Streaming Services

Depending on the legal considerations (specifically the fees a facility or organization must pay to legally play music from original artists), instructors may also choose to make playlists using music streaming services. These services allow users who subscribe to premium plans to have access to a wide variety of music that can be downloaded and played on a device. Some of the major streaming services provide a seemingly infinite number of choices, which allows instructors to

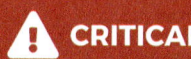

customize their playlists to perfection. In addition, by using the social media sharing capability of some of these services, instructors can get participants to engage with their playlists inside and outside of class. It is also a great way to connect and share with other instructors.

Program Specific Music (Pre-Choreographed and Provided)

In addition to professional fitness music and streaming services, some instructors may acquire music provided by a format-specific program or brand. In this scenario, music is provided to instructors as part of a membership or continuity program. New playlists and choreography specific to the brand are released on a consistent basis to provide affiliated instructors with fresh content.

Instructors who participate in these brand-specific, licensed programs enjoy the benefit of receiving professionally created content and playlists; however, it is designed to be used exclusively in licensed facilities or by individual instructors with proper recognition of the brand. As members of these organizations, it is incumbent on instructors to act ethically by only using the provided music and accompanying movement as dictated by its creators.

Building Your Own Playlist

For instructors who opt to create their own playlists (in lieu of using professionally mixed music), the final step to creating a class that exceeds participant expectations may be structuring each song in it to create a journey that is both physical and emotional. In formats where it is appropriate, this can be accomplished by employing the tactics of energy building, mood shifting, and theming—essentially using music to inspire and motivate every action. Selecting great

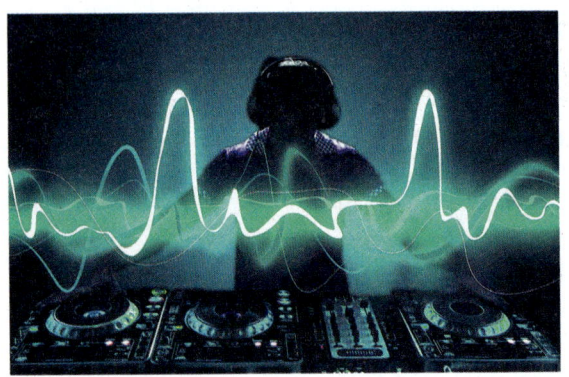

© Billion Photos/Shutterstock

individual songs to accompany each class block, segment, or drill is an important first step. However, equally important is the way that the songs work together in context (Karageorghis, 2017).

Consider how an experienced DJ or musician plays a show. They do not play all their biggest, most powerful hits in the first 20 minutes. Instead, they pace the order of the songs so that fans are engaged throughout, using several songs to build to a peak of explosive energy before shifting to a different sound. This same tactic works well when constructing playlists for group fitness classes. Organize songs so that the energy (and drama) builds during segments of intense work before pulling back into a contrasting recovery song.

For example, imagine a work set featuring three songs; the first song is high energy, the second song is slightly more intense, and the third song is explosive. At the end of that three-song peak, follow it up with a song that has completely different energy, perhaps more playful or calm. Participants will respond naturally

⚙ PRACTICE THIS

Listen to the radio or a streaming service and identify songs with lyrics you think might be motivating or inspirational. Make a list of favorites in a notepad or on a mobile device so that you have them handy when you need them.

to the increase and decrease in intensity when it is signaled in the music. This tactic works on two levels: it supports the effort physically while having a concurrent effect on the participants' mental states.

In addition to the energetic manipulation of the playlist, another powerful tactic can be to infuse the class with a motivational theme supported by some, or all, of the songs. This can be accomplished by using the motivational lyrics in a single song and applying it to the whole playlist. For example, many songs feature the words *strength* or *stronger*. Several of these songs could be peppered throughout a resistance-focused workout at just the right moments, inspiring participants to be strong when it matters most. At the beginning of class, the instructor could acknowledge that the workout is about discovering all the ways in which they are strong. With that message communicated early, participants will be more inclined to connect with it during the difficult moments—almost as if the music and their internal dialogue are one.

 INSTRUCTOR TIP

Lyrics that focus on belief, strength, power, and other athletically inspiring phrases can resonate strongly in the right moment in the right class (Karageorghis, 2017). For example, imagine how useful lyrics like "hit 'em with a one-two," "beast mode," or "I've got the power" might be in a boxing class. And, because song lyrics are often repeated, they can subtly or overtly reinforce themes and imagery, enabling the instructor to cue less.

Selecting music for group fitness is both an art and a science. Although the art, and how it is expressed, is highly individual, there are elements of science that can be applied by all instructors to promote more effective outcomes. How individuals respond to music is a combination of intrinsic (internal) and extrinsic (external) elements. Just as intrinsic motivation is a powerful driver to adhere to an exercise program, the intrinsic elements of song structure, melody, harmony, and lyrics are vital to the exerciser's response. Specifically, the intrinsic elements of tempo, rhythm, and lyrics appear to have the strongest influence on the performance enhancing benefits of music (Karageorghis, 2017). When it comes to motivation, few things can fire up a class like a strong beat combined with powerful lyrics that support the class goal. In practice, that means selecting music with the appropriate tempo for the movement, strong rhythmic qualities, and motivational lyrics that connect with the activity or theme.

In addition to these intrinsic elements, extrinsic factors such as cultural relevance and personal associations (e.g., music that reminds a participant of something meaningful) can also be valuable to forge social connections or induce emotional responses. For example, the iconic theme from the movie *Rocky* (1976) conjures images of training hard and overcoming obstacles. Songs commonly used at sporting events can remind individuals of the feelings they associate with the excitement of a big game. Popular music from a specific generation can remind participants of their formative years. Although it is not possible to know the specific associations or life experiences of every individual, having regional, cultural, and generational awareness can be an important factor in selecting music that will resonate with a majority of participants.

With these influential elements in mind, instructors should try to strike a balance between music that has the appropriate intrinsic qualities to get (and keep) people moving as well as music that is likely to connect with participants emotionally. In other words, unfamiliar music with a great beat and motivating lyrics can be very effective, but, for best results, instructors should also include some popular, recognizable songs that will resonate with their participants on a more personal level.

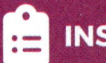 **INSTRUCTOR TIP**

Research indicates that most individuals respond well to music that was popular in their teens and 20s (Karageorghis, 2017). Updated or remixed versions of popular songs from different eras can also be an effective tactic to connect with both older and younger participants.

Although it is not necessary to use these tactics to deliver an effective or challenging workout, they can certainly make the experience more enjoyable. Just as great action movies have moments of tenderness or comic relief, a truly engaging playlist has texture. It should have moments that inspire participants to push their limits and others that enable them to have a period of emotional relief. Without intentional energy shifts, participants may leave the class feeling mentally exhausted instead of invigorated. Like other advanced music application techniques, creating cohesive playlists initially takes more time. But when it comes to participant engagement, the additional effort can be well worth the investment; participants get more out of the experience and, consequently, instructors attract more participants.

When constructing a playlist, the energy of the music should match the energy of the class segment. Given the effects that music can have on both our physical and emotional states, careful consideration should be given to each component of class (**Table 11.5**).

TABLE 11.5 Selecting Music to Match the Intention of Class Components

Component	Music That Matches
Pre-class music	Choose pre-class music intentionally to support the mindset participants should have prior to the workout. If it is an aggressive or high-intensity format, play songs that are energizing. If it is a playful vibe, play songs you might expect to hear at a party or a nightclub. If it is a more subdued format, play music that has a calming vibe. Whatever the format, appropriate pre-class music is an excellent opportunity to get participants in the optimal mental state before the workout.
Movement prep (warm-up)	Although it will vary by format, general considerations for the music in the first few minutes of class should reflect the progressive nature of the movement prep's intensity. If it is too aggressive or fast, it can influence participants to work too hard, too early. It should be energizing and set the tone while leaving room for energy to build in the main body of class.
Main body	Music in the main body of the workout will also vary greatly by format, but, in general terms, it should ebb and flow with the intensity of the work blocks. For example, if the class alternates periods of high intensity and recovery, the energy and/or BPM should shift accordingly. If the intensity is non-stop, the music energy and pace should reflect that as well.
Transition	To signal that the workout is coming to an end, lower intensity and perhaps even accelerate recovery music at the end of class should have a significantly different vibe. Consider a song that has lyrics or a theme that reinforces positive feelings and helps participants transition out of the workout with more spring in their step and an improved mental state.

Music Volume/Decibel Guidelines

As exciting as it can be to move to the sound of thundering bass, to promote health, safety, and longevity (both yours and your participants'), it is important to keep the music volume in classes at safe levels. Over time, prolonged exposure to high-volume music can result in hearing loss or damage, even in younger individuals.

Per the Occupational Safety and Health Administration (OHSA) (2022) workplace safety regulations and the opinion statement provided by IDEA (2014), music volume in group fitness classes should not exceed 85 decibels. In addition, the volume of the instructor's voice should not exceed 95 decibels (to be heard over the music, the voice must be louder, but exposure should not last longer than 1 hour at this level). If an instructor is teaching multiple classes (or participants are attending multiple classes) in a day, it is recommended that some form of hearing protection, such as earplugs, are utilized (IDEA, 2014).

To be compliant with this important recommendation, it is advisable to not only use a sound-level meter but also to provide access to earplugs. Instructors are encouraged to refer to OSHA's noise monitoring regulations for further information and resources.

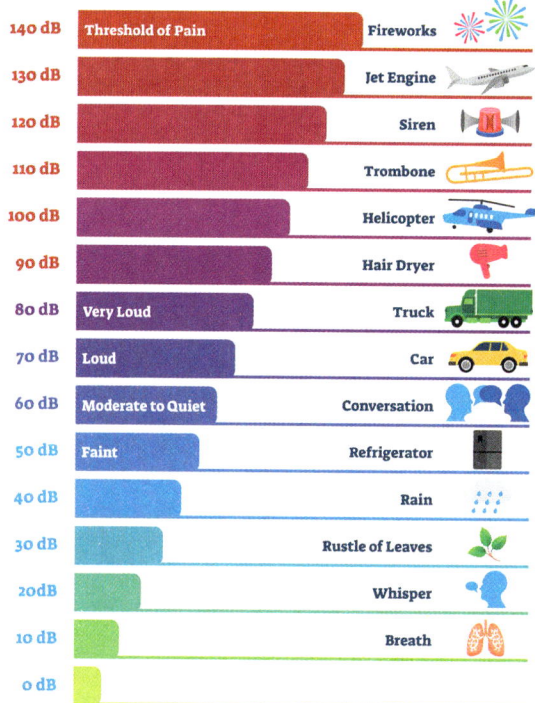

© VectorMine/Shutterstock

⚠ CRITICAL

Many instructors mistakenly equate high volume with high energy in an attempt to create a better class experience. However, when music volume is too loud, it can actually detract from the participant experience by making it harder to hear important cues. And it can be a significant source of distraction and discomfort.

SUMMARY

The power of music to incite movement, to make us feel a wide range of emotions, and to help us connect with each other is undeniable. In the group fitness environment, music can truly make or break the experience. Whether it is helping us dance together in perfect time, pumping us up for a killer interval session, or guiding us to a state of mindfulness, music is an invaluable part of the group fitness experience.

As a Group Fitness Instructor, the ability to effectively select and utilize music has far-reaching effects. It can make a workout easier to follow, more effective, and more fun. It can help some participants work harder, longer, and with less perceived effort and inspire others to (finally) commit to a consistent exercise program. In short, music has the power to make people feel good about exercise, and, as fitness professionals, that is perhaps our most important job.

Although the skills associated with optimal music utilization may come more easily to some, they are skills in which all instructors should invest the time to learn and refine. The reward in participant connection, experience, and success will be worth it.

REFERENCES

Bacon, C. J., Myers, T. R., & Karageorghis, C. I. (2012, Aug.). Effect of music-movement synchrony on exercise oxygen consumption. *Journal of Sports Medicine and Physical Fitness, 52*(4), 359–365.

Biddle, S., Mutrie, N., Gorely, T., & Faulkner, G. E. J. (2021). *Psychology of physical activity: Determinants well-being and interventions* (4th ed.). Routledge.

Bood, R. J., Nijseen, M., van der Kamp, J., & Roerdink, M. (2013). The power of auditory-motor synchronization in sports: Enhancing running performance by coupling cadence with the right beats. *PLoS One, 8*(8), e70758. https://doi.org/10.1371/journal.pone.0070758

Cadwell, K., Gordon, K., Foster, C., Mikat, R., Greany, J., & Porcari, J. (2007). Effect of music tempo on spontaneous exercise intensity. *Journal of Cardiopulmonary Rehabilitation and Prevention, 27*(5), 329. https://doi.org/10.1097/01.hcr.0000291334.93182.3d

Herazo-Beltrán, Y., Pinillos, Y., Vidarte, J., Crissien, E., Suarez, D., & García, R. (2017). Predictors of perceived barriers to physical activity in the general adult population: A cross-sectional study. *Brazilian Journal of Physical Therapy, 21*(1), 44–50. https://doi.org/10.1016/j.bjpt.2016.04.003

Hutchinson, J. C., Karageorghis, C. I., & Jones, L. (2015). See hear: Psychological effects of music and music-video during treadmill running. *Annals of Behavioral Medicine, 49*(2), 199–211. https://doi.org/10.1007/s12160-014-9647-2

IDEA. (2014, June). *IDEA opinion statement: Recommendations for music volume in fitness settings.* https://www.ideafit.com/group-fitness/idea-opinion-statement-recommendations-music-volume-fitness-settings/

IHRSA. (2022). *Music licensing in the United States: A briefing paper.* https://www.ihrsa.org/publications/music-licensing-in-the-united-states/

Jabr, F. (2013). Let's get physical: The psychology of effective workout music. *Scientific American.* https://www.scientificamerican.com/article/psychology-workout-music/

Karageorghis, C. I. (2017). *Applying music in exercise and sport.* Human Kinetics.

Levitin, D. J. (2006). *This is your brain on music: The science of a human obsession.* Dutton/Penguin Books.

Occupational Safety and Health Administration. (2022, September). *Occupational noise exposure.* https://www.osha.gov/noise#:~:text=OSHA%20sets%20legal%20limits%20on,a%205%20dBA%20exchange%20rate

Patania, V. M., Padulo, J., Iuliano, E., Ardigò, L. P., Čular, D., Miletić, A., & De Giorgio, A. (2020). The psychophysiological effects of different tempo music on endurance versus high-intensity performances. *Frontiers in Psychology, 11*, 74. https://doi.org/10.3389/fpsyg.2020.00074

Terry, P. C., Karageorghis, C. I., Curran, M. L., Martin, O. V., & Parsons-Smith, R. L. (2020). Effects of music in exercise and sport: A meta-analytic review. *Psychological Bulletin, 146*(2), 91–117. https://doi.org/10.1037/bul0000216

Terry, P. C., Karageorghis, C. I., Mecozzi Saha, A., & D'Auria, S. (2012). Effects of synchronous music on treadmill running among elite triathletes. *Journal of Science and Medicine in Sport, 15*(1), 52–57. https://doi.org/10.1016/j.jsams.2011.06.003

Wininger, S. R., & Pargman, D. (2003, Spring). Assessment of factors associated with exercise enjoyment. *Journal of Music Therapy, 40*(1), 57–73. https://doi.org/10.1093/jmt/40.1.57

SECTION 4

CLASS INSTRUCTION AND PRESENTATION

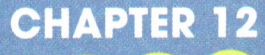

CHAPTER 12

COMMUNICATION

LEARNING OBJECTIVES

The intent of this chapter is to describe different types of communication, explain their value to participants, and explore how you can use inclusive communication to engage, motivate, and build trust with your participants.

After reading this content, students should be able to demonstrate the following objectives:

- **Explain** the value of communication in group fitness instruction.
- **Identify** the types of communication and their uses.
- **Discuss** methods for building rapport and trust with participants.
- **Develop** communication strategies and positive and inclusive coaching techniques that engage and motivate group fitness participants.

Lesson 1: Types of Communication and Learning Preferences

Introduction

Quality communication is central to delivering an engaging and effective group fitness experience. Communication is the path to sharing knowledge, creating community, and ensuring safety in a group fitness setting. Effective communication is developed and practiced. You should dedicate time to improving your communication skills just as you would for developing class plans or learning muscle groups.

Quality communication is not one-size-fits-all. Individuals learn and process information differently. A beginner, for example, may not comprehend a movement cue as quickly as an experienced class participant. Or, one individual might pick up a new movement pattern easily, while another participant needs more practice and repetition. It is the responsibility of the Group Fitness Instructor to evaluate and practice their communication skills, with the goal of delivering effective, positive, motivating, and inclusive messaging to class participants.

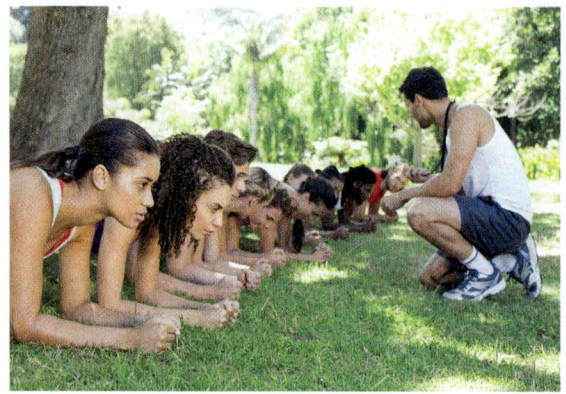
© Wavebreakmedia/Shutterstock

Types of Communication

Human communication takes many forms. For example, people communicate through writing, gestures, vocal tone, and physical movements, to name just a few ways. However, all forms of communication can be categorized into one of two communication types: verbal or nonverbal. Both types are used regularly in a group fitness environment and are critical in maximizing participant engagement. It is important to understand how verbal and nonverbal communication differ so that you can use both forms effectively in your classes.

Verbal Communication

VERBAL COMMUNICATION is defined as interaction through the use of words. Although this concept is simple in definition, everyone experiences the complexities of verbal communication. The message shared between a speaker and listener goes beyond the literal meaning of the words; it also includes meaning encoded by the speaker and meaning received by the listener, which do not always align (Krauss, 2002). The message is also impacted by the environment in which it is received, such as a one-on-one conversation before class versus an instructor leading a large group. An effective instructor must acknowledge these multiple environments and understand how communication skills vary among them. These environments are grouped into four general categories: intrapersonal, interpersonal, small group, and public.

INTRAPERSONAL COMMUNICATION

INTRAPERSONAL COMMUNICATION can be defined as communication with oneself. Intrapersonal communication includes self-talk, visualization, memory, and the use of imagery. Intrapersonal communication is the internal conversation your participants engage in when thinking about their health and fitness, which can motivate (or discourage) them. It is this internal motivation that convinces them to come to class or stay home and that pushes them to take on a new challenge or shy away from discomfort. An instructor can encourage positive self-talk by sharing positive body messaging and by focusing on successes, accomplishments, and benefits by saying the following: "Please take a moment to congratulate yourself for prioritizing yourself today. Your well-being is important, and you deserve this time." Motivational self-talk is a powerful tool and has been shown to increase performance without increasing subjective ratings of effort (Barwood et al., 2015).

INTERPERSONAL COMMUNICATION

INTERPERSONAL COMMUNICATION is communication that takes place between two individuals; it is characterized by a back-and-forth exchange of information while alternating the roles of sender and receiver. Interpersonal communication occurs before and after class, when an instructor is able to engage with attendees one-on-one and build personal connections. Interpersonal communication can provide an excellent opportunity for an instructor to seek out feedback by asking specific questions about a participant's class experience, such as "Was the new cardio segment easy to follow or was it a bit overwhelming today?"

VERBAL COMMUNICATION

Interaction through the use of words, orally or written.

INTRAPERSONAL COMMUNICATION

Communication with oneself, including self-talk, visualization, memory, and the use of imagery.

INTERPERSONAL COMMUNICATION

Communication that takes place between two individuals, characterized by a back-and-forth exchange of information while alternating the roles of sender and receiver.

An instructor can also use interpersonal communication to discuss goals, personal accomplishments, and motivation, such as "How is your training going for the upcoming 5K? Do you feel that attending Sculpt is helping your running speed and endurance?"

Although this type of communication often falls outside of the formal class time, positive interpersonal interactions can strengthen a participant's engagement by creating favorable associations with you and your class. **PROSOCIAL BEHAVIOR** makes a difference in participants' perceptions. At times, we underestimate the value of positive interpersonal interactions. For example, expressing gratitude promotes well-being, but it is easy for people to undervalue communicating gratitude (Kumar, 2022). The next time you have an opportunity, express gratitude to your participants for coming to class; it will have a greater benefit than you may realize.

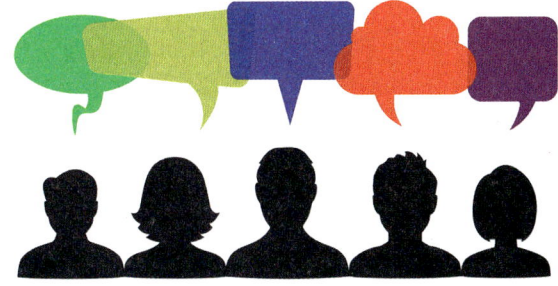
© Pavlo S/Shutterstock

SMALL GROUP COMMUNICATION

SMALL GROUP COMMUNICATION is communication among a group of more than two people, but the number of people involved is small enough to allow all participants to interact. Some group fitness settings are more intimate and allow for more of a conversational style of instruction. For example, an introductory class for new members might have 10 or fewer participants and allow for more back-and-forth interaction, such as "Let's share our favorite type of exercise or movement with the group. Mine is hiking."

Small group communication might also occur before or after class, such as while waiting outside the studio for class to begin. A small group interaction is a great opportunity for casual conversations and building rapport; it could include telling a funny story to a group of participants or asking them about their weekend plans.

PUBLIC COMMUNICATION

PUBLIC COMMUNICATION takes place when one individual addresses a large group. In this type of communication, the sender or receiver roles are often fixed. This is the most common type of communication that occurs in a group fitness setting, with one instructor sharing information with a large group of class participants, such as "Today's workout will focus on strength endurance so we will use lighter weights and perform longer sets." Because this setting creates a unique communication dynamic, it is important to examine it further.

BENEFITS AND CHALLENGES OF PUBLIC COMMUNICATION

In a group fitness setting, public communication is regularly utilized. However, public communication has both benefits and challenges that must be considered to effectively lead and connect with class participants.

In a public communication setting, the roles of sender and receiver are mostly fixed: the instructor as the sender and the class participants as the receivers. This is beneficial in that it creates an organized, predictable template for listening and delivering information. However, these set roles can create a power dynamic that can feel unbalanced and deter feedback. For example, the instructor may ask the entire class for feedback about a movement and not receive any verbal responses because the participants are uneasy about speaking in front of the larger group.

In their role as sender, the instructor provides movement and motivational cues and leads the class to the desired outcome. This dynamic is effective in communicating instructions to a large group of people; however, it takes thought and planning to ensure that the communication is inclusive, unintimidating, and approachable. This can be achieved by focusing on the layers of verbal communication.

PROSOCIAL BEHAVIOR

A social behavior intended to benefit others (like helping, sharing, or cooperating) or society as a whole, including conformity to acceptable social behaviors or rules.

SMALL GROUP COMMUNICATION

An interaction of more than two people but a number small enough to allow all participants to interact.

PUBLIC COMMUNICATION

One individual addresses a large group.

Tone   Verbal tone is how you utilize your voice to communicate a given message. Types of tones are outlined in **Figure 12.1**. An effective Group Fitness Instructor employs a combination of these tones throughout the arc of a class, creating a focused, motivational, engaging, friendly, and welcoming setting.

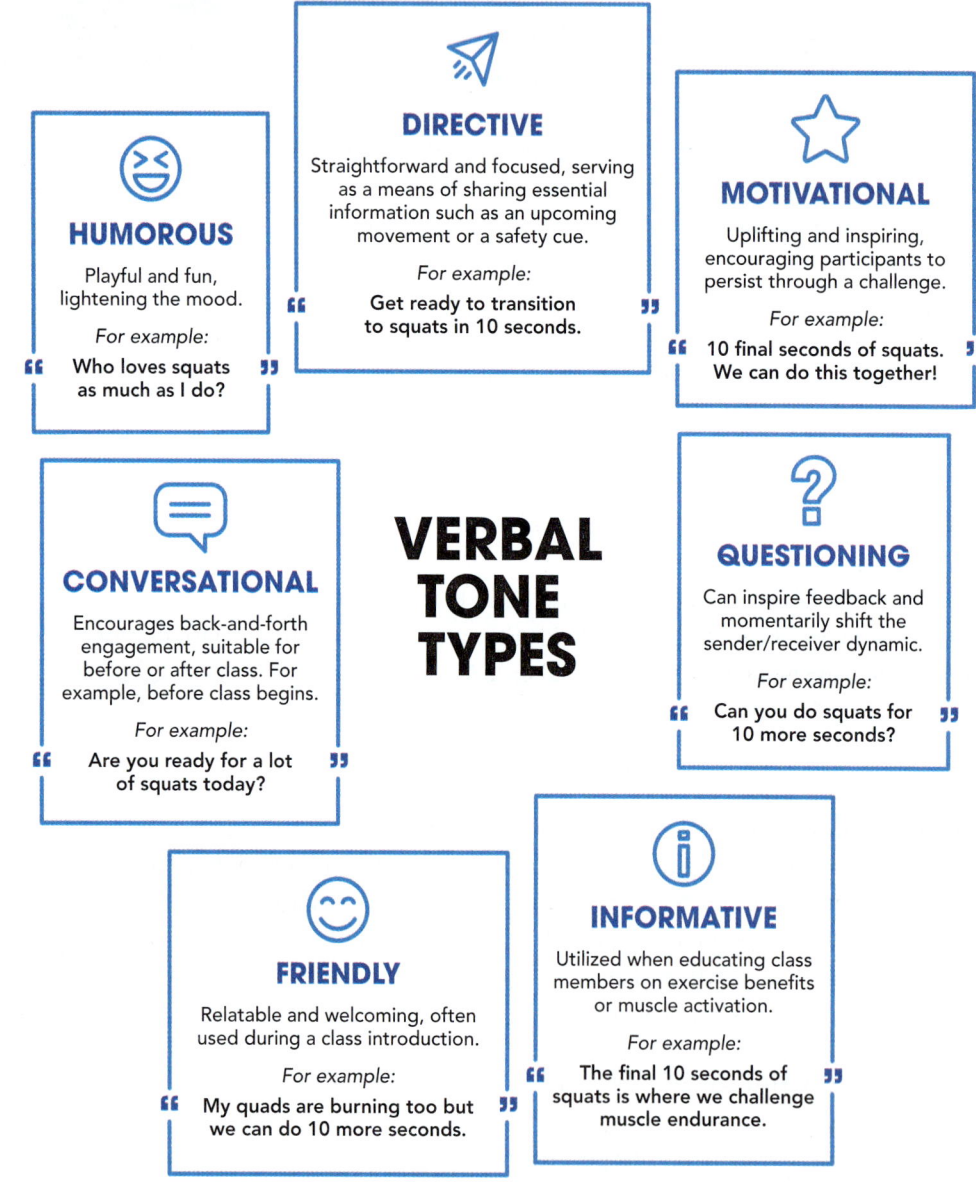

HUMOROUS
Playful and fun, lightening the mood.

For example:
Who loves squats as much as I do?

DIRECTIVE
Straightforward and focused, serving as a means of sharing essential information such as an upcoming movement or a safety cue.

For example:
Get ready to transition to squats in 10 seconds.

MOTIVATIONAL
Uplifting and inspiring, encouraging participants to persist through a challenge.

For example:
10 final seconds of squats. We can do this together!

CONVERSATIONAL
Encourages back-and-forth engagement, suitable for before or after class. For example, before class begins.

For example:
Are you ready for a lot of squats today?

VERBAL TONE TYPES

QUESTIONING
Can inspire feedback and momentarily shift the sender/receiver dynamic.

For example:
Can you do squats for 10 more seconds?

FRIENDLY
Relatable and welcoming, often used during a class introduction.

For example:
My quads are burning too but we can do 10 more seconds.

INFORMATIVE
Utilized when educating class members on exercise benefits or muscle activation.

For example:
The final 10 seconds of squats is where we challenge muscle endurance.

FIGURE 12.1 Verbal Tone Types

⚙ PRACTICE THIS

As you prepare to teach, make an audio that only records the cues you plan to deliver. Listen to the recording and identify the tone category that your communication falls in. Does the tone align with the desired message? If not, practice and adjust to better align your communication.

Speed   Speech rate, or speed, varies among individuals. Some people naturally speak at a faster cadence than others. You have likely met people who talk very slowly and methodically, as well as those who seem to talk at a rapid pace. Understanding where you fall in this spectrum, especially when instructing classes, is helpful in order to adjust your own speech to ensure effective communication.

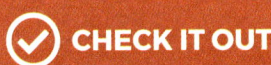

CHECK IT OUT

Yuan, Liberman, and Cieri (2006) found that the average speaking rate ranges from 152 to 170 words per minute. Although there is no specific rate that is recommended for group fitness instruction, the average speaking rate of about 150 words per minute has been found to be the ideal speaking rate for general public speaking and instructing.

When using words to teach a movement, it is best to slow down and insert pauses in your speech. Class participants must be able to clearly hear and comprehend directions and then be allowed time to process those words into physical movement. For those who are familiar with the exercise or accustomed to your communication style, this process may occur quickly, but for those new to the class format or your instruction, a fast speech rate can lead to frustration and a lack of comprehension. The tips in **Table 12.1** can help slow speech rate and enable more effective communication.

TABLE 12.1 Tips for Slowing Speech Rate

Action	How to Use
Breathe.	Pause to take breaths between words, phrases, or sentences.
Reduce filler words.	Reduce the use of non-essential speech, such as "like," "um," "you know?" or any other words you may say often but are not needed.
Prioritize key points.	Focus on emphasizing the essential points critical to execution and safety.
Utilize pauses.	Allow for pauses in speech, giving participants time to process and put your words into action.
Repeat yourself.	Repeat key points to emphasize their importance.
Plan ahead.	Speech rate is often faster and wordier when not planned out. Plan and practice cues ahead of teaching to maintain an appropriate cadence.

Positivity   A participant's long-term success relies on the formation of positive emotions surrounding their fitness experience. Exercisers will experience increased autonomous motivation and rates of exercise in the future as positive past experiences accumulate (Rodrigues et al., 2020). No one wants to feel intimidated, ridiculed, or dismissed. By utilizing a positive communication style, a Group Fitness Instructor can greatly influence the internal emotions participants associate with exercise. Furthermore, a positive instructor can change an experience from something an individual might dread into something they look forward to every day.

In order to create positive emotions, a Group Fitness Instructor should utilize positive phrasing and communication. This can be achieved through the methods highlighted in **Figure 12.2**.

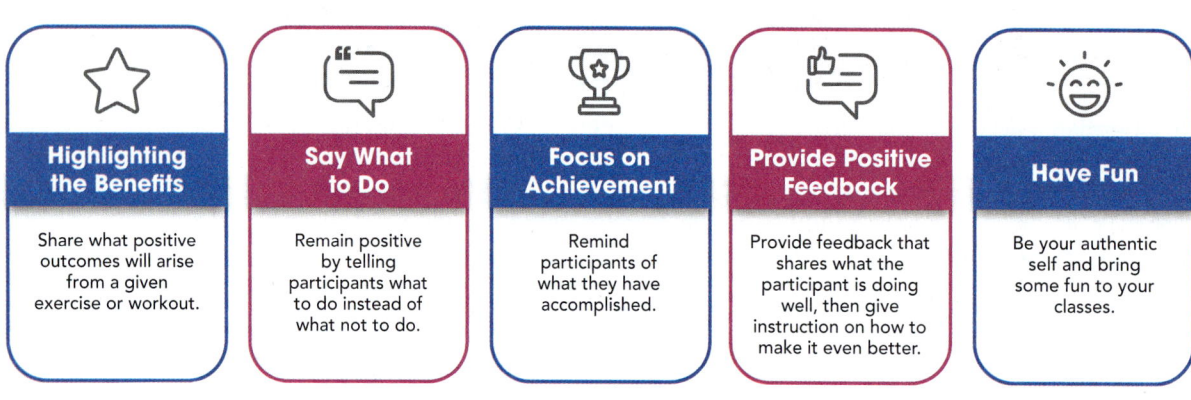

Highlighting the Benefits
Share what positive outcomes will arise from a given exercise or workout.

Say What to Do
Remain positive by telling participants what to do instead of what not to do.

Focus on Achievement
Remind participants of what they have accomplished.

Provide Positive Feedback
Provide feedback that shares what the participant is doing well, then give instruction on how to make it even better.

Have Fun
Be your authentic self and bring some fun to your classes.

FIGURE 12.2 Positive Phrasing and Communication

Nonverbal Communication

> **NONVERBAL COMMUNICATION**
>
> Conveying information without the use of words.

NONVERBAL COMMUNICATION is conveying information without the use of words. It can tell a story just as, if not more, powerfully than words. Nonverbal communication includes facial expressions, body language, eye contact, physical touch, posture, and spacing. Most often, however, verbal and nonverbal communication work together to help ensure that the correct message is given and received. A study found that when verbal and nonverbal communication do not align, the nonverbal message usually overpowers the words being said (Bambaeeroo & Shokrpour, 2017). For example, if an instructor said "Great job!" with a facial expression of frustration, the message would come across as negative. On the other hand, if an instructor said "Great job!" in an enthusiastic voice and a smile on their face, the message would come across as positive. Therefore, it is extremely important for a Group Fitness Instructor to not only understand the types of nonverbal communication, but also be aware of how to use them appropriately to send the correct messages to participants. Nonverbal communication has the capability to repeat your verbal message, contradict your words, substitute for words, and reinforce the meaning of your message. Note that emotional intelligence is intimately linked to nonverbal communication and our ability to understand meaning (Phutela, 2015). This means that the quality of nonverbal communication with participants can either build or undermine the positive relationships formed with instructors. Instructors can use nonverbal communication in a variety of ways when leading a group fitness class, such as through physical guidance, connection tools, posture, and specific coaching.

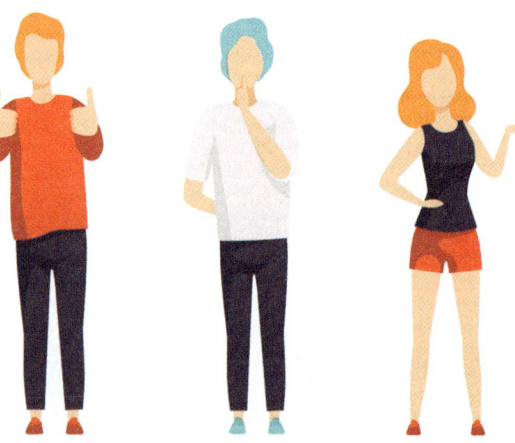

© NotionPic/Shutterstock

PHYSICAL GUIDANCE

Physical gestures are a strong nonverbal tool when communicating with a large group. An instructor can provide guidance through their movements to communicate a variety of information.

The physical demonstration of an exercise often helps participants master a movement, more so than a verbal explanation. For example, seeing a kickboxing combination performed can be much easier to follow than verbal instructions only. Similarly, a simple finger point or hand gesture can keep a group moving in the correct direction, and by counting down the final three repetitions on their hand for the group to see an instructor can help participants anticipate a movement change.

🤖 GETTING TECHNICAL

Theories such as the Information Packaging Hypothesis (Mol & Kita, 2012) and the Lexical Retrieval Hypothesis (Rauscher et al., 1996) claim that gestures also help the speaker conceptualize ideas and form speech. Therefore, gesturing not only benefits the participants, but it also benefits the instructor as it aids them in processing the ideas they want to communicate into words.

CONNECTION TOOL

More subtle nonverbal communication can make a large group seem more intimate and help an instructor connect to individual participants. In a study titled "What Makes Eye Contact Special?" a team of Japanese researchers found that when two individuals make eye contact, the same areas of the brain are simultaneously activated, and the brain becomes primed for socially connecting with others (Koike et al., 2019). Therefore, when you make eye contact with an individual participant, you are priming them to engage and connect. This engagement helps participants understand that they are seen and that their performance is important.

Additional forms of nonverbal communication can also be extremely effective and serve numerous purposes. Consider the various uses of nonverbal communication in **Table 12.2**.

TABLE 12.2 Using Nonverbal Communication

Type of Nonverbal Communication	Possible Uses
Smile	■ Establish a welcoming environment. ■ Communicate positivity.
Nod	■ Communicate approval. ■ Encourage a behavior.
Laugh	■ Lighten the mood. ■ Ease tension.
Close eyes	■ Indicate mindfulness (such as during meditation or stretching).
Breathe	■ Create calm. ■ Demonstrate desired breathing (such as breathing in through the nose and out through the mouth).

POSTURE

According to social scientists, when individuals feel "confident, lively and active they assume an open expansive posture"; however, when they feel helpless, insecure, or disengaged, they assume a closed posture (Zabetipour et al., 2015).

An open posture is characterized by arms at the side, with the chest open and facing directly toward others, and it is complemented by eye contact; positive gestures, such a nodding; and smiling. A closed posture, however, is characterized by rounded shoulders, crossed arms, a lack of eye contact, and not directly facing others. Experienced Group Fitness Instructors strive to present themselves as engaged, welcoming, energized, and confident; therefore, an open posture is preferred.

SPECIFIC COACHING

In some group fitness settings, more specific coaching is needed, such as when teaching a new movement pattern or leading an introductory class. Hands-on coaching can be invaluable in such instances. Research has shown that optimal learning occurs when individuals are given rich inputs from a combination of sensory pathways (Gilakjani, 2011). Hands-on cueing creates proprioceptive feedback, which helps an individual determine and evaluate the posture and movement of their body in space (Moscatelli et al., 2019), which can help improve form and muscle engagement. For example, an instructor can place their hands on the top of a participant's shoulders, reminding them to release tension from their neck and shoulders, or they can place a hand in between an individual's shoulder blades as they guide them to engage their upper back in a row. Instructors can also use touch to improve range of motion, such as placing a hand at hip height as they cue a participant to drive their knee into the instructor's hand, or placing a hand in front of a participant to guide them to punch into the hand for a more powerful jab.

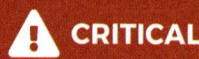

⚠ CRITICAL

It is critical to always ask permission and receive a positive response before cueing a participant with touch.

Learning Styles

People learn in a variety of ways, and many people have been taught about various learning styles, the most common being visual, auditory, and kinesthetic. Often, these learning styles are referred to in finite terms—an individual learns only one way or another. However, multiple research studies, including a study performed by Husmann and O'Loughlin (2019), have found that people are not one kind of learner or another. Instead, humans can learn in a multitude of ways; therefore, it is most effective to layer multiple learning styles when teaching. Instead of assigning learning styles to learners, learning styles should be considered as different ways to present information. Some information is just better presented in one style over the other. For example, teaching a person to swim is not going to happen by giving verbal instruction or showing them a video of someone else swimming. Experiencing the activity of swimming is going to be the most important learning style, regardless of a person's preferred learning style. In group fitness classes, a blending of all three styles specific to the activities at hand will be the ideal way to instruct participants. Consider learning styles as tools in a toolbox. As a Group Fitness Instructor, you should utilize the entire toolbox to communicate with your class.

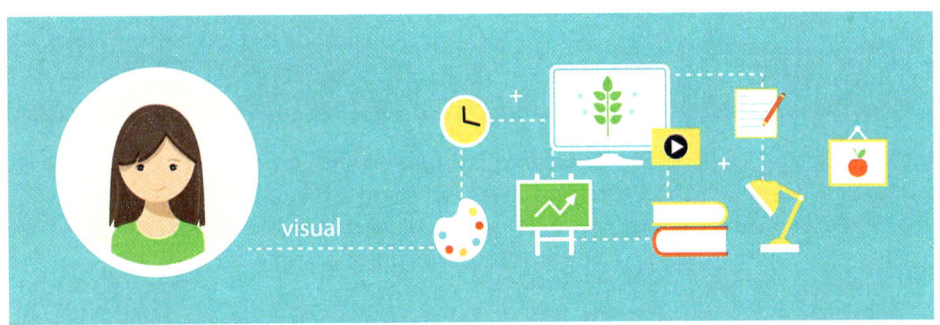

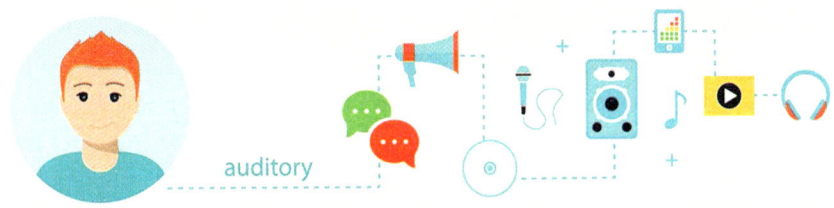

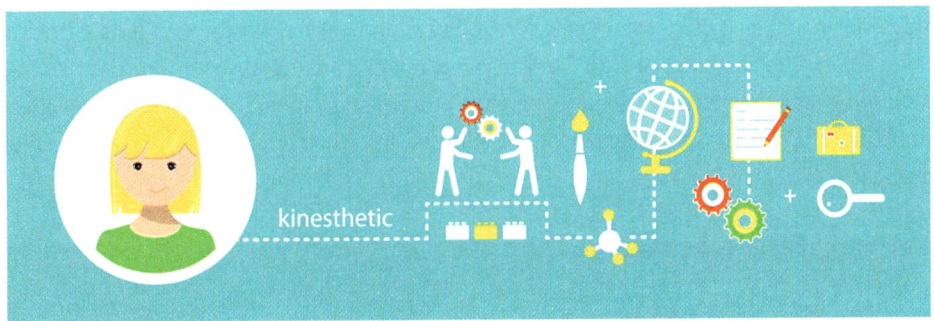

© Batshevs/Shutterstock

When preparing for a class, consider what types of tasks you or your participants need to perform and the best ways to present those tasks for most effective learning. Some tasks lend themselves to certain learning styles more easily, based on the nature of the task. For example, teaching participants to perform a push-up could effectively be taught by providing a visual example showing the correct form and movement. If using resistance bands, allowing for a hands-on (kinesthetic) approach and giving participants the opportunity to try various bands and feel the different levels of resistance will be more effective than just showing them what to do. Additionally, certain tasks that focus more on an individual's specific movements or abilities may require more explanation and verbal teaching (auditory). A Group Fitness Instructor should use a variety of methods to teach and avoid catering to any one specific learning style.

Visual Learning

VISUAL LEARNING is a general term referring to the use of sight to guide learning. Visual learning relies on seeing things in order to learn them, rather than hearing or experiencing them. In a group fitness setting, visual learning occurs by watching the instructor and other participants. A participant will gather information by observing others' form, movement speed, direction, and intensity. Therefore, when teaching a movement pattern or exercise, an instructor should include a physical demonstration. For this reason, it is also important that instructors can demonstrate proper form and range of motion.

VISUAL LEARNING

Utilizing sight to take in information.

Auditory Learning

AUDITORY LEARNING
Deriving information by listening.

AUDITORY LEARNING takes place when an individual derives information by listening. Auditory learning relies on verbal explanations, as opposed to written instructions or visual demonstrations. Clear and concise cueing is vital for auditory learning. Auditory learning is also encouraged by repetition. Because learners are gathering information from spoken words, hearing those words multiple times can be beneficial (Western Governors University, 2020a). Therefore, Group Fitness Instructors should practice saying the same information in a variety of ways. For example, if the movement is core rotation, an instructor could say "Rotate from the trunk, keeping the core engaged" or "As you twist, imagine your spine is a wet towel and you are wringing it dry." Another option is "Begin the movement from your mid-section and engage your obliques." On their own, each cue can be effective, but when offered up as a group, auditory learning is more likely to take place.

Kinesthetic Learning

KINESTHETIC LEARNING
Obtaining information through physical action.

KINESTHETIC LEARNING (or tactile learning) requires active engagement. Kinesthetic learning is hands-on, focusing on a learner trying things out and doing them in order to learn. During tactile learning, learners need to observe and then move (Western Governors University, 2020b). This style of learning aligns well with the movement experience of group fitness, because an individual must do, not only see or hear. A participant not only learns a new exercise by performing it, but they also improve coordination and body awareness through **KINESTHETIC FEEDBACK**. A Group Fitness Instructor should guide participants to translate physical feedback into improved movement. For example, a kinesthetic cue could be "Push yourself away from the floor as you drive out of your squat. Do you feel the back of your legs engage? Those are your hamstrings and glutes activating." A cue such as this instructs participants as to how to feel what they are learning.

KINESTHETIC FEEDBACK

Information about body position and movement as provided by internal feedback mechanisms such as stretch receptors.

Selecting a Learning Style

Although learners may state they have a learning style preference, research has shown that individuals learn by using visual, auditory, and kinesthetic information together (Husmann & O'Loughlin, 2019). Therefore, Group Fitness Instructors should incorporate all three styles into their teaching. An instructor might feel more skilled at delivering one type of learning over another; however, it is the instructor's responsibility to practice all learning styles in order to connect with all class participants. Consider the teaching methods in **Table 12.3** when deciding how to incorporate the various learning styles into your class.

TABLE 12.3 Using Learning Styles as Teaching Methods

Learning Style	When to Use
Visual	▪ When showing a new movement ▪ When showing correct form ▪ When showing a sequence of tasks
Auditory	▪ When explaining a complicated task ▪ When describing a process ▪ When providing context or rationale ▪ When providing feedback
Kinesthetic	▪ When participants need to use a tool or equipment ▪ When you want them to feel a specific feature of a movement ▪ When participants need to be engaged to understand ▪ When providing feedback

Lesson 2: Building Trust and Your Teaching Persona

Building Rapport and Trust

Participants join group fitness classes, in part, to ensure that they maintain proper form, receive an effective workout, and reach their fitness goals. They *also* (and maybe more importantly) join group fitness classes to find a community, to have fun and make friends, and to be motivated and supported. In these cases, the class experience is its own reward and has a significant influence on a participant's well-being. To motivate and support participants, a

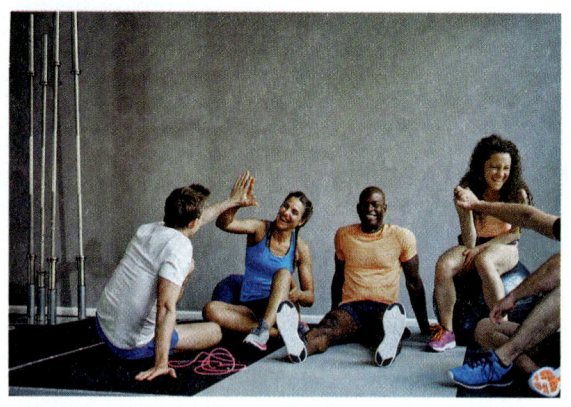

© Ground Picture/Shutterstock

Group Fitness Instructor must build rapport and trust. Research has shown that students learn more when they have access to positive relationships. These relationships provide a foundation for engagement, belonging, autonomy, and learning (The Education Trust & MDRC, 2021). In order to develop positive and trusting relationships, the following areas should be the focus of professional behavior, consistent coaching, participant-centered instruction, and inclusive support.

Professional Behavior

Professional behavior is a form of communicating your respect for a participant's experience, which is a critical aspect of building rapport. By acting professionally, an instructor communicates their respect for participants' time, commitment, and fitness goals. See **Table 12.4** for examples.

TABLE 12.4 Examples of Professional Behavior

Timeliness	Arrive early to class to prepare the space and welcome participants. Timeliness also includes starting and ending class on time.
Preparedness	Arrive to class prepared with the needed equipment (e.g., microphone batteries and wind screens) and in appropriate attire. The choreography should be memorized, the music prepared, and the workout fully planned.
Appropriate communication	Leave outside stress at the door. Focus on the workout and the class participants. Avoid inappropriate topics and language in class.
Adherence to organizational policies	Communicate effectively with local leadership, attend mandatory meetings and trainings, follow facility policies, and obtain subs, when needed.
Social media	Develop a social media presence and online brand that is approachable, appropriate in content, and demonstrates expertise.

Consistent Coaching

Consistency and dependability are essential for building rapport and trust. A study by Zenger and Folkman (2019) showed that leaders are rated as highly functioning when they are role models, set good examples, display follow-through, and are consistent.

In group fitness settings, this includes the following:

- Delivering positive motivation, encouragement, and body image language
- Setting a good example by following a predictable workout structure that is aligned to the published class description
- Following through by giving cohesive verbal and nonverbal cues, ensuring wording and tone align

- Providing consistency in language and communication, such as giving timely, applicable cues that are repeated within the specific class as well as from one class to another, establishing you as a dependable and trustworthy instructor

Participant-Centered Instruction

The primary focus of a Group Fitness Instructor is the participants, and the language used must reflect this. Cues should be participant-focused, establishing that the instructor is there for the participants' benefit and success. Communication should express empathy and establish connection, not set the instructor on a pedestal. For example, the instructor should use *you* or *us* rather than *I* or *me* to shift the focus from the instructor to the participant. **Table 12.5** lists examples of phrases that build participant-focused instruction.

TABLE 12.5 Participant-Focused Cueing

Say This	Avoid This
Can you do five more?	Give me five more.
Can you get another inch lower in your squat?	I need you to go lower in that squat.
You chose to commit to your health today.	I'm glad you came to my class today.
What are your goals today?	I want you to work on . . .
Great effort, you put in the work.	I knew you could do it.

Inclusive Support

Every human being deserves the gift of health. A Group Fitness Instructor has the ability to offer the gift of health by creating an inclusive environment. To create an inclusive environment, Group Fitness Instructors must build rapport and trust. Intimidation, bullying, and shaming do not build trust and have no place in a group fitness environment. Every participant, regardless of body size/shape, background, gender, or ability, must not only feel welcome but successful. When an individual feels successful, they gain confidence; and confidence has been found to be directly correlated to long-term success even among elite athletes (Hays et al., 2009). In addition, when an individual feels accepted as part of a group, social support and increased capacity become incentives for continued participation. Therefore, by building confidence and offering a welcome environment to all, you can create inclusive success.

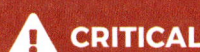 **CRITICAL**

It is your responsibility as a fitness leader to ensure that participants of every size and shape, background, gender identity, and ability not only feel welcomed but successful.

Teaching Persona

All people present themselves to others in specific ways, depending on the environment. A person might be reserved and professional at work yet silly and humorous with family. A group fitness setting is no different. As an instructor, you must consider the persona you are portraying and align it with the type of leader you want to be. The persona you share as an instructor can be considered your personal brand, which should be intentional and authentic and represent your personal strengths (**Figure 12.3**).

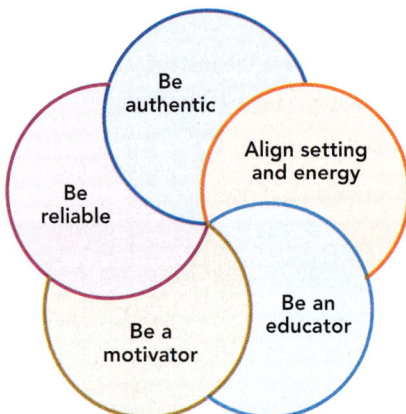

FIGURE 12.3 Teaching Persona

✓ CHECK IT OUT

You can learn more about your personal character strengths by using tools such as the VIA Character Strengths Survey (www.viacharacter.org). Use this survey to identify your top five character strengths then brainstorm how your top strengths can come to life through your teaching persona.

Being Authentic

The most important element to developing a teaching persona is communicating who you are and presenting your authentic self. Rapport and trust cannot be built on a shaky foundation. A Group Fitness Instructor should let their true self shine through, sharing their strengths and challenges with the group. Authenticity also means communicating self-acceptance and trust in the group. By demonstrating trust and self-acceptance, an instructor sets a strong example and encourages the group to do the same. Exercise can be a vulnerable activity, and through authenticity, the instructor can encourage bravery in others. For example, sharing why you chose to become a Group Fitness Instructor, what motivates you, or what type of exercise you enjoy are great ways to express your authentic self. Remember, everything you do is about the *participant* experience, so, when you share, do so with the intention of being relatable and adding value to the class.

Being Relatable

There is a false belief that a Group Fitness Instructor must be the pinnacle of fitness success and that they must make it look easy and effortless. In reality, being honest about the challenges of maintaining an active lifestyle will teach others far more. If a participant is struggling with motivation or being consistent, and they see an instructor portraying fitness as effortless and easy, they may feel like a failure and unsupported. Instead, instructors should strive to build collective empathy among the group. For example, ask "Was it a challenge for anyone else to get to class today?" while smiling and raising your hand. Empathy enables us to share experiences, needs, and goals. It builds "an emotional bridge that promotes prosocial behavior" (Riess, 2017). This prosocial bridge will help participants feel seen, encouraged, and supported, as well as bolster long-term exercise adherence.

Being an Educator

The distinction between expert and educator is essential in understanding the role of a Group Fitness Instructor. As an instructor, you are tasked with being knowledgeable about human movement, training science, teaching methods, and workout building (to name a few) and imparting this knowledge to class participants in an approachable and accessible way. This is the role of an educator. An expert would simply acquire this knowledge but might not focus on sharing it. Therefore, you should consider how you share your knowledge in a manner that is simple to understand and apply, in a way that is friendly and welcoming, and then incorporate your approach as part of your personal brand. This can be accomplished by layering communication. Begin with the essential information of movement

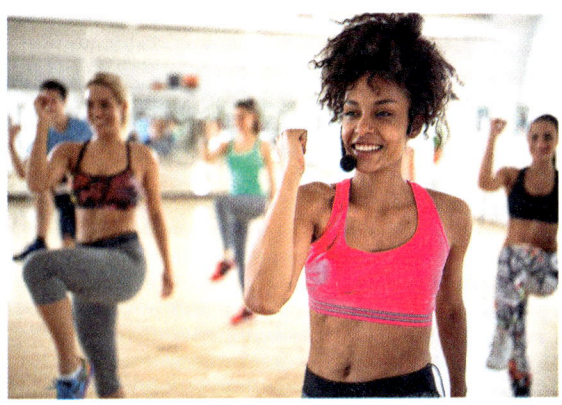
© Lucky Business/Shutterstock

descriptions and safety cues. Then, select one or two additional education areas to focus on that day, for example, teaching the benefits of muscle endurance or monitoring intensity. Share this information in small bits throughout the class, using everyday language and accessible examples. Then, recap the information shared in the transition and offer to answer questions after class. Wrap up by sharing what topic you will focus on in next week's workout. If this example does not feel authentic to your personal brand, select topics that feel true to your passions such as mindfulness, wellness, or music and approach that topic as an educator rather than an expert.

Being a Motivator

How you motivate others is also a key element to your personal brand. Some instructors are more direct and intense with their motivation, whereas others use humor or stories to be more relatable and lighthearted. All motivation should focus on the development of intrinsic motivation, rather than extrinsic motivation, as described in Deci and Ryan's (2012) Self-Determination Theory. Extrinsic motivation is doing something to satisfy an external demand for the purpose of obtaining an external reward or outcome, for example, exercising to improve appearance, to hit a number on the scale, or to fit in with a social group. Extrinsic motivation can be a powerful incentive to act immediately, but that action is usually short-lived and tends to fizzle out quickly. Intrinsic motivation is driven by internal rewards and reflects that a person values a behavior. The motivation to engage in a behavior arises from internal satisfaction rather than external recognition. When intrinsically motivated, a person experiences feelings of enjoyment, personal accomplishment, excitement, and a drive to take on a challenge. That is, a person engages in an activity because it is enjoyable for its own sake and contributes to their holistic, individual well-being. It is the role of the Group Fitness Instructor to emphasize intrinsic motivation over extrinsic motivation.

How can you use communication to accomplish this? You can emphasize intrinsic motivation by using the skills previously outlined: consistent coaching, participant-centered instruction, inclusive support, being authentic, being relatable, and being an educator as you motivate participants. An example of this would be using language like "You've worked so hard today. Allow yourself to feel proud of your effort" (intrinsic motivation), instead of "Keep working hard to burn off all those cookies you want to eat" (extrinsic motivation).

Understanding the Setting

Once a foundation of authenticity and relatability has been established, and the instructor has practiced being an educator and motivator, they should evaluate the setting. Just as verbal and nonverbal communication must align, the instructor's communication style and appearance should also align with the format. The high energy required for a kickboxing class is very different from the calm presence shared in a yoga class. The bright colors worn in a dance format vary greatly from the athletic attire of a HIIT instructor. In addition to energy and attire, the language and style of speech varies by setting. A boot camp format aligns well with quick cues and direct motivation, as this creates a more athletic atmosphere and flows better with the quick pace and intensity of the workout. In contrast, a Pilates class requires more detailed descriptions due to the complexity of the movement patterns and might necessitate offering numerous movement options to accommodate a gentler workout approach. Consider the communication styles in **Table 12.6** that apply to various settings.

TABLE 12.6 Communication Style by Format

	Boot Camp/HIIT	Cardio/Dance	Yoga/Pilates
Instructional approach	▪ Direct ▪ Short/incomplete sentences ▪ Efficient	▪ Quick ▪ Efficient ▪ Nonverbal techniques	▪ Detailed ▪ Complete sentences ▪ Multiple options
Motivational approach	▪ Specific ▪ Clear ▪ Energetic	▪ Fun ▪ Community focused ▪ High energy	▪ Descriptive ▪ Imagery ▪ Storytelling

Lesson 3: Communicating Inside and Outside of the Room

Opportunities for Communication

At first glance, it seems that the opportunity for communication in a group fitness setting is limited to public communication, with the instructor as the speaker and the participants as the receivers. This dynamic offers many benefits, including passing on knowledge on a large scale and using the power of group energy to motivate. However, an instructor should capitalize on additional opportunities for communication in order to form personal connections, build rapport and trust, create an inclusive environment, and foster a social community.

Inside the Room

The framework of a class offers numerous opportunities for the instructor to create moments of connection. Instructors can use nonverbal communication from the front of the room by making eye contact, smiling, nodding, or giving a thumbs-up. Walking around the room and interacting with participants also can be very effective. For example, once a movement is established, the instructor can approach individual participants to offer direct mastery cues. This is an excellent opportunity to use the participant's name and refer to one of their personal goals. Consider the following cues:

- "Tanya, try squeezing your glutes and activating your core as you drive out of that squat. It will help protect your back, which I know is a concern."
- "Powerful burpees, Jacob. Can you pick up the pace? It will help your acceleration speed in your next soccer game."

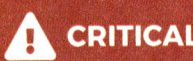

⚠ CRITICAL

If a participant is moving in a way that can result in injury or equipment is being used unsafely, it must be immediately corrected. This is best accomplished by approaching the participant directly. Avoid embarrassing them by calling them out from the front of the room.

Outside the Room

The term *retention* is often utilized when referring to facility memberships. However, to be a successful and sought-after Group Fitness Instructor, you must also focus on *class retention*—the ability to keep participants returning to class week after week and month after month. This is accomplished through a combination of ensuring that participants come out of your class having feelings of accomplishment and belonging and a sense of community. Community can be created through **COMMUNICATION TOUCH POINTS**. Every positive interaction a person has surrounding a specific experience increases their positive perception of that experience, which makes it more likely that they will seek it out again. Group Fitness Instructors benefit from expanding positive touch points beyond the walls of the studio. This includes before and after class, through daily interactions around the facility, and even on social media.

📋 INSTRUCTOR TIP

Remembering participants' names is critical to creating connection; however, it can be a challenge. Experts recommend making eye contact during introductions, repeating the person's name, and trying to connect the name to specific information about the individual (Schumacker, 2018). You can also consider keeping a notebook or using your smartphone to note names, fitness goals, and conversation items to check back in on later; for example, "Welcome back Kristen. How was your trip to Florida?" or "Hi Kevin. How is your 5K training going?" And, if needed, do not shy away from asking a participant to remind you of their name.

COMMUNI-CATION TOUCH POINTS

Moments of interaction that build rapport, trust, and connection through positive communication.

BEFORE CLASS

In addition to being a component of professionalism, arriving early allows an instructor to interact with participants before class begins. If the schedule allows, you should arrive with ample time to set up equipment; prepare the microphone, if applicable; and play pre-class music and still allow 5–10 minutes to welcome participants and interact with the group before the workout begins.

For returning participants, the pre-class interaction can include checking in on how they are feeling today and what their intention is for the upcoming workout. The instructor can also reference back to something the participant did well in the last class and challenge them to focus on continuing their progress today. **Figure 12.4** offers a checklist of a before-class interaction with a new participant.

BEFORE-CLASS CHECKLIST

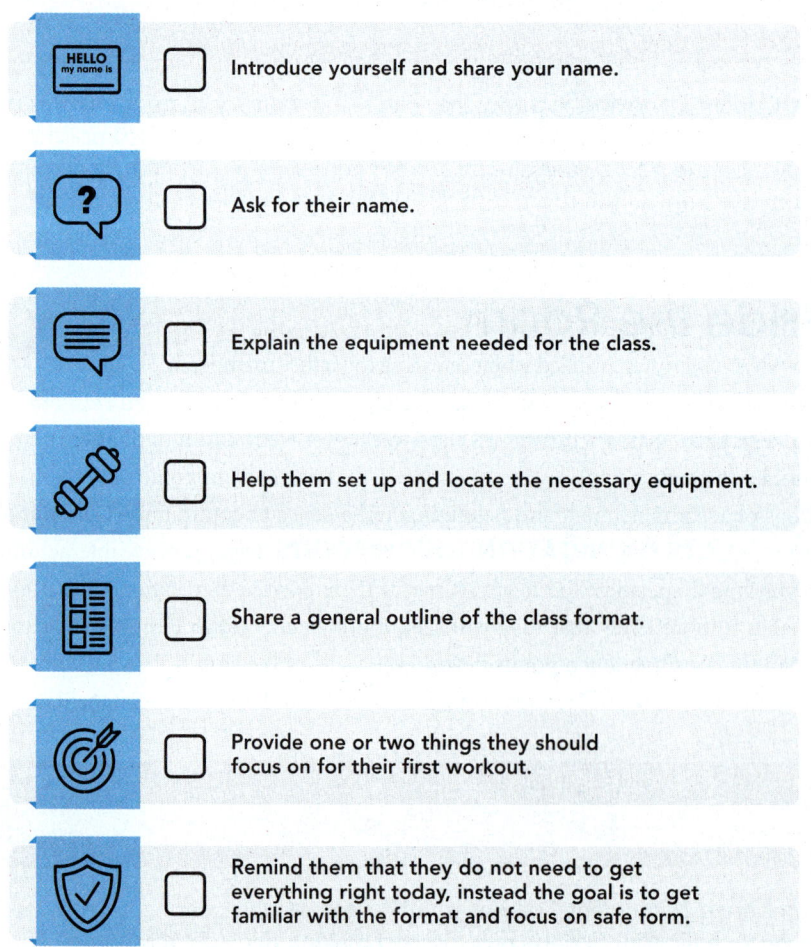

- [ ] **HELLO my name is** Introduce yourself and share your name.
- [ ] **?** Ask for their name.
- [ ] Explain the equipment needed for the class.
- [ ] Help them set up and locate the necessary equipment.
- [ ] Share a general outline of the class format.
- [ ] Provide one or two things they should focus on for their first workout.
- [ ] Remind them that they do not need to get everything right today, instead the goal is to get familiar with the format and focus on safe form.

FIGURE 12.4 Before-Class Checklist

In addition to building rapport between yourself and the participants, it is also beneficial to build connections among the participants. Studies have found that exercise frequency increases when individuals have friends at a health club (Unger & Johnson, 1995). Before-class interactions are a great opportunity to build or reinforce these social connections. As the instructor, imagine yourself as a party host initiating conversations and helping to create connections.

Introduce a new participant to an established participant and try to connect them through a commonality they share. Consider the following example:

- Instructor: "Hi, my name is Kayla. I am your instructor today. What is your name?"
- New participant: "Hi Kayla, I'm Stephanie."
- Instructor: "Welcome, Stephanie. I am so excited that you chose to join us for Kickbox and Core today. Before we get started let me introduce you to Claire. Claire, this is Stephanie. Claire started taking this class about a month ago."

AFTER CLASS

Group Fitness Instructors must also carve out time to re-connect with participants after the class is complete. Research has shown that exercising in a group not only builds social bonds but also increases prosocial behavior (Di Bartolomeo & Papa, 2019); therefore, after class is a prime opportunity to create interactions that boost community. After-class communication can include one or more of the following topics:

- Assess successes. Help individuals focus on the successes they experienced in the class they just completed. Ask questions such as "Where did you feel strongest in the workout today?" or "What was the most fun for you today?" Or comment directly on an area of improvement such as "Your endurance has really grown over the past month" or "You did all your push-ups from your toes today. Great job!"
- Ask for feedback. Communication only builds community if it is a two-way street. Therefore, instructors must not only give feedback, but they must also ask for it in return. When asking for feedback, use specific yet open-ended questions, such as "I am trying to focus on my motivational instruction. How do you like to be motivated?" Asking for feedback in this manner may also help spark continued conversation.
- Make future plans. After class is the ideal time to remind individuals that health is an ongoing journey. Ask what they will do in the rest of their day to recover (e.g., meditate, hydrate, rest, or stretch). Ask how they plan to move tomorrow and the rest of the week. Let them know that you look forward to seeing them in class again next week. Making future plans displays your trust in participants' ability and capacity to own their well-being and engage in activities that support it.

Virtually

In order to expand communication touch points, you should also consider virtual and digital communication options. This can be as simple as sending out pre- or post-class emails to participants (with the permission of both the members and facility management). You could also include a quick summary of the workout and some suggestions for additional classes that week. You could also issue a call-to-action social media post, such as "I am teaching a new 30-minute Core Blast workout today at noon. Can't wait to see you there," or you could advertise more-involved offerings such streaming classes or an on-demand class platform.

SUMMARY

Group fitness offers the opportunity to create a sense of fellowship among participants and make them feel like they have a fitness home. Effective communication is vital to creating a welcoming, safe community. Communication comes in many different forms, but no matter the form, Group Fitness Instructors should communicate thoughtfully and intentionally with the goal of building rapport, trust, comfort, and community. Instructors must also keep in mind that no single type of communication or learning stands alone. Communication is layered and built upon in order to facilitate a positive group fitness experience. Instructors should encourage intrinsic motivation through consistent coaching, participant-centered instruction, and inclusive support and by being authentic, relatable, and an educator. An instructor should also maximize all opportunities to communicate and connect with participants before, during, and after class, as well as through technology, when appropriate. These lessons in communication are the foundation of cueing, which is the next layer to success.

REFERENCES

Bambaeeroo, F., & Shokrpour, N. (2017). The impact of the teachers' non-verbal communication on success in teaching. *Journal of Advances in Medical Education & Professionalism, 5*(2), 51–59.

Barwood, M. J., Corbett, J., Wagstaff, C. R. D., McVeigh, D., & Thelwell, R. C. (2015). Improvement of 10-km time-trial cycling with motivational self-talk compared with neutral self-talk. *International Journal of Sports Physiology and Performance, 10*(2), 166–171. https://doi.org/10.1123/ijspp.2014-0059

Deci, E. L., & Ryan, R. M. (2012). Self-determination theory. In P. A. M. Van Lange, A. W. Kruglanski, & E. T. Higgins (Eds.), *Handbook of theories of social psychology,* Volume 1, 416–436. Sage. https://doi.org/10.4135/9781446249215.n21

Di Bartolomeo, G., & Papa, S. (2019). The effects of physical activity on social interactions: The case of trust and trustworthiness. *Journal of Sports Economics, 20*(1), 50–71. https://doi.org/10.1177/1527002517717299

Gilakjani, A. P. (2011). Visual, auditory, kinesthetic learning styles and their impacts on English language teaching. *Journal of Studies in Education, 2*(1), 104–113. http://doi.org/10.5296/jse.v2i1.1007

Hays, K., Thomas, O., Maynard, I., & Bawden, M. (2009). The role of confidence in world-class sport performance. *Journal of Sports Sciences, 27*(11), 1185–1199. https://doi.org/10.1080/02640410903089798

Husmann, P. R., & O'Loughlin, V. D. (2019). Another nail in the coffin for learning styles? Disparities among undergraduate anatomy students' study strategies, class performance, and reported VARK learning styles. *Anatomical Sciences Education, 12*(1), 6–19. https://doi.org/10.1002/ase.1777

Koike, T., Sumiya, M., Nakagawa, E., Okazaki, S., & Sadato, N. (2019). What makes eye contact special? Neural substrates of on-line mutual eye-gaze: A hyperscanning fMRI study. *eNeuro, 6*(1), 0284-18.2019. https://doi.org/10.1523/ENEURO.0284-18.2019

Krauss, R. M. (2002). The psychology of verbal communication. In N. J. Smelser & P. B. Baltes (Eds.), *International encyclopedia of the social and behavioral sciences.* Pergamon.

Kumar, A. (2022). Some things aren't better left unsaid: Interpersonal barriers to gratitude expression and prosocial engagement. *Current Opinion in Psychology, 43*, 156–160. https://doi.org/10.1016/j.copsyc.2021.07.011

Mol, L., & Kita, S. (2012). Gesture structure affects syntactic structure in speech. *Proceedings of the Annual Meeting of the Cognitive Science Society, 34*, 761–766.

Moscatelli, A., Bianchi, M., Ciotti, S., Bettelani, G. C., Parise, C. V., Lacquaniti, F., & Bicchi, A. (2019). Touch as an auxiliary proprioceptive cue for movement control. *Science Advances, 5*(6). https://doi.org/10.1126/sciadv.aaw3121

Phutela, D. (2015). The importance of non-verbal communication. *IUP Journal of Soft Skills, 9*(4), 43–49.

Rauscher, F. H., Krauss, R. M., & Chen, Y. (1996). Gesture, speech, and lexical access: The role of lexical movements in speech production. *Psychological Science, 7*(4), 226–231. https://doi.org/10.1111/j.1467-9280.1996.tb00364.x

Riess, H. (2017). The science of empathy. *Journal of Patient Experience, 4*(2), 74–77. https://doi.org/10.1177/2374373517699267

Rodrigues, F., Teixeira, D. S., Neiva, H. P., Cid, L., & Monteiro, D. (2020). Understanding exercise adherence: The predictability of past experience and motivational determinants. *Brain Sciences, 10*(2), 98. https://doi.org/10.3390/brainsci10020098

Schumacker, L. (2018, September). There's a reason you forget someone's names immediately after meeting them. *Insider*. https://www.insider.com/why-do-i-forget-peoples-names-2018-9

The Education Trust & MDRC. (2021, March). *The importance of strong relationships*. https://edtrust.org/resource/the-importance-of-strong-relationships/

Unger, J., & Johnson, C. A. (1995). Social relationships and physical activity in health club members. *American Journal of Health Promotion, 9*(5), 340–343. https://doi.org/10.4278/0890-1171-9.5.340

Western Governors University. (2020a, August). *Auditory learning style explained.* https://www.wgu.edu/blog/2020/08/auditory-learning-style.html

Western Governors University. (2020b, August). *What is tactile learning?* https://www.wgu.edu/blog/what-tactile-learning2008.html

Yuan, J., Liberman, M., & Cieri, C. (2006). *Towards an integrated understanding of speaking rate in conversation.* http://itre.cis.upenn.edu/myl/llog/icslp06_final.pdf

Zabetipour, M., Pishghadam, R., & Ghonsooly, B. (2015). The impacts of open/closed body positions and postures on learners' moods. *Mediterranean Journal of Social Sciences, 6*(2), S1. https://doi.org/10.5901/mjss.2015.v6n2s1p643

Zenger, J., & Folkman, J. (2019). The 3 elements of trust. *Harvard Business Review.* https://hbr.org/2019/02/the-3-elements-of-trust

CHAPTER 13

THE ART OF CUEING

LEARNING OBJECTIVES

The intent of this chapter is to identify various cueing techniques, establish their purpose in group fitness, and explain how to effectively deliver them. This chapter will also review proper exercise technique, safe body mechanics, and how to build your own cues.

After reading this content, students should be able to demonstrate the following objectives:

- **Discuss** the role of cueing in group fitness instruction.
- **Identify** the different types of cues and their appropriate uses.
- **Describe** effective, safe mechanics and body alignment for various exercises and movements.
- **Discuss** the process for building and delivering group fitness cues.

Lesson 1: Verbal Cueing

Introduction

Cueing is a powerful tool that, when done well, allows a Group Fitness Instructor to positively influence participant performance, helping them to develop confidence and healthy habits that can last a lifetime. Cueing is not simply words; it is a vital balance of education, motivation, and connection that comes together as an art form, creating an environment in which goals are set and achieved.

The art of cueing is the unifying factor that brings the instructor's knowledge of human movement, exercise and training, the components of a workout, and positive communication to life. A well-cued class flows, feels intentional yet natural, and draws the group in. It supports form, safety, movement, motivation, and fun. Great cueing builds community and belonging and breaks down barriers of intimidation and exclusion. When mastered, the art of cueing is an amazing culmination of words and actions.

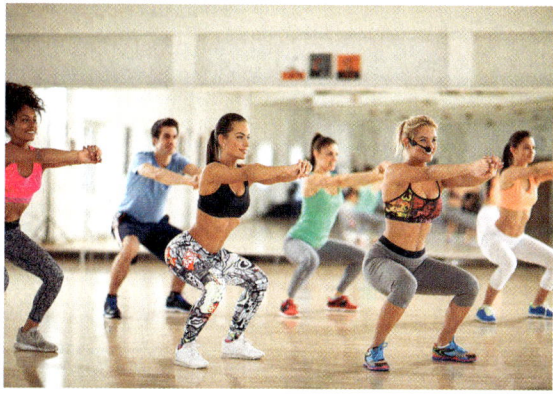

© Lucky Business/Shutterstock

Great cueing requires practice, intention, and feedback. Cueing is very different from common speech. It requires specific timing and rhythm and word choice and repetition, and it should connect to all styles of presenting information, including visual, auditory, and kinesthetic.

In this chapter, you will be introduced to a layered approach to cueing. This approach is meant to create consistency and predictability for class participants, as well as a defined order of operations to master the art of cueing. You will learn three interconnected cueing concepts: **VERBAL CUEING PROGRESSION**, **THREE-DIMENSIONAL CUEING**, and **PERSONALIZED CUEING** (**Figure 13.1**). As you begin your group fitness instruction journey, first focus on building your skills within the verbal cueing progression. Once you are able to deliver verbal cues with confidence, you can integrate three-dimensional cueing and personalized cueing. Each of these three elements supports one another, and together they create a complete experience.

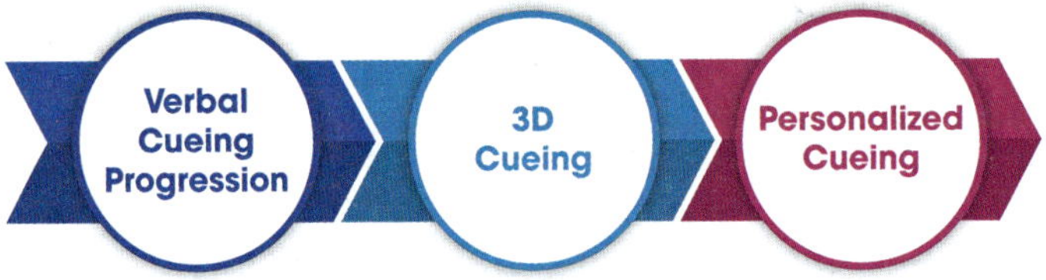

Verbal Cueing Progression → **3D Cueing** → **Personalized Cueing**

FIGURE 13.1 Cueing for Success

Verbal Cueing Progression

The verbal cueing progression is the first step to comprehensive cueing. This progressive approach categorizes types of verbal cues and lays them out in the order in which they should be delivered (**Figure 13.2**) based on the Schema Theory of Motor Learning (Schmidt, 1975). According to the Schema Theory an individual must first receive a generalized motor program (GMP), which is a set of movement commands that explains the desired result. The verbal cueing progression outlines these cues as movement cues. Those commands are then adapted to suit the specific situation, incorporating feedback for improvement, addressed here as mastery cues (Wulf, 2012). Finally, motivation cues are layered in to encourage adaptation and progress.

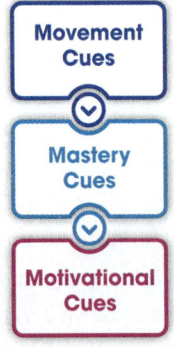

FIGURE 13.2 Verbal Cueing Progression Matrix

Movement Cues

Movement cues are the foundation for successful cueing. They are the first step of the verbal cueing progression (**Figure 13.3**). They establish the movement expectation as well as explain safe execution. Movement cues develop the GMP.

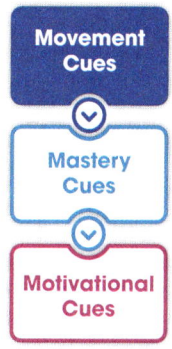

FIGURE 13.3 Verbal Cueing Matrix: Movement Cues

Every set, work block, or interval begins with a movement cue. The simplest movement cue describes what, how, and when (**Figure 13.4**). Note that movement cues are not only helpful; they are required. An instructor should not progress to mastery or motivational cues until the movement cues are understood and being executed safely.

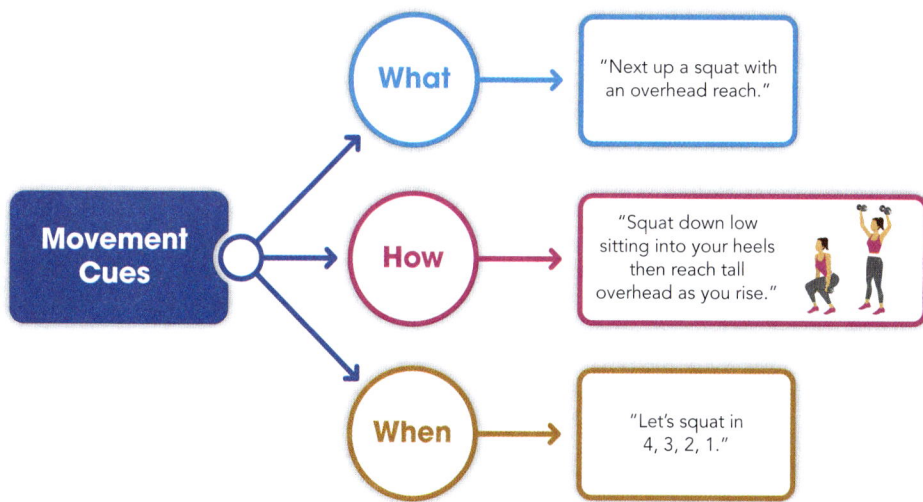

FIGURE 13.4 Movement Cue Breakdown

WHAT CUES

Begin by stating the name of the upcoming exercise or movement pattern. For example, "Next, we will move into a lower body sequence of hamstring curls, side shuffles, and jogging in place." It is beneficial to consistently call exercises or movement sequences the same thing; consistent naming patterns have been shown to help participants learn over time, because they present a predictable and recognizable path to follow (Deci & Ryan, 1985). It is also best to utilize common exercise names that do not rely on jargon or overly scientific wording. Overly complicated or technical names can be intimidating and reduce comprehension. The goal is for the name to be easily recognizable and remembered. Some examples are outlined in **Table 13.1**.

TABLE 13.1 Common Exercise Name Usage

Common Exercise Names to Use	Complex Exercise Names to Avoid
Side raise	Shoulder abduction
Hamstring curl	Knee flexion
Bicep curl	Elbow flexion
Single-leg bridge	Supine unilateral bridge
Side shuffle	Frontal plane shuffle
Jog in place	Static jog

Also consider teaching and naming movement combinations within the body of a class so that you can reference back to those names for easier cueing; for example, tell the class to perform "the jab combo," and then teach them a combination of three right jabs followed by one left jab and a squat. Every time you return to this combination during the workout, you would cue "the jab combo" to build consistency and exercise recognition.

HOW CUES

After naming the exercise or movement pattern, you then describe how to execute that movement. How cues should tell what body part to move where. For example, consider the following cues:

- **Squat:** "Reach hips back as you lower them to knee height. Drive out of your mid-foot to return to standing."
- **Side shuffle:** "Four side steps to the right and four side steps to return to center."
- **Mountain climbers:** "From a straight-arm plank position, alternate driving one knee to your chest."

How cues should focus on key words and be simple and to the point. Keep in mind that participants must hear the cue, understand it, and process it into movement in a very short period of time. Overcomplicating how cues just results in confusion.

WHEN CUES

The last component of the basic movement cue refers to timing. When cues must communicate when the movement should begin and how long or how many repetitions are expected. Participants should be given time to prepare for a movement change. For formats that include repetitions or are timed to music, when cues should be given approximately 4 counts prior to the movement change. Counts refer to either 4 counts of music (when counting in an 8-count pattern) or four repetitions of an exercise. For example, if cueing by repetitions and the class is performing 16 lunges on the right leg, when there are 4 lunges remaining, the instructor can say "Switch legs in 4, 3, 2, 1" or "Four more reps and then switch." Or, if cueing to an 8-count music pattern, when you reach the final 8 counts before the movement change, internally count 1, 2, 3, 4; give the next movement cue during 5, 6, 7, 8; and then change the movement at the start of the next 8 count.

If leading a class format that is driven by time, such as a boot camp class that includes timed intervals, the instructor should aim to deliver transition cues approximately 10–15 seconds prior to the transition. For example, "15 seconds left of mountain climbers and then we switch to a plank hold."

Once the new movement begins, it is also helpful to share how many repetitions the group should complete, or, if teaching an interval format, for example, let them know how long the interval will last.

Consider the following example that puts the what, how, and when cues together: "Up next, Shuffle Jacks. That's four side shuffles and two jacks. In 4, 3, 2, 1." (*Give time to complete.*) "Great, let's do eight more." The key is to keep it simple, easy to understand, and to the point.

⚙️ PRACTICE THIS

Timing of cues takes practice and repetition. Begin by turning on music, preferably with 32-count phrasing, and count the 8 counts aloud for an entire song. If using group fitness–formatted music, you will hear a musical change every 32 counts (4 × 8 counts), such as vocals or drums.

Next, pick a simple cue. "Step touch side to side" is an easy one to start with. Practice saying these words during the 5, 6, 7, 8 of the 8 count.

Once you have practiced the verbal cue a number of times, get up and practice it with movement. Begin with squats, then cue "Step touch side to side" on the 5, 6, 7, 8 of the music and then begin a step touch on the next 1 count.

If this timing feels rushed or overwhelming, work in a countdown to your cueing as shared in the earlier example. Give the upcoming movement cue on the 1, 2, 3, 4 counts and then count down the final 4 counts aloud to help the class (and you) master the timing. "Step touch side to side in 4, 3, 2, 1."

If you decide to cue earlier, it is essential to include a countdown; otherwise, the class will not know when to change the movement or change the movement too early.

Safety Cues

The other key piece to movement cues, beyond the basic what, how, and when cues, are safety cues. Safety cues address the AFAA 5 Questions (**Figure 13.5**). They are meant to keep participants safe from injury or harm. For this reason, an instructor may not progress until safety cues have been addressed (**Figure 13.6**).

Safety cues include the following:

- Contraindications cues such as "Those with shoulder injuries should not press overhead."
- Alignment cues such as "In a squat, your knees should track forward not toward each other as this can put excessive pressure on your knee joint."
- Equipment cues such as "Make sure your clips are securely attached to your bar."
- Directional cues such as "Everyone shuffle to the right."
- Spatial cues such as "Be aware of those around you."

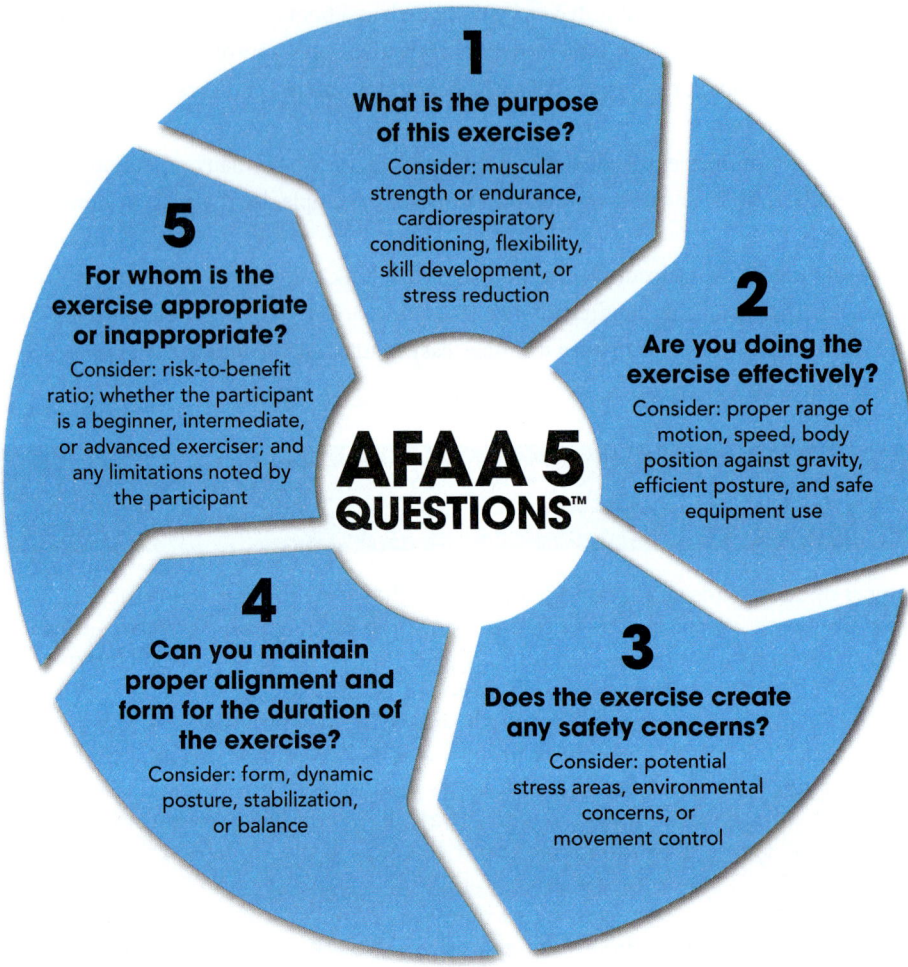

FIGURE 13.5 AFAA 5 Questions™

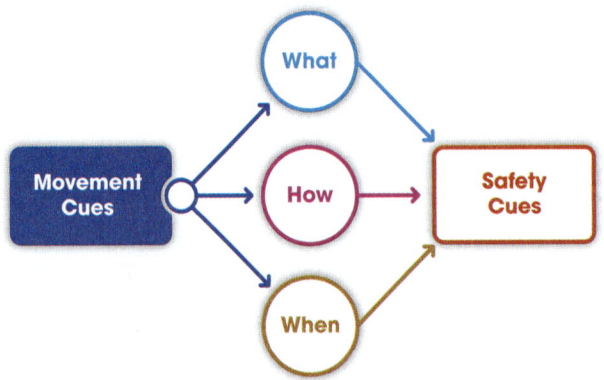

FIGURE 13.6 Movement Cues: Safety Cues

Mastery Cues

The next step of the verbal cueing progression is mastery cues. Mastery cues allow participants to understand the focus and benefits of an exercise more fully as well as provide feedback to improve their movement (**Figure 13.7**).

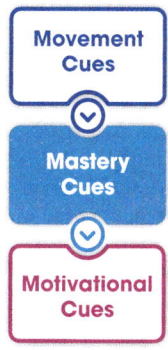

FIGURE 13.7 Verbal Cueing Matrix: Mastery Cues

Once participants are moving in the correct way safely, the instructor can focus on bringing more depth and precision to the movement. Mastery cues are used to drive results, progress participants, and build autonomy.

DRIVING RESULTS

Many exercises are nuanced and layered. Understanding those nuances and layers will enhance a participant's execution of an exercise. For example, at first glance, a squat seems very simple. It is just like getting in and out of a chair, which we all do every day. So, we must know how to do it correctly, right? Getting out of a chair is one thing, but performing a squat over multiple repetitions for the purpose of building strength and endurance is another. Common squatting mistakes include bending too far forward at the hips and knees knocking. The proper form facilitates safe performance of an exercise as well as proper engagement of muscle groups (i.e., working the right muscles at the right time) to optimize effectiveness. The instructor can use movement cues to ensure that participants grasp the basic movement pattern of a squat and then focus on mastery cues to drive further results. **Table 13.2** provides some mastery cues that can improve common squatting issues.

TABLE 13.2 Driving Results

Desired Outcome	Cueing Example
Posterior chain activation (glutes and hamstrings)	"Let your knees and hips bend at the same time as you descend, and then drive through your mid-foot and think about pushing into the ground as you stand."
Core activation	"Pull your navel toward your spine as if you are tightening an imaginary belt."
Upper body alignment	"Keep your chest lifted and core engaged."
Full range of motion	"Focus on your hips and knees moving at the same time and stick to a range that is pain-free and doable."

Note that mastery cues can be invaluable but potentially overwhelming to new exercisers. Therefore, they do not need to be included to drive results for every single movement. Emphasize a few areas that will benefit the most participants in a given workout and try to weave in cues that reinforce that focus throughout class. For example, you may choose to focus on core engagement for a given class and offer core-focused mastery cues for a handful of select exercises. Or you may choose to focus on range of motion for a given class and frame your mastery cues around the full range of motion for each exercise. Mastery is an ongoing process and should be taught as such. It certainly does not happen overnight or in one class.

PROGRESSIONS AND REGRESSIONS

Mastery cues are also an effective way to offer progressions and regressions to account for the variety of abilities and needs in a given group fitness class. The class format and difficulty level should be well-established on the group fitness schedule. General guidelines for prerequisites and safety should be clearly outlined; however, an instructor must anticipate a gathering of various levels, abilities, and experience in every group setting. Therefore, they must be prepared to demonstrate progressions and regressions for every exercise.

Recall that progressions are mastery cues given to advance an exercise by adding to its challenge level to maintain a desired intensity. When offering progressions, an instructor can encourage participants to add more weight or move faster (when applicable), or they can focus on the complexity of the movement. By making a movement more complex, an instructor can also advance the intensity and offer a new dynamic challenge. When progressing intensity through movement complexity, an instructor can challenge balance, add an additional pattern (e.g., an overhead press to a lunge), or add resistance to a movement that would normally not incorporate it (e.g., add band resistance to a sidestep or jab).

Progression cues should be delivered in a manner that does not portray them as better than other options. The goal is to avoid making participants feel pressured into taking a harder option

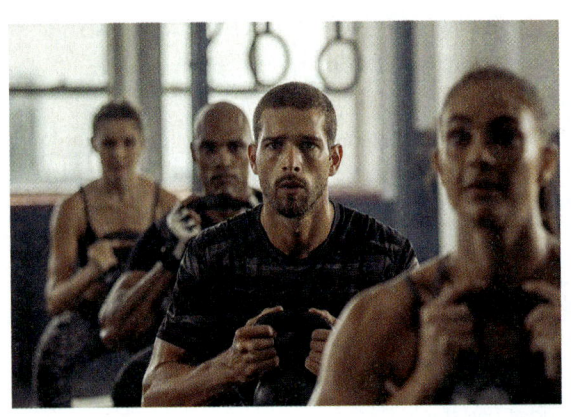

© Ground Picture/Shutterstock

when it might not be appropriate. This is best accomplished by offering progression cues as part of an exercise sequence or additional options to increase effectiveness. Often, this is successfully done with questions to build a frame of reference.

Begin by referencing the desired result: "This is the most challenging interval of the workout." Then, ask participants if their experience matches the desired result: "Are you breathing hard? Feeling challenged to get through it?" Lastly, use the answer to those questions as a guide to the next steps: "If you answered yes, hold on and continue to push through. Just 30 more seconds. If you want an extra challenge, try adding a jump to your squats." This technique avoids establishing a more fit group or a better group; it simply delivers results.

⚙ PRACTICE THIS

Remember that regressions do not mean that an exercise becomes easier. It makes them more effective. Sometimes performing a movement correctly is the hardest challenge.

Regressions are movement cues given to make an exercise simpler to execute correctly and/or to accommodate specific needs. Just as you progress a movement through complexity, an instructor can regress a movement by reducing complexity. This includes adding stability to a participant's platform or points of contact (e.g., placing a hand on a ballet barre), removing a layer of a movement pattern, or focusing on fewer mastery cues and instead on foundational movement cues.

The focus and technique of delivering regression mastery cues match that of progression cues. Reference the desired result, ask a question to establish if the current experience matches the desired result, and then use the answer to determine next steps, for example:

> "We are still in the warmup phase of our workout. Your effort should feel comfortable and sustainable. Is the weight already challenging? If you feel outside of your comfort zone, put the bar down and continue with bodyweight squats. We have plenty of challenging efforts ahead."

Offering progression/regression cues is one way to support participants in developing autonomy and competence because it helps them take ownership of the workout and builds their confidence.

BUILDING AUTONOMY AND COMPETENCE

AUTONOMY describes peoples' need to feel that they can directly affect a successful outcome and that their actions make a difference. People must know that they can control their own behaviors and, therefore, their likelihood of achieving a goal, such as knowing that they can take action to improve their health by attending a group fitness class. Autonomy could even be described as a basic human need, and your contribution as a Group Fitness Instructor can be a big one in a participant's life.

Competence is the idea that people gain confidence through mastery. When you take on a new skill and can improve and feel competent, you are more likely to take further action and not give up. When an individual is challenged and successfully meets that challenge, then they are motivated to take on other challenges. For example, attending a new group fitness format and successfully completing the workout can boost confidence to return to that class and try new formats.

If an individual feels that they are in an environment where their autonomy and competence are being diminished, it will likely decrease their intrinsic motivation. Recall that intrinsic motivation is the internal motivation to engage in a behavior, reflecting a valuing of the behavior. That is, a person engages in a behavior because the behavior itself is its own reward. However, environments that support and encourage autonomy and competence have been shown to increase intrinsic motivation (Deci & Ryan, 1985). Intrinsic motivation is desirable in a group fitness setting because intrinsic motivation leads to more sustainable behavior change. If an individual is motivated to exercise by extrinsic drivers, such as appearance, social pressure, or directions from their physician, their chances of long-term exercise adherence are lower than those who are motivated intrinsically. Therefore, Group Fitness Instructors should strive to boost both autonomy and competency to boost intrinsic motivation (Hagger & Chatzisarantis, 2007). This does not mean that extrinsic motivators are bad or not useful. They are part of life. It does mean, however, that being intrinsically motivated yields better long-term adherence and outcomes. As a Group Fitness Instructor, you should not underestimate your role in helping others reach their potential, not only from a fitness standpoint but also a personal one.

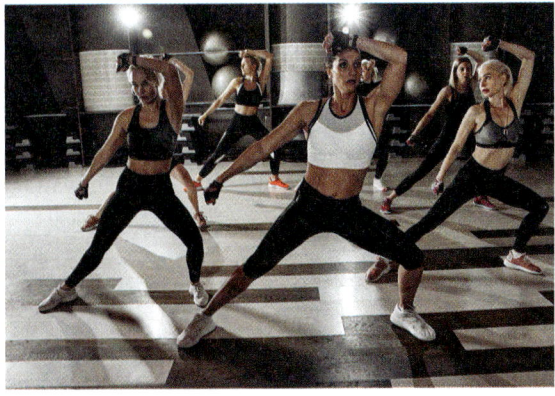

© Ivan_kislitsin/Shutterstock

Self-Determination Theory outlines the importance of motives in predicting behavior (Gaesser et al., 2020). As your participants' goals change and they celebrate wins and set new goals, you can support their intrinsic motivation by recognizing their success, no matter how big or small. This will help them to maintain the upward spiral and remind them of their competence.

Although this topic centers around the concept of motivation, it is directly related to how instructors teach and cue because autonomy and competence are both founded on the idea of mastery. If an instructor can encourage participants to play an active role in their own success and then lead them to do so by teaching the skills needed for mastery, then the need for autonomy and competence is met.

An instructor can build participants' intrinsic motivation through autonomy and competence by thinking of themselves as an empathetic educator rather than as an expert. You should approach your role as an instructor simply as someone who currently holds applicable knowledge, and whose goal is to share that knowledge with others, leaving ego at the door.

The following are some simple ways to take on the role of educator rather than an expert:

- **Avoid jargon, slang, or inside jokes.** Use of jargon, slang, or inside jokes establishes the idea of "insiders" and "outsiders." If you do not understand the joke or the slang being used, then you are an outsider, and your feelings of autonomy and competence are quickly diminished. Instead, use common language that is universally understood and promotes inclusion.
- **Avoid finite terms or unchangeable ideas.** For example, by describing someone as sedentary, it implies a permanent characteristic, such as having brown eyes or being 6 feet tall. In contrast, saying a person currently lives a sedentary lifestyle or has lost connection with the joy of movement implies the possibility of change and encourages the idea of autonomy. The individual has control over the choice to be sedentary and, therefore, can choose to change it when they are ready.
- **Create moments of success.** Recall that when an individual is challenged and successfully meets that challenge, they are motivated to take on other challenges. However, if an individual takes on a new challenge and fails, they are less likely to be motivated to show up for the next challenge. Therefore, mastery cues must set participants up for success. Overwhelming the group with too much information or overcomplicated mastery cues can lead to frustration and diminish autonomy and competence. Instead, pick a focus, explain that focus in simple terms, and then layer on motivational cues.

Motivational Cues

Participants are now moving safely with more precision and expertise and are ready for the final layer of cues in the verbal cueing progression: motivational cues. Motivational cues reinforce the skills and advancements learned through movement and mastery cues, as well as encourage participants to continue learning (**Figure 13.8**).

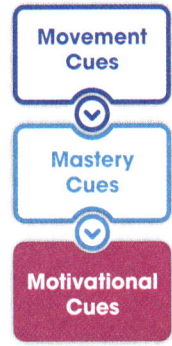

FIGURE 13.8 Verbal Cueing Matrix: Motivational Cues

Motivational cues come in many different forms, including dissociative and associative cues (**Table 13.3**). The cognitive concept of association and dissociation was first examined in marathon runners in a study conducted by Morgan and Pollack (1977). They found that competitive marathon runners relied on associative strategies, turning focus inward to focus on feedback cues from the body; whereas non-competitive runners relied more on dissociative strategies, turning focus outward to not be distracted by internal bodily cues and discomfort. Many studies since have reinforced these findings, including a study that applied these findings to a general exercise population (Lind et al., 2009), which found dissociative strategies can be more effective in reducing the rate of perceived intensity at low to moderate exercise intensities, where they prove less effective at higher intensity levels in which associative cues become more effective. Therefore, it is most effective to utilize dissociative strategies in formats or workout segments that demand less intensity, such as a recovery phase or the beginning of class. However, when the work demands more intensity, such as during a high-intensity interval, focusing on the effort at hand is most appropriate.

TABLE 13.3 Forms of Motivational Cues

Dissociative Cues	Associative Cues	
▪ Humorous	▪ Empowering	▪ Time focused
▪ Personal	▪ Encouraging	▪ Competitive
▪ Visual imagery	▪ Inspiring	▪ Respiration and breathing
▪ Future thinking	▪ Relating	▪ Perceived exertion

DISSOCIATIVE CUES

A **DISSOCIATIVE CUE** is a cue that turns participants' focus outward and offers distraction from internal feedback or discomfort. In a group fitness setting, dissociative cues are used to shift focus externally through tactics such as entertainment, fun and enjoyment, and imagery, while taking the mind off of discomfort. Dissociative cues are best utilized during low to moderate exercise intensities when the effort is not all-consuming and the individual is able to think about other things (Lind et al., 2009). This strategy has been found to be especially effective for beginner exercisers, because they often shy away from exercise due to the anticipation of

DISSOCIATIVE CUE

Cues that turn the focus outward to offer distraction from internal cues or discomfort.

discomfort and a dissociative strategy may decrease their subjective rating of perceived exertion (Lind et al., 2009).

Dissociative cues work well as motivational cues because safe and correct movement has already been established through movement and safety cues. In this way, it is now safe to draw participants' attention elsewhere as long as movement integrity holds. Take a closer look at the dissociative cues provided in **Table 13.4**.

TABLE 13.4 Dissociative Cues

Type of Dissociative Cues	Description	Example
Humorous	Using a humorous story or joke to lighten the mood, add fun, and reduce intimidation	"Let me tell you about all the things I did wrong in my first ever group fitness class …"
Personal	Sharing a personal story or struggle to motivate and relate to the group	"Exercise was not always a part of my life. Let me share how I changed that …"
Imagery	Using visually descriptive language that draws participants to a desirable place or time	"Close your eyes and imagine you are riding down a beautiful beach."
Future thinking	Drawing attention to future benefits, goal achievement, and outcomes, making the current challenge worthwhile	"Think about what you want your health and wellness to feel like 1 year from today."

This type of planned distraction can keep participants motivated; however, it cannot be the only motivational tactic employed. You should also integrate associative cues to encourage a mind–body connection. The brain is the "body's command center" and is deeply intertwined with the operations of the rest of the body (Menesez, 2020). Our thoughts, feelings, beliefs, and attitudes can affect our physical functioning and performance. Accordingly, an instructor can utilize associative cues to encourage the mind and physical body to work in sync to overcome challenging workout segments.

ASSOCIATIVE CUES

ASSOCIATIVE CUES are cues that turn the focus inward to concentrate on the feedback received from the body. This can be anything from breathing rate, to muscle fatigue, to perceived exertion, to mental state. It is essential that a participant never ignores internal cues, especially if they are conveying pain that can lead to injury. Associative feedback is also essential to proper exercise execution and muscle activation.

Associative cues can be used as motivation when they provide essential strategies for overcoming temporary physical or mental challenges/discomforts. Take a closer look at the associative cues in **Table 13.5**.

ASSOCIATIVE CUES

Cues that turn the focus inward to concentrate on the feedback cues from the body.

TABLE 13.5 Associative Cues

Type of Associative Cue	Description	Example
Empowering	Using language to increase self-efficacy, competence, and autonomy	"Lean into the challenge to become stronger."
Encouraging	Showing empathy and providing motivation at the same time	"It isn't easy, but it's worth it. Keep it up!"
Inspiring	Energizing participants and connecting them to a goal or outcome	"Ten more hard reps and you will walk out of here stronger than you walked in."
Relating	Letting participants feel like they are part of a team and that they are not alone	"We're a team. Let's get through this last set together."
Time focused	Pushing through to the end of an effort	"30 seconds left then you get a 2-minute break. Finish strong!"
Competitive	Encouraging competition as a group (but not between individuals)	"Let's hold this plank 15 seconds longer than we did last week."
Respiration	Focusing on breathing to encourage effort or recovery	"Take some deep breaths to reset your heart rate and prepare for the next push."
Perceived exertion	Using the RPE scale or referencing how an effort should feel to encourage individual performance	"This is your most challenging effort. Can you push just beyond your comfort zone?"

Once intensity reaches highly challenging levels, most participants switch to cognitive association, meaning they benefit more from focusing on the effort at hand rather than using distraction tactics, and their focus shifts inward to concentrate on feedback from the body (Lind et al., 2009). A role you can play as an instructor is to guide the association to positive thoughts and outcomes. For example, an instructor can use a cue like "Your body is probably letting you know that it is working really hard and feeling some fatigue. We are getting stronger as we wrap up these last 30 seconds."

⚙ PRACTICE THIS

Now it is your turn. Write your own examples for the different types of dissociative and associative cues listed in Tables 13.4 and 13.5.

Three-Dimensional Cueing

Three-dimensional cueing refers to the integration and intersection of the three content delivery styles: visual, auditory, and kinesthetic learning. Visual learning is guided by sight, auditory learning is guided by sound, and kinesthetic learning is guided by doing. Recall that individuals do not solely learn through one style but instead gather and process information through all three. Therefore, it is essential that group fitness cueing incorporates all three types.

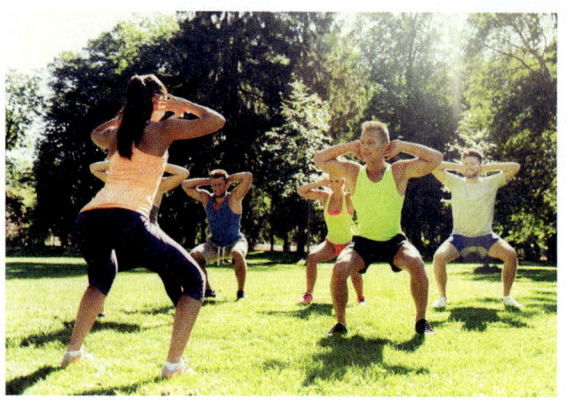

© Ground Picture/Shutterstock

Visual Cueing

VISUAL CUEING relies on the use of physical movement to communicate information. This communication most often comes in the form of movement demonstrations or informational gestures.

VISUAL CUEING

The use of physical movement to communicate information.

MOVEMENT DEMONSTRATION

Visual demonstration uses physicality to teach movement. Participants internalize the details of a movement by watching the instructor perform the movement first. Therefore, it is important that instructors move with precision and demonstrate excellent form in order to reinforce correct visual learning. Even if an instructor verbally cues correct form, an incorrect physical demonstration can lead to poor form in participants (Krauss, 2002).

PRACTICE THIS

Physical demonstration should be evaluated visually. Do not assume that you have good form. Instead, record yourself completing a number of common movement patterns and critique your form with an open mind or ask an experienced instructor to provide feedback.

INFORMATIONAL GESTURES

Gestures can be very helpful when communicating directional or numeric information, and they can reinforce verbal cues or sometimes allow an instructor to omit verbal cues. Directional cues can come in the form of pointing right or left, indicating the way in which you want the group to move. They can also be gesturing to move forward or back within a space. Directional cues can also indicate range of motion or rhythm, such as a flat hand moving downward to indicate the depth or timing of a squat.

Numeric gesturing can be used to count down remaining repetitions on your hands. Gestures can indicate time remaining in an interval by visually counting down or time passed by counting up.

Auditory Cueing

AUDITORY CUEING relies on verbal communication to share information. In addition to following the verbal cueing progression, auditory cues should be clear, succinct, and consistent. As a Group Fitness Instructor your goal is to simplify sometimes new and complex ideas into easy-to-follow directions.

An instructor can create clarity with simple and direct language:

Say this … "Take four steps to the right."
Not this … "How about we move to the right."

They can be succinct by eliminating filler words:

Say this … "Face sideways for shuffles."
Not this … "Next we will face the side of the room and shuffle."

They can be consistent by repeating the same movement names, giving the same directional cues, and following the same verbal cueing progression every time.

© Kzenon/Shutterstock

Kinesthetic Cueing

KINESTHETIC CUEING utilizes physical movement and physical feedback to communicate information. This is accomplished by giving participants time to try out a movement. In its simplest form, this can be "Here is what a push-up looks like. Now you try." Or you can take this technique further by integrating progressions and regressions: "Try out a push-up with your hands on a step. Now try it with knees down or try it with your hands on the floor from your toes. Select a challenging option where you can maintain good form."

Kinesthetic cueing can also tap into physical feedback to inform movement. For example, "If you power that jump from the balls of your feet, do you get more height?" or "If you draw your belly in, do you feel less discomfort in your lower back?"

Although three types of cueing were just described separately, an effective Group Fitness Instructor integrates all elements to create three-dimensional cueing. Consider the examples in **Table 13.6** that put all three dimensions together.

TABLE 13.6 Three-Dimensional Cueing Examples

An instructor demonstrates a side-stepping lunge as they say "Eyes on me. Take a wide step to the right. Bend the right knee and sit the hips back. Step back to center. Now you try."
An instructor points to the right and says, "eight side shuffles." Then, they follow up with "If you get lower, do you feel your quads?"
An instructor says, "Show me what full range of motion looks like in a squat" as they demonstrate a squat with hips lowering to knee height. Then, they follow up with "Did you feel your quads and glutes working?"

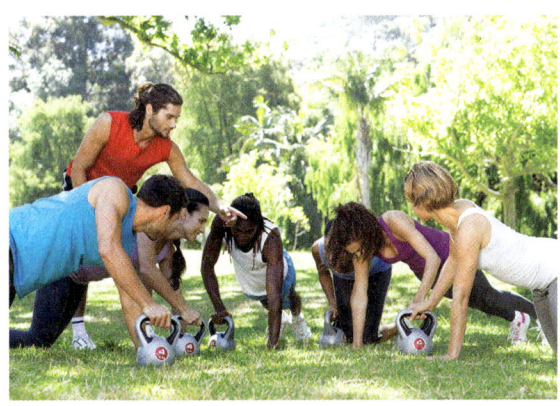

© Wavebreakmedia/Shutterstock

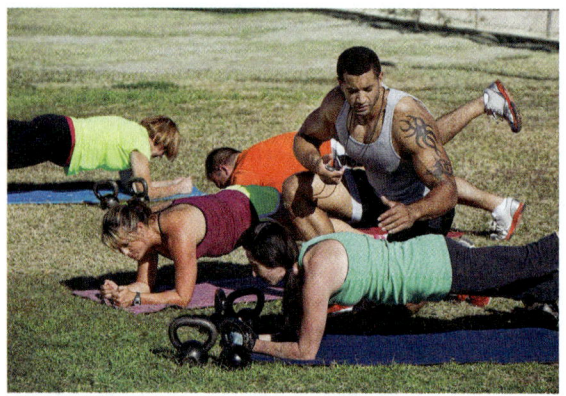
© CREATISTA/Shutterstock

Personalizing Cues

The final step in the cueing plan is personalization. In a general setting, it is rare to have several moments to give personal cues, but there are circumstances in which personal cues are not only beneficial but sometimes required, such as for safety, to provide feedback, or to give hands-on guidance.

Cueing for Safety

The first area to address regarding personalized cues is safety. The priority in all group fitness settings is safety and, if an instructor sees something unsafe, they must correct it immediately. Safety concerns include an unsafe movement, incorrect use of equipment, or unsafe equipment setup (e.g., an unsecured step riser). When addressing unsafe equipment use or setup, an instructor should immediately approach the individual and assist in fixing the problem. In the case of an unsafe movement, an instructor may first give a general cue, addressing the full class, because the cue may also remind others to check their form. However, if this does not correct the problem and the unsafe movement might lead to injury, the instructor should approach the individual. When approaching an individual to provide a safety cue, it is recommended that the instructor move their microphone away from their mouth or cover it with a hand to ensure that the individual is not embarrassed in any way. Then, kindly let them know what you see and the risk of the incorrect movement and guide them on how to correct it, such as with a verbal correction and a physical demonstration. For example, "Rebecca when you round your back in a deadlift, you risk injuring your back. Let's lighten up the weight and focus on hinging from your hips and keeping your chest lifted. Let's try it together." Then, proceed to demonstrate correct form and give them feedback until the movement is safe.

POSITIVE FEEDBACK

Feedback that communicates approval of a behavior and motivates an individual to continue the current behavior.

CONSTRUCTIVE FEEDBACK

Feedback that provides information regarding an individual's actions that can be used to improve performance and build successful behaviors.

Giving Feedback

Some group fitness formats lend themselves more to personalized feedback than others. A large kickboxing class of 50 people might pose a difficult environment to connect with individuals; however, a small core class of 10 can allow for one-on-one moments during the workout. Either way, there is immense value in moments of positive personal connection.

It is important to focus on providing positive feedback. Negative feedback, such as shaming or teasing, even if the instructor believes they are doing it in a friendly manner, can be extremely detrimental to a participant. Our brains are hard-wired for connectedness, and when we feel rejection, our brain perceives it in the same way it processes physical pain (Eisenberger et al., 2003). For this reason, instructors should focus on constructive and positive personalized feedback as a means of decreasing feelings of rejection and increasing positive emotions. **POSITIVE FEEDBACK** communicates approval of a behavior and motivates an individual to continue the current behavior, for example, "Great intensity, Jorge! Keep it up." **CONSTRUCTIVE FEEDBACK** provides information regarding an individual's actions that can be used to improve performance and build successful behaviors. **Table 13.7** provides methods for offering constructive and positive feedback when giving personal feedback in a group fitness setting.

TABLE 13.7 Methods for Offering Feedback

Method	Feedback
Timing	Leaving the front of the class during a tricky section of choreography or when changing the exercise is not ideal. Instead, connect with individual participants for personalized feedback during a time when you are less needed at the front of the class: during a break in sets, during core work, during the cool down, or once the group is moving correctly with confidence.
Catch them doing something right	A great opportunity for positive connection is immediate recognition.[a] Catch someone doing something right and compliment them on it. "Wow, those push-ups look great, Sheena. Great job keeping your core tight." Be specific about what they are doing well ("keeping your core tight") so they know how to repeat the behavior in the future.
Correct with encouragement	Corrective feedback is meant to create a positive change.[b] If a correction is needed, first highlight something the individual is doing well and then tell them the correction that is needed and what benefit the correction will provide. "Damien, awesome intensity on those cardio intervals today. Can you lift your hips a bit higher in your plank? We don't want your back to hurt."
Consider the individual	Not all participants want feedback in a public setting. Some might prefer that you speak to them privately before or after class. If you are not sure, ask. Approach the individual before or after class and ask "Jackie, I have really enjoyed having you in class the past 2 weeks. Because I don't know you well, do you mind if I ask what type of feedback you prefer? Do you prefer if I give you some tips during class or connecting afterward?"

[a] Nelson, B. (2005). *1001 ways to reward employees*. Workman.
[b] Rabinowitz, P. (2022). Providing corrective feedback. In *Organizing for effective advocacy*. https://ctb.ku.edu/en/table-of-contents/advocacy/encouragement-education/corrective-feedback/main

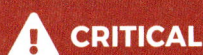

⚠ **CRITICAL**

Hands-on cues can be helpful, especially for kinesthetic learning; however, there are specific considerations when utilizing these types of cues:

- An instructor must ask permission and receive positive confirmation before touching participants. Never assume someone is comfortable being touched. While this may seem awkward, it can be accomplished quite easily such as by saying, "Are you okay being cued with touch?"
- Only touch individuals where appropriate and for a specific purpose.

Hands-On Cues

Hands-on cues can help participants be more mindful of their movements. They help increase awareness of posture, alignment, and muscle engagement (Cook et al., 2020).

Hands-on cues can be used for the following purposes:

- **Focus muscle activation.** A hands-on cue can help an individual engage the correct muscles during a movement, for example, a hand placed between a participant's shoulder blades to encourage upper back activation during a row.

- **Guide range of motion.** A hands-on cue can be effective when correcting range of motion, for example, placing your hands at a participant's wrists to show them where to begin an overhead shoulder press.
- **Encourage intensity.** A hands-on cue can help boost intensity, for example, having a participant punch into your hands to deliver a more powerful jab or reach your outstretched hand to encourage them to jump higher.

Cueing for Success

Cueing for success is a three-part approach to mastering the art of cueing (**Figure 13.9**). The road map begins with the verbal cueing matrix, which outlines the three foundational steps to cueing: movement cues, mastery cues, and motivational cues. Verbal cues should follow this specific order—movement, mastery, and motivational—because they progressively build on one another to create group success. Once verbal cues are practiced and effectively delivered, an instructor can layer in the various styles of learning to deliver three-dimensional cues through auditory cues, visual cues, and kinesthetic cues. Lastly, an instructor focuses on personalized cues.

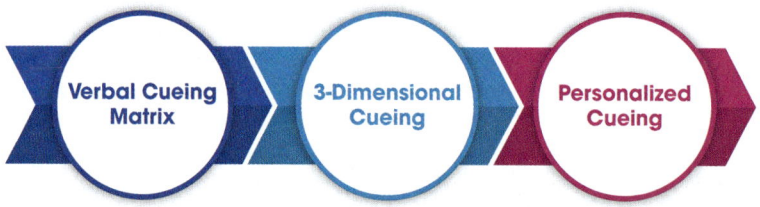

FIGURE 13.9 Cueing for Success

Prior to layering in personalized cues, a new instructor should spend time delivering verbal cues and three-dimensional cues with consistency and efficiency. The conscious brain can only handle a portion of high-order information (i.e., applying cues and feedback or analyzing and evaluating movement) at a time (Wu et al., 2016), and that is true for both the instructor and the participant. Mastering verbal cueing and three-dimensional cueing will take time and practice. Once these cues flow easily and clearly, then personal feedback can be layered in. Cueing must also be practiced and evaluated on an ongoing basis. Ask for feedback from participants and fellow instructors, attend other instructors' classes, and record yourself to personally evaluate your progress and areas for improvement.

Lesson 3: Applied Anatomy and Cueing

Applied Anatomy

Now that the framework for successful cueing has been laid out, the next step is to put it into action. A variety of common positions and movements are integrated into a group fitness workout, such as prone, supine, split-stance, kneeling, pushing, pulling, squatting, hip-hinging, and overhead movements. It is important to have strong knowledge of proper form for these positions because they are the foundation for many common exercises executed in a group fitness setting.

Prone

The term *prone* describes the position of your body when oriented face down (**Figure 13.10**). This position is often used for core strength and endurance (e.g., planks) and posterior chain (back of the body) exercises (e.g., back extensions or cobras). Prone exercises require core strength, control through the spine and hips, and coordination; therefore, they may not be appropriate for all individuals. To correctly execute a prone exercise, individuals should engage their abdominals and maintain length in their spine. Additionally, the lower back and hips should not sag toward the floor or jut toward the ceiling. To maintain alignment of the neck and head, once movement begins, eyes should turn toward the floor. See **Table 13.8** for prone position cues.

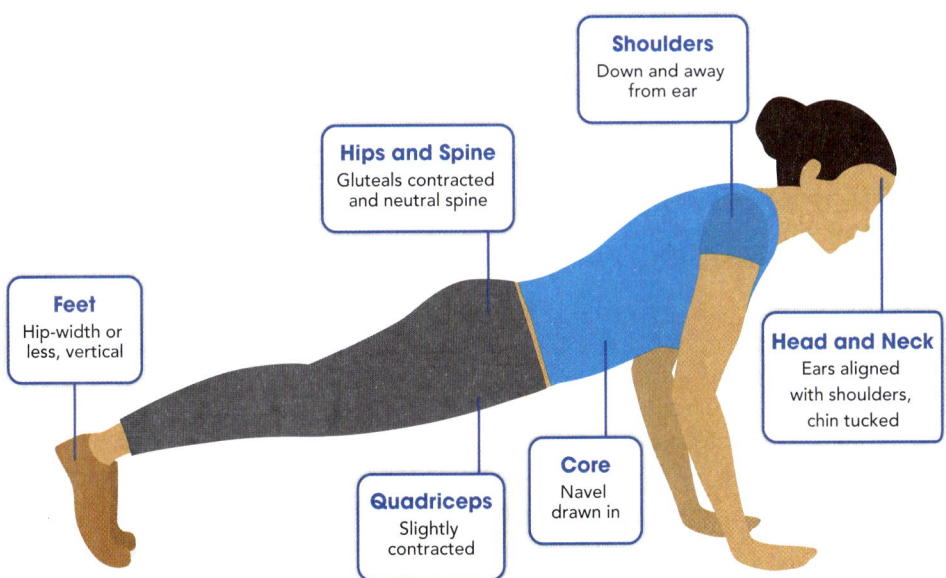

FIGURE 13.10 Prone Position

TABLE 13.8 Cueing for Prone Position

Verbal			
Movement Cue	**Safety Cue**	**Mastery Cue**	**Motivational Cue**
"Take a face-down position."	"Prone exercises may not be appropriate for spinal instability, spinal arthritis, or facet joint problems."[a]	"Gently draw your navel away from the floor to support your spine and maintain posture."	"Exercises in the prone position help you build a stronger back, which is critical to your overall movement health."

Three-Dimensional		
Visual	**Auditory**	**Kinesthetic**
The instructor demonstrates laying on the stomach with the core engaged.	"Lay on your stomach with an engaged core to begin the next exercise."	"Lay on your stomach and draw your navel up and away from the floor by engaging your core."

(continues)

TABLE 13.8 Cueing for Prone Position (*continued*)

Personalized		
Safety Cue	**Feedback Cue**	**Hands-On Cue**
"This position should be avoided if it is uncomfortable for your back."	"This position looks uncomfortable for you. Would you like to try changing to a hands and knees position?"	Place a hand on their lower back and say, "Draw your belly up toward my hand."

[a] Perolat, R., Kastler, A., Nicot, B., Pellat, J.-M., Tahon, F., Attye, A., Heck, O., Boubagra, K., Grand, S., & Krainik, A. (2018). Facet joint syndrome: From diagnosis to interventional management. *Insights Imaging, 9*(5), 773–789. https://doi.org/10.1007/s13244-018-0638-x

👍 HELPFUL HINT

Achieving a neutral spine is a common cue in group exercise. And at times, it can be challenging to clearly explain. Recall that a neutral spine is an alignment where the vertebrae are properly stacked to maximize safety and results. A neutral spine is best achieved as a combination of different positions from hips to head. The pelvis should be level and neither anteriorly nor posteriorly rotated relative to the spine. If a participant thinks of their pelvis as a bucket of water, the water should not spill out of the front (anterior) or back (posterior). This can be accomplished by drawing in the navel (core activation) and contracting the gluteals. These two cues in combination will take the hips and lumbar spine into neutral and reduce the common movement fault of an excessively arched lower back. For the thoracic spine, instructing participants to pull their shoulders back and down away from the ears in combination with core activation will encourage ideal posture. For the cervical spine (head and neck), instructing participants to keep their chin from jutting forward and aligning their ears over their shoulders will create ideal posture in this checkpoint. Although this may seem like a lot of cues, they can quickly be delivered as "neutral spine is glutes tight, navel in, shoulders back, and chin tucked." Once participants understand what it means, simply cueing "neutral spine" will suffice.

Supine

The term *supine* refers to being positioned face up (**Figure 13.11**). When in supine position, an individual may have their knees bent or legs extended flat on the floor, depending on the exercise. The knees-bent position provides more lower back support and may be more appropriate for those with lower back pain. Supine exercises often target the abdominals and core, including crunches and bicycles. The supine position is also used for posterior chain (e.g., bridges) and anterior chain (front of the body) exercises (e.g., chest press). When in supine position, maintain abdominal engagement to support the spine. Additionally, keep the shoulders back and away from the ears. See **Table 13.9** for supine position cues.

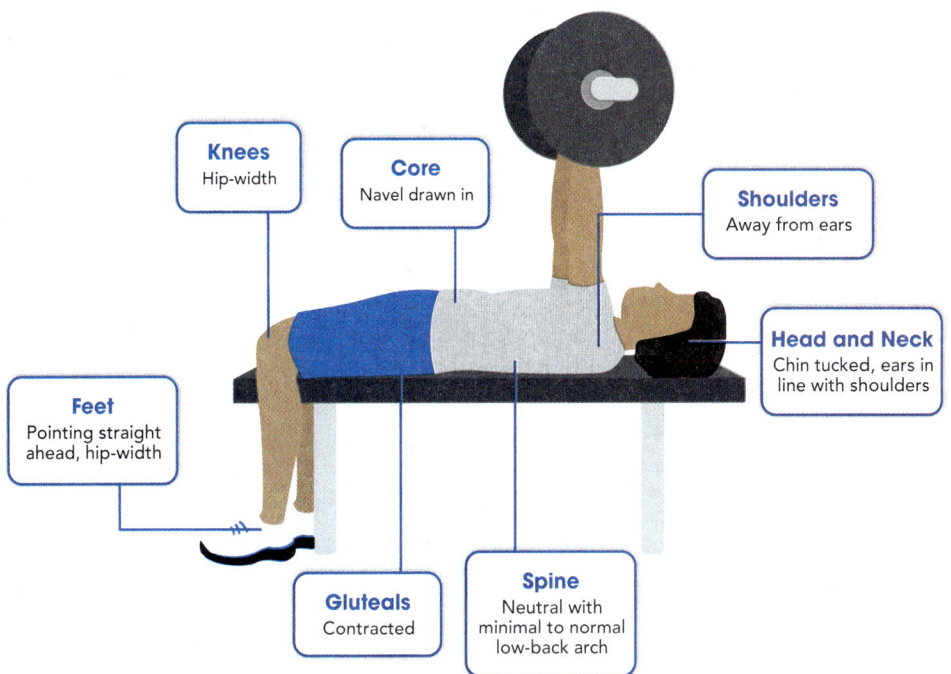

Knees
Hip-width

Core
Navel drawn in

Shoulders
Away from ears

Head and Neck
Chin tucked, ears in
line with shoulders

Feet
Pointing straight
ahead, hip-width

Gluteals
Contracted

Spine
Neutral with
minimal to normal
low-back arch

FIGURE 13.11 Supine Position

TABLE 13.9 Cueing for Supine Position

Verbal			
Movement Cue	**Safety Cue**	**Mastery Cue**	**Motivational Cue**
"Lay on your back."	"Supine position may not be appropriate for pregnant women,[a] those with congestive heart failure, or severe acid reflux."[b]	"Find neutral spine by taking a deep breath and letting your body relax into the floor."	"Supine exercises promote core engagement, which will help you move with strength and safety."

Three-Dimensional		
Visual	**Auditory**	**Kinesthetic**
"Lay on your back with shoulders relaxed and a neutral spine" (instructor demonstrates).	"Lay on your back and take a deep breath as you relax into the floor."	"Lay on your back and maintain the same long spine you have when you are standing. There should be a small space between your low back and the floor. Can you feel that?"

Personalized		
Safety Cue	**Feedback Cue**	**Hands-On Cue**
"Bend your knees if this position is uncomfortable for your back."	"I see your back arching. Can you take a deep breath, draw in your navel, and release the tension in your lower back?"	Place a hand underneath their lower back and say, "Draw your navel toward my hand."

[a] American College of Obstetricians and Gynecologists. (2022, March). *Exercise during pregnancy: Frequently asked questions.* https://www.acog.org/womens-health/faqs/exercise-during-pregnancy?utm_source=redirect&utm_medium=web&utm_campaign=otn

[b] Lindberg, S. (2019, April). *How does supine position affect health?* Healthline. https://www.healthline.com/health/supine-position

Split-Stance

When in split-stance, one foot is in front of the other with feet hip-width apart (**Figure 13.12**). When using split-stance for upper body exercises, step one foot back 6–12 inches. This can provide a balance challenge as well as reduce lower back discomfort in some individuals. When in split-stance, the core should remain engaged to avoid excessive arching (a slight arch is normal) of the

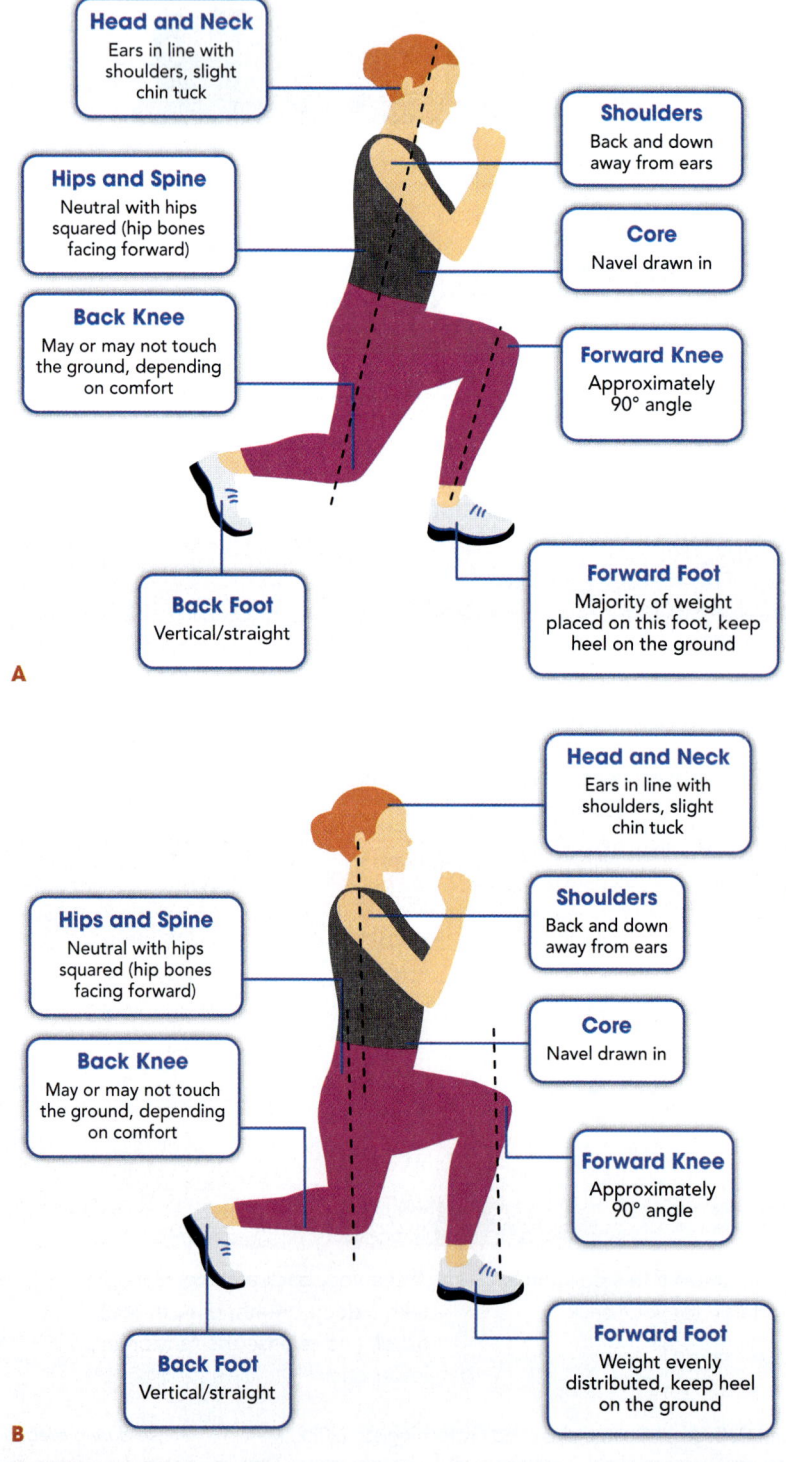

Head and Neck
Ears in line with shoulders, slight chin tuck

Shoulders
Back and down away from ears

Hips and Spine
Neutral with hips squared (hip bones facing forward)

Core
Navel drawn in

Back Knee
May or may not touch the ground, depending on comfort

Forward Knee
Approximately 90° angle

Back Foot
Vertical/straight

Forward Foot
Majority of weight placed on this foot, keep heel on the ground

A

Head and Neck
Ears in line with shoulders, slight chin tuck

Shoulders
Back and down away from ears

Hips and Spine
Neutral with hips squared (hip bones facing forward)

Core
Navel drawn in

Back Knee
May or may not touch the ground, depending on comfort

Forward Knee
Approximately 90° angle

Back Foot
Vertical/straight

Forward Foot
Weight evenly distributed, keep heel on the ground

B

FIGURE 13.12 (A) Split-Stance: Gluteal Dominant, (B) Split-Stance: Quadriceps Dominant

back and keep hips squared to avoid discomfort in the knees, hips, and back. A split-stance is often used in step-up and lunging exercises. When executing a lunge, one foot steps back with a longer stride as the hips remain square (if hips rotate or the low back arches excessively, reduce stride length). A lunge stride should also allow for the front knee to bend without the front heel lifting off the floor to eliminate pressure in the front knee. See **Table 13.10** for split-stance position cues.

TABLE 13.10 Cueing for Split-Stance Position

Verbal			
Movement Cue	**Safety Cue**	**Mastery Cue**	**Motivational Cue**
"Step one foot back 6–12 inches for upper body work or longer for lunges."	"The feet remain hip-width apart for stability and safety."	"Engage your glutes and core to keep the hips facing forward."	"Split-stance challenges balance and strengthens your legs."

Three-Dimensional		
Visual	**Auditory**	**Kinesthetic**
"Step one foot back while keeping the hips facing forward, a neutral spine, and the chest lifted" (instructor demonstrates).	"Step one foot back as you keep your hips and shoulders facing the front of the room."	"Step one foot back. Do you feel wobbly or strong and steady? If wobbly, try bringing your back foot forward a little."

Personalized		
Safety Cue	**Feedback Cue**	**Hands-On Cue**
"You should feel stable in this stance before you add movement."	"Take your feet a bit wider and you will feel more stable."	Stand in front of the participant and cue them to turn their shoulders and hips to face you.

 INSTRUCTOR TIP

Lunges can be used to emphasize either the quadriceps or the gluteals, depending on the participant's position. To emphasize the gluteals, participants should take a slight forward lean with the trunk with more weight placed on the forward foot. The front heel should stay in contact with the ground. To emphasize the quadriceps, participants should maintain a vertical trunk and a vertical forward shin with weight evenly distributed across both feet.

Kneeling

Kneeling is the position in which one (i.e., half-kneeling) or both knees (i.e., tall kneeling) touch the ground (**Figure 13.13**). When kneeling, the hips should align over the knees. Avoid pushing the hips forward as this may cause excessive arching of the spine and lower back discomfort. The participant should think about stacking their head, shoulders, hips, and knees. The kneeling position helps develop strength, while challenging balance and core stability. With this balance challenge, individuals should focus on core engagement, including the gluteals, adductors (inner thighs), and abdominals. Proficient engagement of the core (navel drawn in) and gluteals will assist in keeping the body in alignment from head to knee. See **Table 13.11** for kneeling position cues.

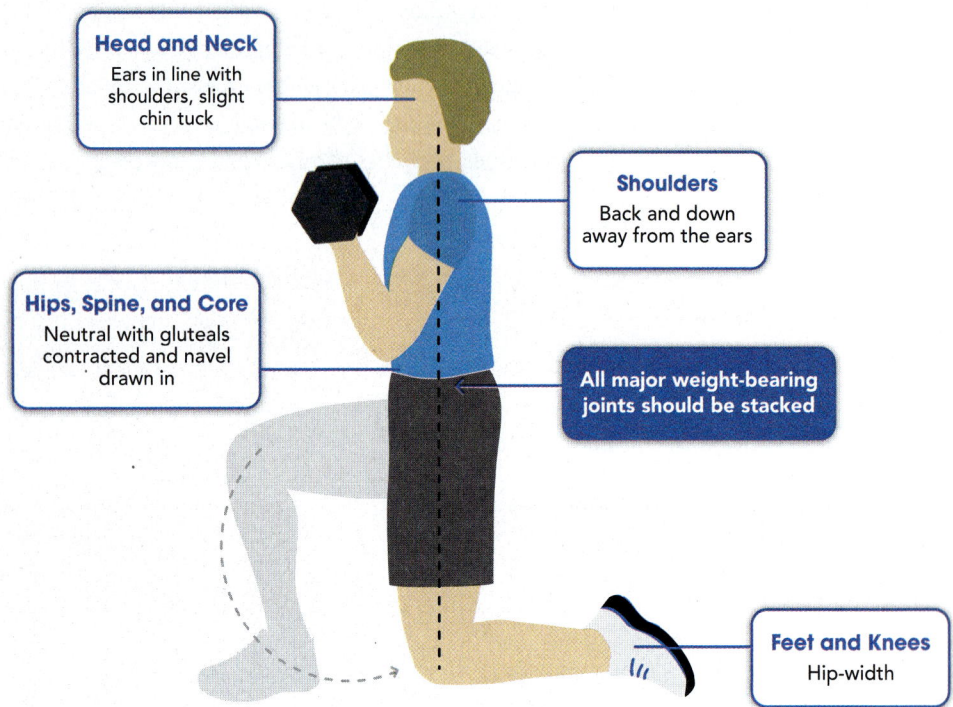

Head and Neck
Ears in line with shoulders, slight chin tuck

Shoulders
Back and down away from the ears

Hips, Spine, and Core
Neutral with gluteals contracted and navel drawn in

All major weight-bearing joints should be stacked

Feet and Knees
Hip-width

FIGURE 13.13 Kneeling Position

TABLE 13.11 Verbal Cueing for Kneeling Position

Verbal			
Movement Cue	**Safety Cue**	**Mastery Cue**	**Motivational Cue**
"Lower down one knee at a time to a kneeling position, ending with your hips over your knees."	"You might want to use a mat under your knees when kneeling. Kneeling may not be appropriate for those with knee injuries, arthritis, or recent surgery."	"Keep the knees and feet hip-width apart to ensure proper alignment and to reduce stress on the knees."	"Work your backside during kneeling exercises by squeezing your glutes and engaging your core."
Three-Dimensional			
Visual	**Auditory**		**Kinesthetic**
"Kneel down one knee at a time, align the hips over the knees, with the knees and feet hip-width apart" (instructor demonstrates).	"Come to kneeling, placing a mat underneath your knees if you like."		"As you kneel, activate the back side of your legs by contracting your glutes."
Personalized			
Safety Cue	**Feedback Cue**		**Hands-On Cue**
"If kneeling is uncomfortable, you can perform this exercise standing."	"Can you push your hips forward a bit so they are over your knees?"		Place a hand on the top (or just above) of their head and say, "Lengthen your spine and push my hand right through the ceiling."

Pushing

Pushing refers to exerting force to move something away from the body, such as a chest press or triceps extension, or exerting a force to move your body away, such as a push-up (**Figure 13.14**). Pushing movements often target the chest, shoulders, and triceps. Pushing can also occur in a number of positions, including seated, standing, prone, and supine. In any pushing position, shoulders should remain positioned away from the ears, the upper back should be engaged to reduce rounding, and the core should be strong to eliminate overarching of the lower back. It is common for the chin to jut forward during pushing movements. A slight **CHIN TUCK** can be helpful (envision pushing the back of your head to the back of the room) to maintain position of the head and neck. See **Table 13.12** for pushing position cues.

CHIN TUCK

A neutral position of the head and neck (cervical spine) where the chin is level and head is pulled straight back so the ears are aligned over the shoulders.

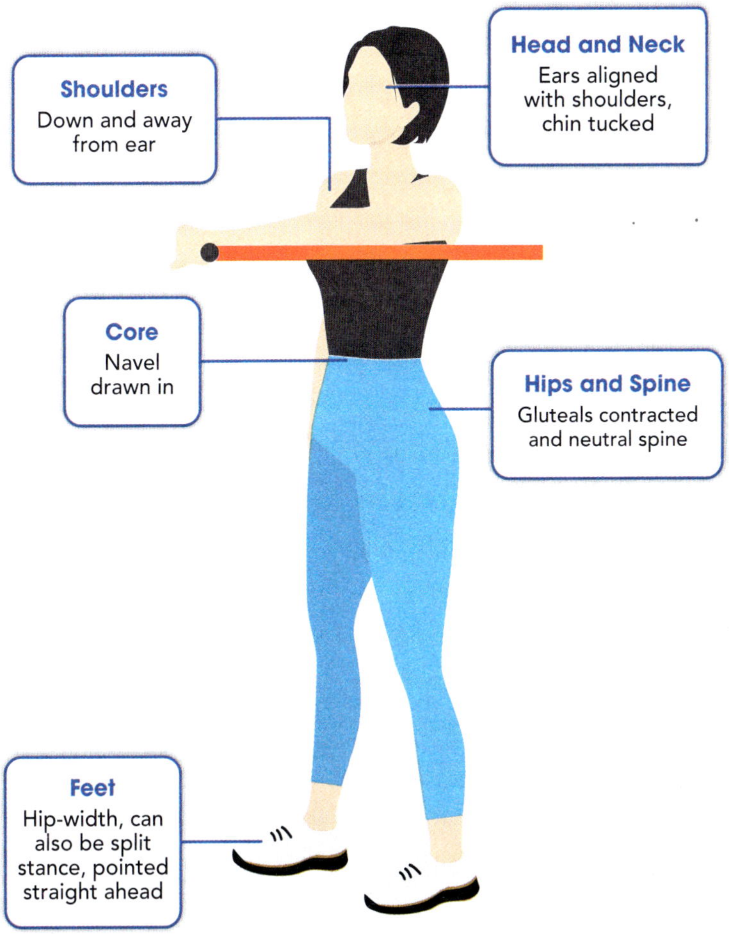

Shoulders
Down and away from ear

Head and Neck
Ears aligned with shoulders, chin tucked

Core
Navel drawn in

Hips and Spine
Gluteals contracted and neutral spine

Feet
Hip-width, can also be split stance, pointed straight ahead

FIGURE 13.14 Pushing Position

TABLE 13.12 Cueing for Pushing Position

Verbal			
Movement Cue	**Safety Cue**	**Mastery Cue**	**Motivational Cue**
"Begin with bent arms. Extend the arms to drive the resistance away from you."	"Keep the elbows soft at the extended position to avoid hyperextension of the elbows."	"Pull the shoulders down away from the ears."	"We use a pushing movement pattern throughout our day. Let's practice doing it here with strength and great form."

(continues)

TABLE 13.12 Cueing for Pushing Position (*continued*)

Three-Dimensional		
Visual	**Auditory**	**Kinesthetic**
"Relax the shoulders and maintain a neutral spine. Avoid pushing the chin forward or hyperextending the elbows" (instructor demonstrates).	"Push the weight away from your body as you keep your core strong."	"Focus on your chest doing the work as you push that weight away from you."
Personalized		
Safety Cue	**Feedback Cue**	**Hands-On Cue**
"Tuck your chin in slightly to avoid over-extending your neck."	"Let's adjust your range of motion a bit. Can you extend your arms a bit further while keeping your elbows soft and shoulders relaxed?"	Place a hand in front of the participant and ask them to reach for your hand (without hyperextending the elbow or rounding their shoulders).

Pulling

Pulling refers to exerting force to move something toward the body, such as a row or biceps curl (**Figure 13.15**). The primary muscles engaged in an upper body pull include the back muscles,

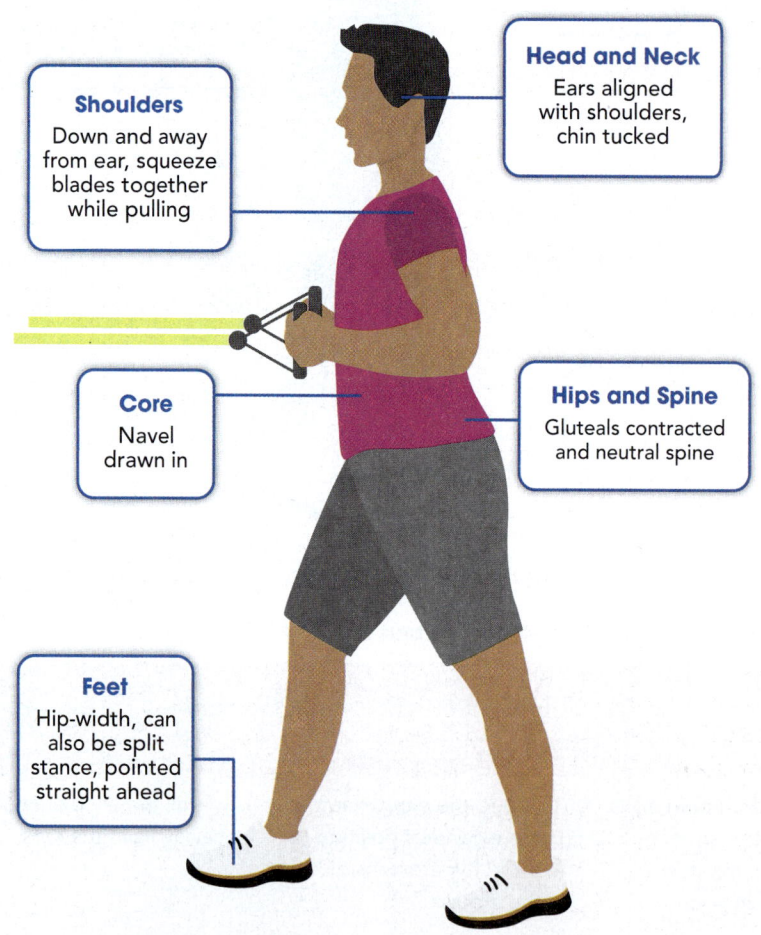

Shoulders
Down and away from ear, squeeze blades together while pulling

Head and Neck
Ears aligned with shoulders, chin tucked

Core
Navel drawn in

Hips and Spine
Gluteals contracted and neutral spine

Feet
Hip-width, can also be split stance, pointed straight ahead

FIGURE 13.15 Pulling Position

biceps, and the middle and lower trapezius. The technique cues are very similar to pushing movements. While pulling, focus on shoulder depression and core engagement. Proper neck and head position should also be focused on when pulling with the chin slightly tucked, eyes looking ahead, and the neck long. See **Table 13.13** for pulling position cues.

TABLE 13.13 Verbal Cueing for Pulling Position

Verbal			
Movement Cue	**Safety Cue**	**Mastery Cue**	**Motivational Cue**
"Begin with the arms extended. Bend the arms to pull the resistance toward you."	"Focus on maintaining a straight spine to avoid arching of the lower back."	"Focus on engaging your upper and mid back as you pull."	"Strong backs support strong posture."

Three-Dimensional		
Visual	**Auditory**	**Kinesthetic**
"Relax your shoulders and maintain a neutral spine. Avoid pushing the chin forward or over-extending the back" (instructor demonstrates).	"Pull the weight toward your body as you focus on your upper and mid back."	"Think about pulling from your elbows and shoulder blades instead of your hands."

Personalized		
Safety Cue	**Feedback Cue**	**Hands-On Cue**
Draw in your navel to keep a neutral spine.	Focus on squeezing your shoulder blades together to activate your upper back, rather than pulling with your arms.	Place a hand in between their shoulder blades and cue them to squeeze your hand as they pull.

Squatting

A squat movement begins in a standing position (**Figure 13.16**). The individual then lowers their hips to approximately knee height by bending their knees and pushing their hips back simultaneously. They then rise, driving out of their mid-foot, and return to standing. A squat is a complex exercise that requires coordinated flexion of the hip, knee, and ankle joints on descent and extension of the hip, knee, and ankle joints when standing up. Areas of form focus include a lifted (open) chest and straight spine as well as reaching the hips back and loading into the heels and mid-foot. It is common to lower the hips to a position parallel to the knees; however, some participants may find it more comfortable to stop short of that point. See **Table 13.14** for squatting position cues.

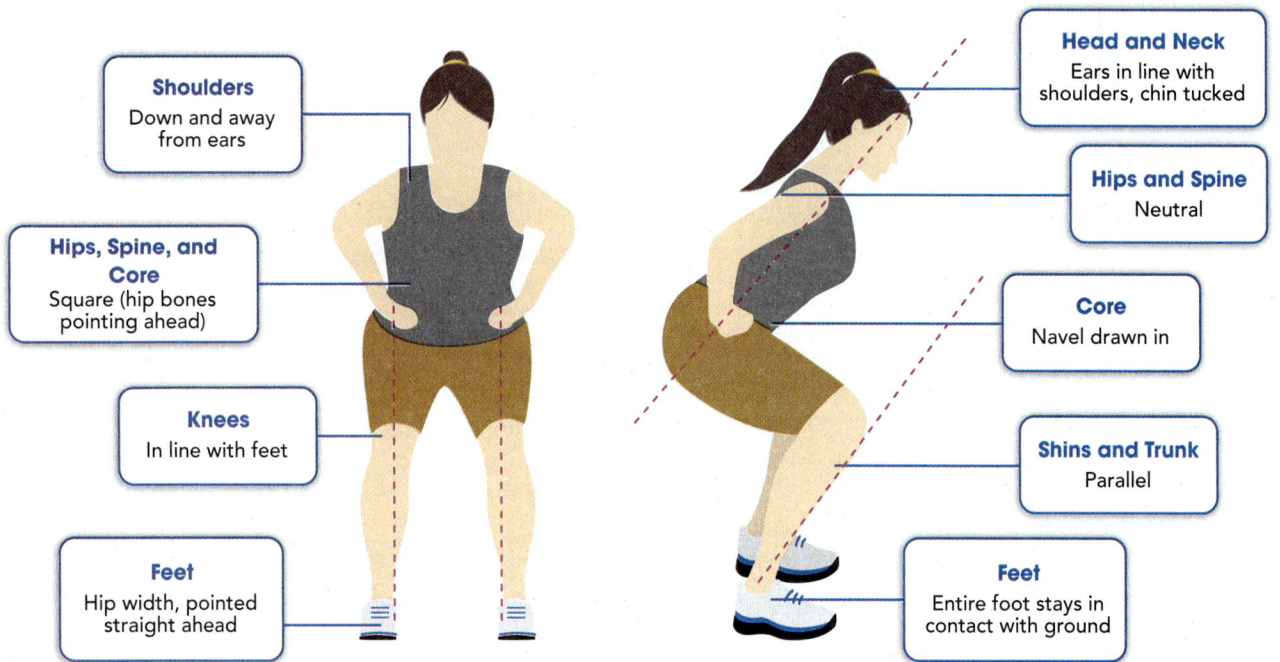

FIGURE 13.16 Squatting Position

TABLE 13.14 Cueing for Squatting Position

Verbal			
Movement Cue	**Safety Cue**	**Mastery Cue**	**Motivational Cue**
"Stand with the feet hip-width apart. Bend at the knees while lowering the hips to knee height as if sitting in a chair. Sit into your heels as you lower. Drive out of your heels and mid-foot to return to standing."	"The knees align with the toes. Do not allow them to cave in toward each other."	"Engage through your hamstrings and glutes and drive out of your hips to rise."	"Squats are the ultimate lower-body exercise, targeting quads, hamstrings, and glutes."

Three-Dimensional		
Visual	**Auditory**	**Kinesthetic**
"Ensure the knees are aligned with the toes and keep the heels on the ground. Push the hips back, lowering the hips to knee height, maintaining a neutral spine" (instructor demonstrates).	"Reach your hips back like you are sitting in a chair as you keep your core strong and eyes focused ahead of you."	"Think about driving the top of your head right through the ceiling as you rise."

Personalized		
Safety Cue	**Feedback Cue**	**Hands-On Cue**
"Keep your chest open and core strong to support your lower back."	"I see your knees moving inward as you squat. Engage your glutes to encourage your knees to track in line with your toes."	Place a chair or step behind the participant and ask them to tap their glutes to the chair before rising.

The cue of a lifted chest can sometimes be misinterpreted as pointing the ribs to the front of the room while arching the low back. However, the cue refers to the shoulders being back and down with the chest being open. Sometimes saying "Shoulders back and chest open" may be easier to understand.

Hip Hinging

When hip hinging, an individual bends forward from the hip joint (**Figure 13.17**). When hinging, the hips are the axis of rotation. The hip hinge engages the posterior chain, including the hamstrings, gluteals, and lower back. Proper hip hinging also requires a strong core to support a straight spine. Hip hinging is most commonly seen as deadlift variations. The most common mistake when hip hinging is rounding of the spine. The spine is to remain straight when executing a hip hinge, with the chin slightly tucked and the shoulders pulled back and down. See **Table 13.15** for hip-hinging position cues.

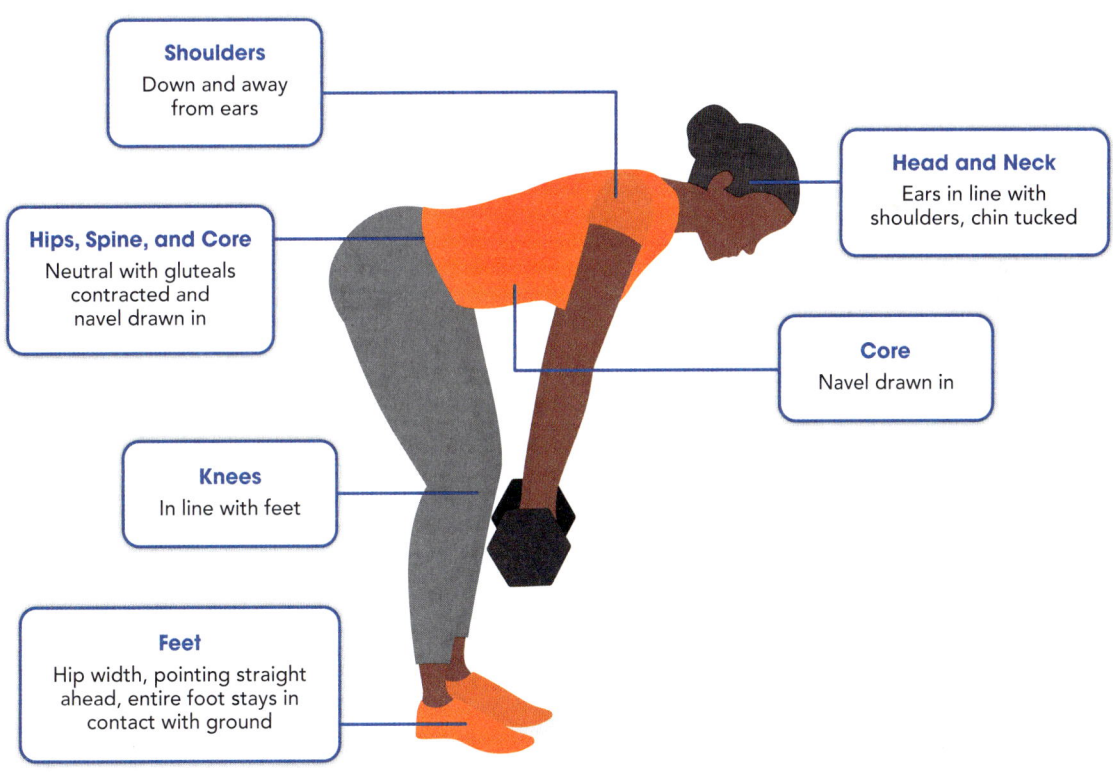

Shoulders
Down and away from ears

Head and Neck
Ears in line with shoulders, chin tucked

Hips, Spine, and Core
Neutral with gluteals contracted and navel drawn in

Core
Navel drawn in

Knees
In line with feet

Feet
Hip width, pointing straight ahead, entire foot stays in contact with ground

FIGURE 13.17 Hip-Hinging Position

TABLE 13.15 Cueing for Hip-Hinging Position

Verbal			
Movement Cue	**Safety Cue**	**Mastery Cue**	**Motivational Cue**
"Stand with the feet hip-width apart and a slight bend in the knees. Hinge forward from the hip joint without bending the knees further. Maintain a flat back, engaged core, and straight spine. Range of motion ends when hamstrings stretch and prior to the back rounding. Drive through heels and mid-foot and engage the glutes as you return to standing."	"A neutral spine is critical for executing a proper hip hinge. Hip hinging might not be appropriate for some back injuries."	"Focus on the back of your legs contracting as you rise."	"Hip hinging is all about the back of your legs and glutes. Let's build strong glutes and hamstrings."

Three-Dimensional		
Visual	**Auditory**	**Kinesthetic**
"Maintain a flat back, engaged core, and long spine. Keep the neck neutral" (instructor demonstrates).	"Fold from your hips with a long spine and strong core."	"You should feel this hinge in the back of your legs and glutes rather than your back. Think about pushing your hips forward as you stand."

Personalized		
Safety Cue	**Feedback Cue**	**Hands-On Cue**
"Draw the shoulder blades together and away from the ears to keep the upper back from rounding."	"Think about this movement only coming from your hips. Do not allow your knees to bend further as you hinge."	Place a dowel or your forearm on their upper back. As they hinge, cue them to keep their upper back in contact with the dowel.

Overhead

Overhead movements can include pushing, pulling, and static exercises, such as an overhead press, overhead triceps extensions, or overhead medicine ball carry (**Figure 13.18**). When the arms are extended overhead, excessive arching of the lumbar spine is common. Much like kneeling movements, participants should think about stacking their head, shoulders, hips, and knees. Abdominal and gluteal engagement can counteract an overextended spine and keep the lower back safe from injury. Keeping the shoulders away from the ears (i.e., no shrugging) and proper head and neck position must also be considered. See **Table 13.16** for overhead position cues.

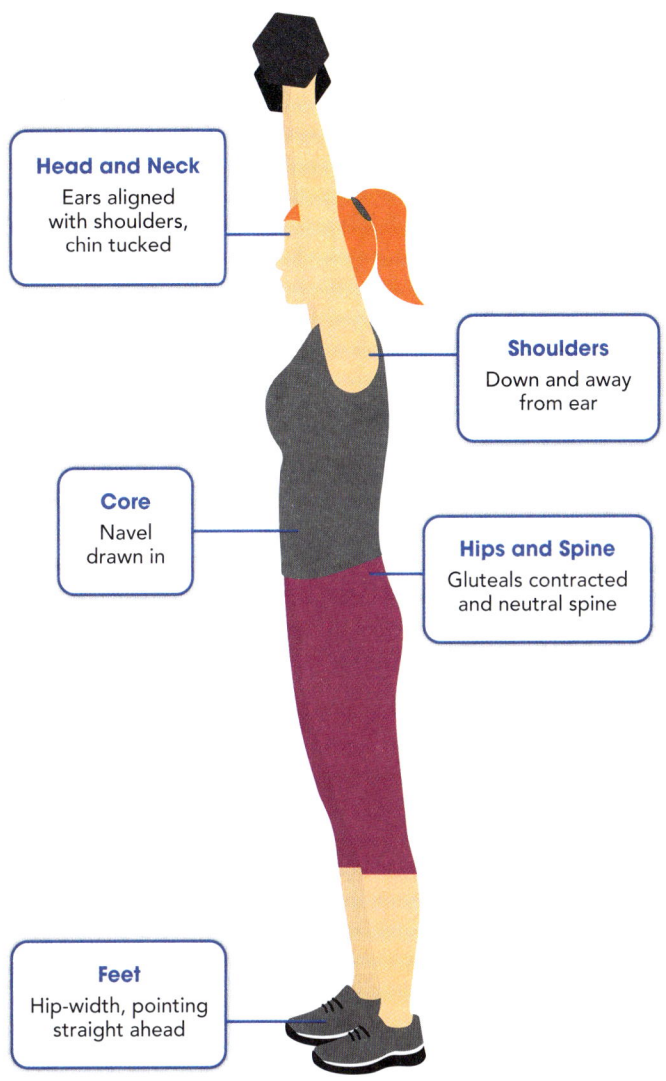

Head and Neck
Ears aligned with shoulders, chin tucked

Shoulders
Down and away from ear

Core
Navel drawn in

Hips and Spine
Gluteals contracted and neutral spine

Feet
Hip-width, pointing straight ahead

FIGURE 13.18 Overhead Position

TABLE 13.16 Cueing for Overhead Position

Verbal			
Movement Cue	**Safety Cue**	**Mastery Cue**	**Motivational Cue**
"With a strong core and neutral spine, extend your arms overhead."	"Avoid hyperextension on the elbows and overextending the lower back. Behind the neck presses should be avoided.[a] Overhead movements may not be appropriate for those with shoulder, neck, or back injuries."	"Relax your shoulders down away from your ears."	"Let's build strong shoulders and strong posture by focusing on standing tall and engaging your core and glutes."
Three-Dimensional			
Visual	**Auditory**		**Kinesthetic**
"Keep the shoulders down, the chin tucked, and the core engaged with a neutral spine" (instructor demonstrates).	"Let's see a smooth strong movement as you press the weight overhead."		"Draw your navel toward your spine as you press overhead."

(continues)

TABLE 13.16 Cueing for Overhead Position *(continued)*

Personalized		
Safety Cue	Feedback Cue	Hands-On Cue
"If you have any shoulder injuries, I will provide an alternative exercise for you."	"To reduce back discomfort, stay strong through your core and glutes as you drive overhead."	Place your hand on the top of the participant's shoulders and cue them to draw the top of their shoulders down away from your hands.

[a] Durall, C., Manske, R., & Davies, G. (2001). Avoiding shoulder injury from resistance training. *Strength and Conditioning Journal, 23*(5), 10–18. https://doi.org/10.1519/00126548-200110000-00002

Landing

Jumping and landing require much of the same joint motions (hip, knee, and ankle flexion/extension). Jumping involves acceleration, whereas landing involves deceleration of the body's weight against gravity. It is important to assess how well participants land because it imposes higher forces on the body and can be considered more challenging than jumping. It will also affect the quality of jumping motions because every subsequent jump is only as good as the landing that precedes it. Many movements require proper landing, including jumps, hops, agility drills (e.g., ice skaters), and many lower body power exercises (**Figure 13.19**). Landing can occur in multiple directions and with changes in elevation. Good cues for safe and effective landings encourage absorption of forces in soft tissues and soft, symmetrical contact with the ground. See **Table 13.17** for landing movement cues.

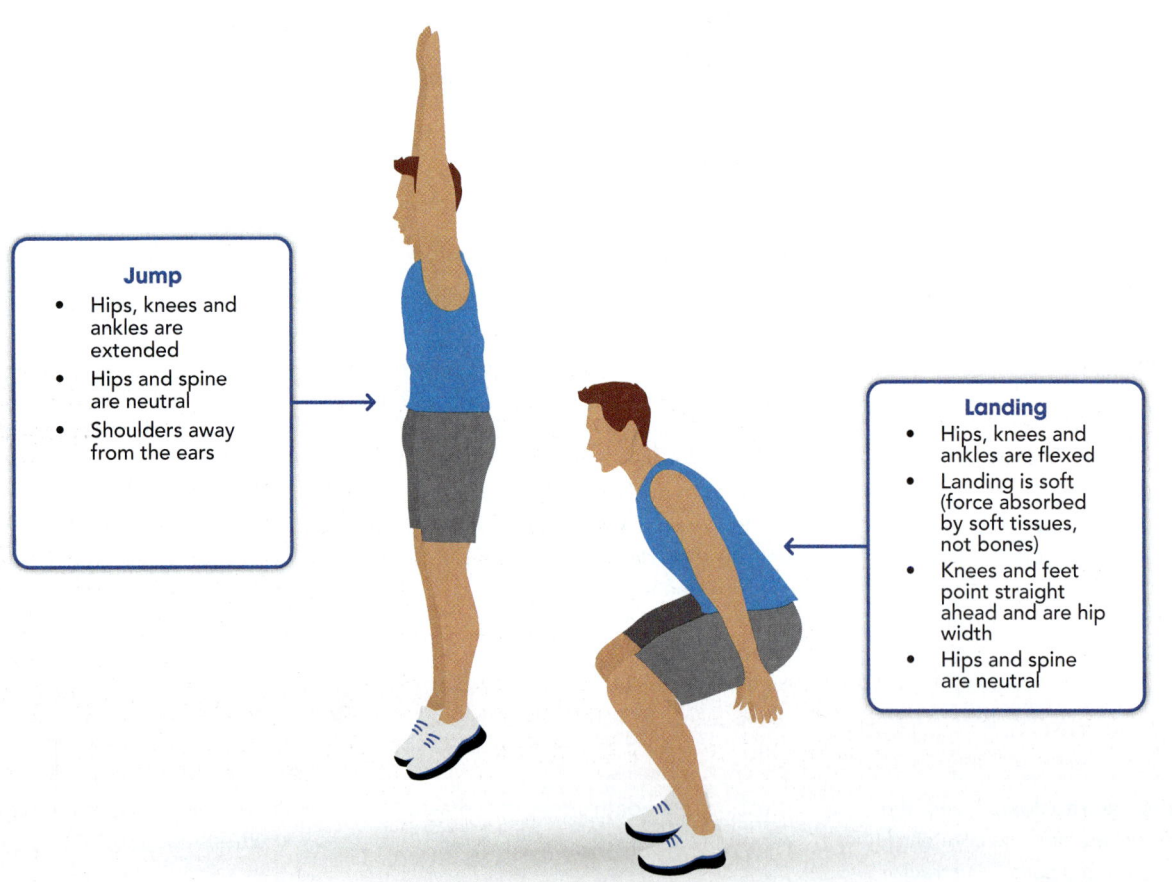

Jump
- Hips, knees and ankles are extended
- Hips and spine are neutral
- Shoulders away from the ears

Landing
- Hips, knees and ankles are flexed
- Landing is soft (force absorbed by soft tissues, not bones)
- Knees and feet point straight ahead and are hip width
- Hips and spine are neutral

FIGURE 13.19 Landing

TABLE 13.17 Cueing for Landing

Verbal			
Movement Cue	**Safety Cue**	**Mastery Cue**	**Motivational Cue**
"Land with the balls of the feet touching first and your hips and knees bending to absorb the impact."	"Be sure to land quietly and jump only to a height you can comfortably land from."	"Try to contact the ground with both feet at the same time. Land with the feet and knees pointing forward and avoid the knees caving in or bowing out."	"Your ability to land well reduces fall and injury risks in everyday life and helps create powerful legs."

Three-Dimensional		
Visual	**Auditory**	**Kinesthetic**
"The hips, knees, and ankles all flex at the same time to absorb your weight" (instructor demonstrates).	"Listen to your landing, and land softly so you barely hear your shoes hitting the floor."	"Feel your leg muscles, not bones, absorb the impact. Landings should feel soft, not stiff."

Personalized		
Safety Cue	**Feedback Cue**	**Hands-On Cue**
"If you have any back or lower body injuries, we can accomplish the same benefits without leaving the ground."	"Reduce the height of your jump to soften your landing."	Place your hand on the quads and say, "You should feel the landing in your muscles, not bones."

Building a Cue

The groundwork for verbal progression, three-dimensional, and personalized cues has been established. Now is the time to build a complete cueing experience. As a new Group Fitness Instructor, the first priority is to master the verbal cueing progression: movement, mastery, and motivational cueing. Table 13.18 provides cueing examples for a deadlift.

TABLE 13.18 Deadlift Verbal Cueing Examples

Cue Type	Cue Example	Notes
Movement	"Next, we'll perform a lower body movement: the deadlift."	Remain consistent with the exercise name.
Mastery	"Focus on engaging your glutes and hamstrings to stack your upper body on top of your hips."	Remember to offer the participants an opportunity to get the initial movement down first. Offer progressions or regressions once the base movement is established.
Motivational	"Keep working it. The deadlift is one of the best exercises to strengthen your lower body!"	Offer motivational cues that support intrinsic motivation by focusing on autonomy and competence.

Practice consistently delivering these three levels of cueing in order, keeping in mind safety, consistent naming of exercises, and delivering specific information (e.g., specific motivational cues rather than simply saying "Great job!"). Once competent with the verbal cueing progression, begin incorporating three-dimensional cues within your movement, mastery, and motivational cues, layering in visual and kinesthetic cueing in addition to auditory cueing. Let us continue with the deadlift example in **Table 13.19**.

TABLE 13.19 Three-Dimensional Cueing Examples

Cue Type	Cue Example	Notes
Visual	"Please look at the position of my back as I hinge forward. Notice I keep my shoulder blades pulled together."	Participants are focusing on what you are demonstrating.
Auditory	"Set your feet hip-width apart and prepare to hinge at your hips."	Participants are focusing on what you are saying.
Kinesthetic	"As you drive to the top and push your hips forward, you should feel your glutes and hamstrings engage to initiate the movement."	Participants are focusing on what they are feeling in their bodies.

Once auditory, visual, and kinesthetic cues have been layered into your verbal cueing progression, you are ready to move onto personalized cueing. It is most important to get participants moving correctly prior to giving personalized feedback; therefore, personalized cues often work best in a second or third set of an exercise. For the deadlift example, in the first set of deadlifts, you first provide movement cues. Once participants have grasped the general movement pattern, you add mastery and motivation cues, utilizing all three dimensions of cueing. That will be plenty of information to process for the first set of 15 deadlifts, for example. After a period of rest or when returning to deadlifts later in the workout, you can incorporate personal cues to help participants get even more out of their deadlift. **Table 13.20** provides some examples of personalized cues for a deadlift.

TABLE 13.20 Personalized Cueing Examples

Cue Type	Cue Example	Notes
Safety	"I'm noticing that this movement looks uncomfortable for you. Can I offer you an option that might be more comfortable?"	Try offering the group a general cue first and, if there is still a safety concern, approach the individual discreetly when the time is right.
Feedback	"Your lower body form looks great! Can I help you with upper body form to make sure your lower back isn't uncomfortable?"	Remember to offer positive and constructive feedback.
Hands-on	"Is it okay if I put my hand between your shoulder blades? As you hinge forward and stack back up, keep squeezing your shoulder blades together to pinch my hand."	Ask for permission before touching the participant, and let them know where you will be placing your hands.

Now it is your turn. Select two to four common group fitness exercises, such as a biceps curl or push-up, and map out examples of verbal cues, three-dimensional cues, and personalized cues.

SUMMARY

By understanding different types of cues, and how to craft them appropriately, you will not only prepare yourself to be a successful Group Fitness Instructor, but you will also help your participants be successful as well. Cueing will help your participants better understand how their body moves, how it should move, why it needs to move that way, and what can happen when they make incorrect movements. Cues can keep your participants safe and provide them with motivation. They can also guide individuals through various types of learning and stages of their personal development and enrichment. Conversely, using cues incorrectly or using poorly crafted cues can result in many problems, including injuries, discouragement, or disengagement. With the knowledge you have been provided, you have the tools necessary to create and use cues that contribute to the success of your participants.

REFERENCES

Cook, G., Burton, L., Kiesel, K., Rose, G., & Bryant, M. (2020). *Movement: Functional movement systems: Screening, assessment, corrective strategies.* On Target.

Deci, E. L., & Ryan, R. M. (1985). *Intrinsic motivation and self-determination in human behavior: Perspectives in social psychology.* Springer. https://doi.org/10.1007/978-1-4899-2271-7_3

Eisenberger, N. I., Lieberman, M. D., & Williams, K. D. (2003). Does rejection hurt? An FMRI study of social exclusion. *Science, 302*(5643), 290–292. https://doi.org/10.1126/science.1089134

Gaesser, V. J., Maakestad, W. M., Hayes, E. S., & Snyder, S. J. (2020). Motivational coaching improves intrinsic motivation in adult fitness program participants. *International Journal of Exercise Science, 13*(5), 1167–1178.

Hagger, M. S., & Chatzisarantis, N. L. D. (Eds.). (2007). *Intrinsic motivation and self-determination in exercise and sport.* Human Kinetics.

Krauss, M. (2002). The psychology of verbal communication. In N. Smelser & P. Baltes (Eds.), *International encyclopedia of the social and behavioral sciences.* Elsevier. http://www.columbia.edu/~rmk7/HC/HC_Readings/IESBS.pdf

Lind, E., Welch, A. S., & Ekkekakis, P. (2009). Do "mind over muscle" strategies work? Examining the effects of attentional association and dissociation on exertional, affective and physiological responses to exercise. *Sports Medicine, 39*(9), 743–764. https://doi.org/10.2165/11315120-000000000-00000

Menesez, L. (2020, August). *What is the mind–body connection?* Florida Medical Clinic. https://www.floridamedicalclinic.com/blog/what-is-the-mind-body-connection/

Morgan, W. P., & Pollack, M. L. (1977). Psychological characterization of the elite distance runner. *Annals of the New York Academy of Sciences, 301*, 382-403. https://doi.org/10.1111/j.1749-6632.1977.tb38215.x

Schmidt, R. A. (1975). A schema theory of discrete motor skill learning. *Psychological Review, 82*(4), 225–260. https://doi.org/10.1037/h0076770

Wu, T., Dufford, A. J., Mackie, M.-A., Egan, L. J., & Fan, J. (2016). The capacity of cognitive control estimated from a perceptual decision making task. *Scientific Reports, 6*, 34025. https://doi.org/10.1038/srep34025

Wulf, G. (2012). Motor schema. In N. M. Seel (Ed.), *Encyclopedia of the sciences of learning* (pp. 2350–2352). Springer. https://doi.org/10.1007/978-1-4419-1428-6_870

CHAPTER 14

MONITORING PARTICIPANTS AND ADAPTING TO CLASS DYNAMICS

LEARNING OBJECTIVES

The intent of this chapter is to provide an overview of monitoring techniques that can be used to assess participants' exercise technique, form, and intensity and to describe how to appropriately provide modifications to ensure the success of your participants. This module will also explore unexpected events in the group fitness setting and how to best resolve them.

After reading this content, students should be able to demonstrate the following objectives:

- **Identify** methods for monitoring participants' exercise movement, form, and posture.
- **Identify** appropriate modifications, progressions, or regressions based on observations made during monitoring.
- **Identify** methods for monitoring exercise intensity.
- **Discuss** considerations for offering group fitness classes outdoors.
- **Identify** methods for responding to unexpected variables in the group fitness setting.

Lesson 1: Monitoring Participants

Introduction

Group fitness is a dynamic environment in which no two classes are alike. Instructors must plan, practice, execute, and adapt. Instructors will encounter participants with a wide range of conditioning, unexpected environments, technical difficulties, and outside distractions, all of which

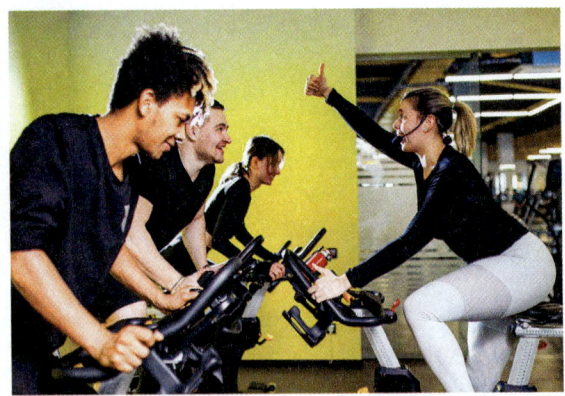
© Yurakrasil/Shutterstock

need to be handled with confidence and expertise. This ever-changing environment requires constant monitoring and modification. In this chapter, you are given the tools to develop the skills to monitor participants, translate the feedback received, and make modifications to create a seamless positive feedback loop—a system in which the Group Fitness Instructor's actions (coaching/cueing) facilitate positive change and improvement in participant's behavior (i.e., form, effort, etc.).

Positive Feedback Loops

Feedback loops are a circular system in which outputs are routed back into a system as an input, creating a cause–effect sequence (Heick, 2022). Feedback loops can be seen in all types of systems, from computers to geoscience. They are also essential tools in human learning. In a learning feedback loop, the system, in this case, the human brain, utilizes an output as an input to affect future behavior. As shown in **Figure 14.1**, an action (or output) is monitored, analyzed, and learned from, creating an input or data point. The information gathered then modifies the next output, creating a continuous loop of learning. In the case of a **POSITIVE FEEDBACK LOOP**, the input is utilized to improve on and create beneficial effects on future behavior.

> **POSITIVE FEEDBACK LOOP**
>
> A system in which output is used as an input to improve on and create beneficial effects on future behavior.

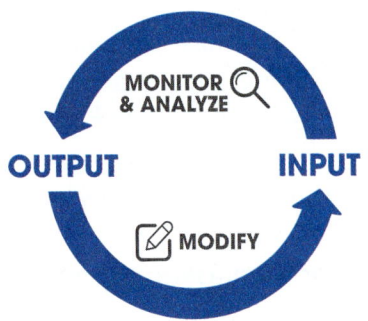

FIGURE 14.1 Feedback Loop

When applied to a group fitness setting, a positive feedback loop is a team effort between the instructor and participant. One example is when an instructor provides feedback on exercise form. The participant executes a movement (the output). The instructor observes and analyzes the participant's form and provides corrective feedback (the input). The participant then utilizes this feedback to modify their current and future form, creating a new and improved output, completing the loop.

Research has demonstrated that feedback that provides specific information relating to a given task can have significant effects on learning and achievement (Hattie & Timperley, 2007). However, note that the relationship between the feedback-giver and the feedback-receiver is critical (Wiliam, 2017). As leaders of the group fitness experience, building rapport and trust is as essential as being specific for effective feedback. Once a trusting relationship is established, an instructor can utilize positive feedback loops to produce beneficial improvements in participant behavior and outcomes. Here is an example of basic positive feedback in action:

> "When I go to bed early (input), I feel well rested (output). Therefore, I am going to focus on going to bed an hour earlier (modification), which results in my feeling well rested more often (future output)."

Consider the following example for within the group fitness environment:

A participant is performing a side plank (action/output). The instructor observes that the participant is holding most of their weight in their shoulder, creating undue stress in the shoulder joint (information gathered from observation). The instructor cues the participant to slightly raise their hips and engage their glutes, adductors, abdominals, and obliques (input). The participant follows the instructor's cues and feels the stress release from their shoulder and more targeted core engagement (modification). They then remember this feedback to positively affect their form when performing a side plank in the future (future output).

For an effective positive feedback loop to occur, successful Group Fitness Instructors hone their observation and feedback skills. Strong knowledge of proper form and muscle activation is needed to provide accurate and specific feedback. In a large group, the instructor must constantly be on the lookout for needed corrections and opportunities for improvement.

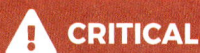 **CRITICAL**

Notice that in the plank example the observation is of a positive benefit: *core engaged = stronger abdominal muscles*. This positive observation leads to a positive modification: *Do more of that*. This can also occur as a negative feedback loop, an observation that leads to a negative outcome: *My back hurts when I squat*. This leads to a negative input: *Squatting is bad*, which leads to a negative modification and future output: *I am not going to squat anymore*.

Without the guidance of a qualified instructor, participants can easily fall into negative feedback loops, which affect their long-term emotions and attitudes toward exercise. Consequently, it is the role of the Group Fitness Instructor to guide participants into positive feedback loops through learning and problem solving, rather than critiquing and focusing on errors or negative outcomes. Authors Connie Moss and Susan Brookhart (2019) call the moment when a student takes feedback, makes changes, and moves closer toward improvement and desired outcomes the "golden second opportunity." Our interactions with participants should strive to create these types of experiences.

Monitoring Participants

To start a positive feedback loop in motion, an instructor should constantly monitor participants and look for opportunities to provide positive feedback. Within the scope of a class, there are many areas for an instructor to monitor. These areas can be categorized by their focus and include safety, movement comprehension, intensity, and engagement.

Safety

Recall that safety is the instructor's highest priority. You must monitor participant form, range of motion, equipment, and the surrounding environment and be aware of injuries, discomfort, and movement contraindications. By closely monitoring form, an instructor can recognize fatigue or intensity that is too high or low and reduce overall participant risk.

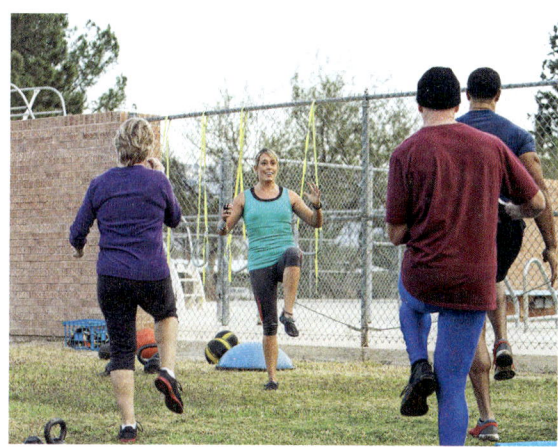

© CREATISTA/Shutterstock

For example, if a regular class participant with normally excellent form is dropping their hips and arching their back while holding a plank, this might indicate overtraining, fatigue, or muscle and joint discomfort. If a new class participant is struggling to extend their arms in an overhead press, this might indicate that the weight is too heavy, they do not have the necessary flexibility, or they are experiencing discomfort, and alternative movement options are required. It is your job as an instructor to intervene to ensure that movement is safe at all points during a workout.

 INSTRUCTOR TIP

Common form errors to monitor include, but are not limited to:

- **Prone positions:** Hips and back sagging toward the floor; chin jutting toward floor.
- **Supine positions:** Lower back excessively arching without core activation (often appears as ribs extending toward the ceiling).
- **Upper body exercises:** Shoulders rounding forward and/or shrugging, chin jutting forward, and excessive lower back arch (particularly during overhead movements).
- **Lower body exercises:** Heels lifting off the floor (front heel in split stance positions) and knees collapsing inward or bowing outward.

The surrounding environment must be monitored for obstacles and potential risks. Equipment left around the room can cause participants to trip. Small children running into the group fitness space can be dangerous. A water bottle spilled on the floor can pose a slipping hazard. If anything like this should occur, you should pause class to fix the situation and ensure everyone's safety.

Equipment must also be observed for safety. Equipment can be broken or incorrectly used, which can lead to injury. The instructor should check all equipment prior to class and then continuously monitor its use throughout the workout.

Common equipment items to monitor include, but are not limited to:

- Step platforms not properly placed on risers
- Worn bands
- Bar clips not properly secured
- Slippery mats and floors
- Underinflated stability balls
- Faulty locking mechanisms on indoor cycles or other equipment with multiple adjustment points

Safety feedback should be given immediately and not withheld until after class or until the situation is repeated. Any malfunctioning or broken equipment should also be removed from the workout area or labeled as out of order and reported to the proper staff.

Movement Comprehension

Incorrect form does not always mean a lack of fitness, bodily discomfort, or a lack of coordination. Sometimes participants simply do not understand what is being asked of them; maybe an exercise description did not make sense, or a cardio combination was not clear. The instructor

Even in a safety situation, you can create a positive feedback loop. Begin by bringing attention to the concern; explain why it is unsafe, which can maximize the learning opportunity; and then teach the participant how to fix the issue in the present moment, which will lead to future positive modifications.

For example, an instructor may say something like this: "Violet, the safety clips on your bar are not secured. This can be dangerous as the weights may fall off and injure you or someone else. Here is how to secure the clips."

should monitor for feedback that may indicate that the participant does not understand, such as incorrect form, standing and watching, or doing the wrong exercise or pattern.

If you suspect a lack of comprehension, monitoring and analyzing might require explaining the exercise or movement pattern in a new way. For example, if you relied on verbal cues the first time around, try utilizing a different approach, such as describing the movement using imagery or including a physical demonstration. If this corrects the issue, then you have gathered valuable information for what style of communication is best for those instructions. If this does not correct the issue, then perhaps a lack of comprehension is not the culprit, and the instructor may need to consider modifying the exercise altogether, or the effort demanded. Either way, the outcome is creating a positive feedback loop for you as an instructor. You have utilized the output the group is providing to modify your cueing behavior for future success.

Intensity

Every group fitness class is driven toward a specific outcome. Whether the goal is building total-body strength, increasing cardiorespiratory conditioning, improving flexibility, or strengthening the mind–body connection, intensity is a key component to achieving the goal. Therefore, an instructor should establish and teach a protocol for monitoring intensity. Training intensities are often grouped into training zones, which can be monitored in multiple ways. Common methods found in the group fitness setting include the rate of perceived exertion (RPE), heart rate monitoring, and talk tests, which are used alone or in combination to delineate and monitor training zones.

RATING OF PERCEIVED EXERTION

Rating of perceived exertion (RPE) is a subjective measurement of physical activity intensity. Exercisers rate their physical effort on a scale of 1–10 based on factors such as breathing rate, sweating, muscle fatigue, and the amount of time they are able to persist at the current level of intensity (Centers for Disease Control and Prevention, 2022). RPE provides a means of assessing intensity without the use of formulas or wearable devices, and, even though it is subjective, it is closely rated to objective measures of intensity such as lactate threshold and heart rate across a wide range of demographics and fitness levels (Scherr et al., 2013). Thus, RPE serves as an effective and reliable means to gauge training intensity in a group fitness setting.

In addition to the scale numbers 1–10, the RPE scale provides brief descriptions of the effort that accompanies each number. As a Group Fitness Instructor, you can expand on these descriptions to allow for more understanding and personalization of the information. For example, at an RPE of 6, an exerciser may feel that they are beginning to feel uncomfortable, their breathing

The original RPE scale was the Borg 6–20 scale. The Borg 6–20 scale is the research standard, but it can be somewhat confusing because it starts at a score of 6 (rather than 1 or 0) and has 15 different choices. The reason behind the 6–20 scale is that each value corresponds to a heart rate, and most adult heart rates range between 60 BPM and 200 BPM. Subsequently, a Borg score of 6 corresponds to a heart rate of 60 BPM, whereas a Borg score of 12 corresponds to a heart rate of 120 BPM. However, for simplicity and ease of use, AFAA recommends that group fitness professionals use the newer 1–10 RPE scale with their participants.

rate has increased, and they are now sweating. A description of feelings helps the RPE scale become more relatable. A simple number might not be meaningful to participants, but when that number is related to how they will feel, it becomes understandable. **Table 14.1** expands on the RPE scale to include examples of descriptive words that help communicate the desired result.

TABLE 14.1 Rating of Perceived Exertion Scale with Descriptors

RPE	Effort	Descriptors
10	Maximal	Feels impossible to keep going, cannot maintain
9	Really, really hard	High intensity, can barely breathe, can only continue for 30 seconds or less
8	Really hard	Uncomfortable, on the edge, maximum 1–2 minutes of effort at this level
7		Challenging, breathing hard, moving out of comfort zone
6	Hard	Strong working effort, sweating, starting to feel uncomfortable
5	Moderate	Effort level a person could maintain for an hour
4		Breathing rate is increasing, starting to work
3	Easy	Warm-up effort, preparing to work, easily maintainable
2	Really easy	Walking into class, breathing easily
1	At rest	Awake but still, not active to very light

⚙ PRACTICE THIS

Work out using the RPE scale and come up with your own descriptions of how each effort feels.

Utilizing RPE in a class setting requires education and understanding. Begin with a brief description of the RPE scale in the class warm-up as it relates to the goals of the workout. For example:

"In cycling class today, we are going to work on improving our cardiorespiratory performance. We'll keep our effort in check using a 1 to 10 scale. One represents rest and 10 is your all-out, maximal effort. We are going to focus on working at a 6 to 7, which should feel challenging and begin to take you out of your comfort zone. Throughout the workout, I will ask you to check in on your rating to be sure you are reaching your goals."

Then, continue to cue RPE throughout the body of the workout using a variety of methods to describe the desired effort, including how hard they should be breathing, the length of time they could continue the effort, and any other descriptions you like to use. For example:

"For the next 3 minutes, we will hold our intensity at a 7. This should feel hard; you will be breathing heavily and pushing to get to the end of the effort, but you will be a stronger rider when we get there."

MONITORING HEART RATE

Heart rate reflects your body's cardiorespiratory response to work. Simply put, as intensity increases, heart rate increases until a maximum, unsustainable level is reached. An individual's heart rate can be affected by numerous factors beyond exercise intensity (**Table 14.2**). Some of these factors are internal and others external. Instructors should familiarize themselves with factors that can affect heart rate in order to have a better understanding of intensity.

TABLE 14.2 Factors Affecting Heart Rate Beyond Exercise Intensity

Internal Factors	
Hydration	Dehydration can cause heart rate levels to elevate.
Fuel	Different exercise intensities use different forms of fuel. If the body does not have enough fuel specific to the required energy system, heart rate can increase.
Sleep	A lack of sleep can lead to elevated heart rate.
Medical conditions	Many medical conditions and medications can result in an atypical heart rate response. Therefore, it is important that participants with any medical conditions consult a physician prior to starting an exercise program.
Emotional state	Emotions such as anxiety and stress can affect heart rate.
External Factors	
Temperature	Hot conditions can cause heart rate to increase; cold conditions can decrease the heart rate.
Humidity	High humidity can increase heart rate.
Elevation	At higher altitudes, heart rate may increase due to the lower air pressure.
Caffeine and other drugs	Caffeine is a stimulant that can increase heart rate. Some drugs, such as beta-blockers, can decrease an individual's heart rate, making a physician's evaluation critical.

USING FORMULAS TO ESTIMATE HEART RATE ZONES

Several methods have been developed that use heart rate to delineate training zones and measure intensity. One method involves determining the **MAXIMAL HEART RATE (HR$_{MAX}$)**. Maximal heart rate is the fastest rate an individual's heart can beat in 1 minute. Maximal heart rate can be tested in a few ways, including maximal exercise testing and submaximal exercise testing; both require a controlled testing environment under the supervision of a trained professional, such as in a medical or laboratory setting. As an alternative to heart rate testing, a standardized formula can be used to estimate HR$_{max}$. Although not as accurate as controlled maximal heart rate testing, standardized formulas offer a starting point and a more accessible option in a fitness setting. Arguably the most commonly used HR$_{max}$ formula is 220 – Age = HR$_{max}$. Heart rate training zones can also be created using talk tests. This process will be explained later.

It is important to note that the HR$_{max}$ formula was never intended to be used as a tool to design cardiorespiratory fitness programming, because maximal heart rate varies significantly among individuals of the same age (Kolata, 2001).

Additional, more applicable formulas have been developed to estimate HR$_{max}$ and training zones, including the **TANAKA FORMULA** and **HEART RATE RESERVE (HRR)** (also known as the Karvonen method). These methods create **HEART RATE TRAINING ZONES** divided by percentages of HR$_{max}$. The Tanaka formula is deemed more accurate than Haskell's calculation of 220 – Age (Roy & McCrory, 2015). It can be used to create HR training zones by simply multiplying the desired **TARGET HEART RATE** percentage by the calculated HR$_{max}$. However, HRR may be the most appropriate in the fitness setting because it also considers the individual's **RESTING HEART RATE (HR$_{REST}$)** in addition to their HR$_{max}$. If a training target heart rate calculation is desired, use the Tanaka formula to create HR$_{max}$, then plug that into the HRR formula to determine the target heart rates for the training zone categories. It is common to see target heart rate ranges divided into three, four, or five zones depending on the population and training needs. **Table 14.3** shows examples of heart rate training ranges divided into different zones.

Group fitness professionals should never use mathematical formulas as an absolute, because a person's heart rate response to exercise is dependent on many additional factors that a formula does not account for. However, these formulas are simple to use and can be easily implemented as a general starting point for measuring cardiorespiratory training intensity and are best used in conjunction with RPE and/or talk tests. Heart rate can be monitored through several methods. The most common methods are chest straps, which utilize electrodes to measure heart rate, and optical sensors, which utilize light to measure pulse at the wrist (optical sensors are found in many smartwatches or fitness wearables). Both can be very effective to measure intensity in a group fitness setting if participants are wearing them and participants know their personal heart rate ranges. Heart rate can also be measured manually by taking your pulse at the radial artery at your wrist (on the thumb side) or the carotid artery at your neck. However, this method can slow down the flow of a class, is not always executed correctly by participants, and still requires an understanding of heart rate ranges. For this reason, experienced Group Fitness Instructors use a combination of strategies to communicate and observe effort, including RPE and talk tests.

TALK TEST

A **TALK TEST** is another method used to gauge exercise intensity. In the past, the talk test was used as an informal method of determining light versus moderate workload (i.e., the ability to speak comfortably). As a Group Fitness Instructor, you can expand upon early versions of the talk test and apply the concept in a class setting. Essentially, you will assess an individual's training zone by observing and listening to them. **Table 14.4** provides an example of talk test categories and how they relate to effort. Fortunately for the exercise community, research has

---

MAXIMAL HEART RATE (HR$_{MAX}$)

The fastest rate an individual's heart can beat in 1 minute.

TANAKA FORMULA

A formula used to estimate an individual's maximal heart rate: HR$_{max}$ = 208 – (0.7 × Age). Percentages of HR$_{max}$ are used to create training zone estimates.

HEART RATE RESERVE (HRR)

Also called the Karvonen method; a formula used to calculate exercise target heart rates that takes into account maximal heart rate and resting heart rate: [(HR$_{max}$ – HR$_{rest}$) × Desired intensity percentage] + HR$_{rest}$ = Target heart rate.

HEART RATE TRAINING ZONES

Often calculated as a percentage of maximal heart rate. Heart rate values are divided into functional ranges used to gauge intensity and develop particular forms of cardiorespiratory fitness.

TABLE 14.3 Heart Rate Training Zone Examples

Five Training Zones		Four Training Zones		Three Training Zones	
HR Training Zone	Target HR Range as Percentage of HR_{max}	HR Training Zone	Target HR Range as Percentage of HR_{max}	HR Training Zone	Target HR Range as Percentage of HR_{max}
1 (Very light)	50–59%	1 (Light)	50–59%	1 (Low)	65–74%
2 (Light)	60–69%	2 (Moderate)	60–69%	2 (Moderate)	75–84%
3 (Moderate)	70–79%	3 (Hard)	70–79%	3 (High)	85%+
4 (Hard)	80–89%	4 (Maximum)	80–89%		
5 (Maximum)	90–100%				

TABLE 14.4 Descriptive Talk Test

Effort	Description
Warm-up and recovery effort	Easily holds a conversation
Moderate effort	Can say a few sentences at a time
Hard effort	Can say a few words at a time
Maximum effort	Prefers not to speak

TARGET HEART RATE

A predetermined exercising heart rate.

RESTING HEART RATE (HR_REST)

The number of heart beats per minute when at complete rest.

TALK TEST

A self-evaluation of intensity associated with the ability to talk while exercising.

shown that changes in an individual's ability to speak and breathe signal when their fuel metabolism shifts in response to exercise intensity. These studies have also shown a strong relationship between the talk test and exercise heart rate (Foster et al., 2008; Jeans et al., 2011; Persinger et al., 2004; Quinn & Coons, 2011; Recalde et al., 2002; Reed & Pipe, 2016). This means that the talk test is a valid and reliable way to monitor and create exercise training zones.

GETTING TECHNICAL

Talk tests work because of an exercise science concept called ventilatory threshold (VT) points. These are points during increasing exercise intensity where a person's ability to comfortably speak and breathing rate shift. These "breathing shift points" align with fuel system changes (e.g., shifting from aerobic to anaerobic metabolism). Ventilatory threshold 1 (VT1) is when breathing becomes audible with some signs of rib cage elevation as intensity increases. At VT1, the body is shifting from metabolizing primarily fat to an equal mix of carbohydrates and fat as fuel sources. Ventilatory threshold 2 (VT2) is noted when an individual prefers not to speak or will only provide a one-word answer. At VT2, metabolism has shifted to using primarily carbohydrates for almost all energy demands. Working just below VT2 is considered a person's maximal sustainable effort (i.e., as hard as a person can exercise for more than a few minutes) and may be considered as a point where an exerciser could provide just a few words before needing to take a breath.

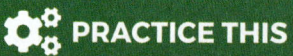
Work out using the talk test and come up with your own descriptions of how each effort feels.

USING TALK TESTS TO CREATE TRAINING ZONES

Figure 14.2 shows how talk tests and VT markers can be used to create zones. Heart rate and RPE can be combined with the talk test in marking transitions from one zone to another. Once an exerciser matches the description of the zone, they simply note their heart rate or RPE and use those to mark ranges. For example, an exerciser may be breathing harder and audibly and notice that speaking is becoming challenging. They would be considered to be in training Zone 2. They can take their heart rate or assign an RPE at that point and use it as an indicator of being in Zone 2 in the future. New participants can be encouraged to work at an intensity that is challenging, but doable because there are benefits from the light intensity at the onset of training (Swain & Franklin, 2002).

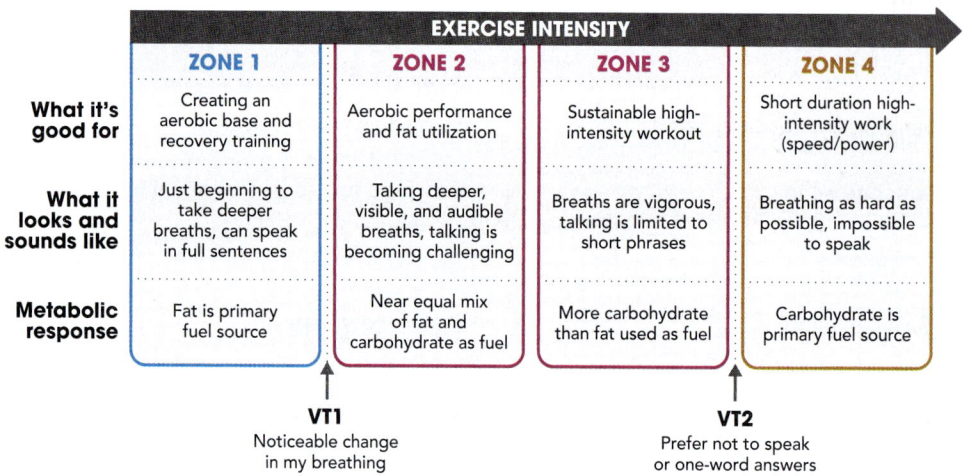

FIGURE 14.2 Training Zones Based on Talk Test

KEY TAKEAWAYS FOR MONITORING INTENSITY

The following are the key takeaways for monitoring exercise intensity:

- Heart rate, RPE, and talk tests are all different ways to monitor intensity and create training zones.
- Zones created based on heart rate formulas are estimates and a good starting point, but they do not consider the wide variance in heart rate response among individuals.
- RPE is a simple and valid way to gauge intensity.
- RPE and talk tests correlate well with physiological responses to exercise such as heart rate, making them valid ways to create zones and gauge intensity.
- A talk test can be used to create training zones alone or in combination with RPE and heart rate.
- A Group Fitness Instructor can use these methods to create work blocks with specific intensities in mind, easily describe how different training zones should feel to their participants, and identify which zone they are in.

Engagement

All participants come to group fitness classes with their own set of experiences, goals, expectations, and ability levels. No matter how well planned your class is, some participants may disengage for various reasons. It is important to understand how to recognize disengagement and use strategic actions to keep participants engaged throughout the workout. An instructor can monitor engagement levels by observing participants' verbal and nonverbal behavior. **Table 14.5** outlines indications of engagement compared to signs of disengagement (Goman, 2022). If participants appear disengaged, an instructor should focus on positive ways to reconnect them to the group and the workout (**Figure 14.3**).

TABLE 14.5 Engaged Versus Disengaged Listeners

Signs of Engagement	Signs of Disengagement
Eye contact	Eyes looking downward or around the room
Open posture with eyes up, shoulders open, hands at side, and slight lean in toward the speaker	Closed posture with arms crossed, head down, and shoulders rounded
Offering verbal responses to the instructor	Talking to other participants when the instructor is speaking
Nodding, smiling, and laughing	Not offering gestures of approval
Following cues and instructions	Ignoring cues and not following along
Facing you head-on when receiving instructions or feedback	Facing away or busy with other tasks when receiving instructions or feedback
Mirroring of instructor's body language	Not matching the instructor's body language

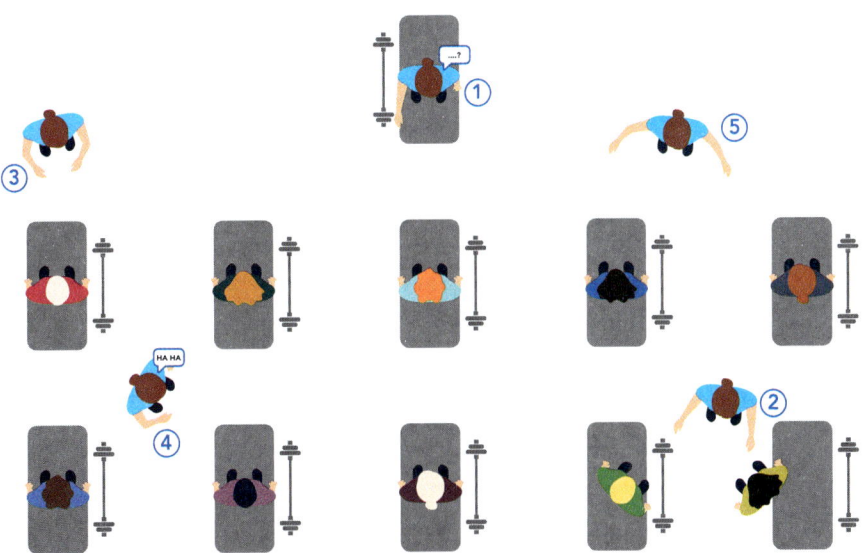

1. **Ask questions** – Pose questions to the group that require them to answer aloud.
2. **Pair up** – Include a partner or group drill/exercise such as partner band work or circling up for a group plank hold.
3. **Let them choose** – Provide the group with two options for the next set and let them choose what they will do next.
4. **Lighten the mood** – Tell an appropriate joke or story to lighten the mood and reenergize the class.
5. **Give them space** – Let participants know they are free to have their own experience and to listen to their bodies.

FIGURE 14.3 Engaging Participants

Lesson 2: Modifications

Providing Modifications

Once an instructor has monitored the group and gathered feedback, it is time to decide what to do with that information. A **MODIFICATION** is an alteration to an exercise or movement, including progressions, regressions, and alternative movement selections. A modification offers a path to improve an individual's performance. The following are questions you can consider to determine if a modification is needed.

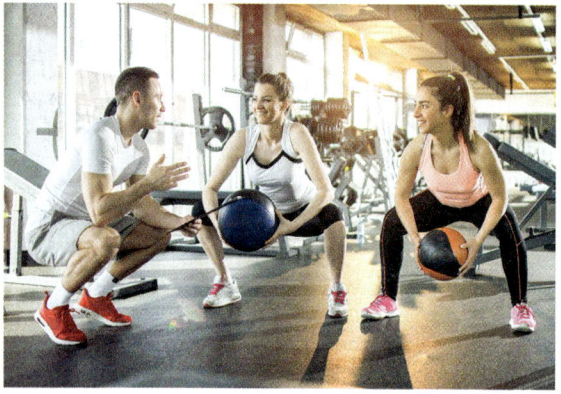

© Bojan Milinkov/Shutterstock

What Is the Priority?

You will gather a lot of information over the course of a class. There is neither the time nor the need to correct everything at once. Therefore, you must prioritize. The first priority is always safety. If something unsafe is being observed, it must be addressed immediately. Next is the class vision or objective. Modifications should align with the focus and goal of the workout. A yoga instructor might not concern themselves with heart rate zones, and a dance format might not focus on movement precision. However, a boot camp class might be very engaged with RPE, and a strength training class might focus on range of motion and form. It might also be beneficial to select a specific focus for the day. For example, a core class might focus on breathing for a given workout or a beginner class might emphasize engagement over intensity during the first week it meets.

Is the Modification a Necessity or an Enhancement?

An instructor must remember that learning takes place over time (Wiliam, 2017). With that in mind, not everything needs to be addressed immediately. Therefore, it is prudent to determine if a modification is a necessity or an enhancement. If it is needed to ensure safety, execute the proper form, or progress to the next section of the class, then it is a necessity, and a modification should be made. However, if the modification is an enhancement, such as an advanced way to perform an exercise or an advanced choreography option, then it is worth selecting a few enhancements per class rather than overwhelming the group with too many modifications to avoid cognitive overload (Morse, 2004).

 INSTRUCTOR TIP

Enhancements should be included as part of the workout planning process. When developing a workout, include a few enhancements, or advanced movement options, to offer in the workout. By pre-planning these, you will ensure that you do not overwhelm the class with too many options.

Is the Modification Needed by the Entire Group or by Select Individuals?

While monitoring participants, you will see areas that can be improved for the entire group and areas of modification for select individuals. For example, you might observe most of the class can slightly increase the depth of their squat, and you might notice that one participant is putting their weight into their toes when squatting to a lower depth. Both observations require modifications that are valid and should be addressed; however, they should be addressed in different ways. For example, you may give the group a challenge (progression) by asking them to hold the bottom of their squat static, and then encourage everyone to lower their hips by half an inch, and then another half an inch, until their range of motion is correct. However, for the one participant, it may be best to approach them individually during the squat section of class and ask them to sit their hips back a bit further and shift their weight into their heels.

These general questions are part of analyzing what has been observed. The answers become input, which then leads to modifications and future outputs.

Progressions

A progression is a modification that increases the demand of an exercise or movement combination (Miller, n.d.). Progressions are appropriate for participants who have mastered both the form of an exercise and require increased demand to achieve the desired intensity. A progression can come in several forms, including cardiorespiratory intensity, weight or resistance, compound movements, and base of support.

CARDIORESPIRATORY INTENSITY

Each class participant will possess a unique level of cardiorespiratory fitness. By utilizing one or a combination of the intensity measurements discussed earlier, an instructor can standardize the workout goals; for example, challenging all participants to work at a 7 on an RPE scale or noting that everyone should feel near, but not fully, breathless.

In order for all participants to achieve the same intensity goal, some participants might need to progress an exercise or movement pattern. For example, Michael might achieve an RPE of 7 by walking forward and back in a cardio dance format; however, Tanya might need to run up and back to achieve an RPE of 7. Accordingly, the instructor can offer a running progression as an option to achieve the desired intensity.

To create a positive feedback loop in this example, the instructor first observes the class for signs of intensity, including breathing challenge and form. Next, they reinforce the goal and create a learning opportunity by explaining what an RPE of 7 should feel like and the benefits of the intensity level. Then, the instructor offers progressions to those who are not yet at an RPE of 7. Here is an example of this in action:

> "Let's walk up and back. The goal is to reach a 7 on a 1 to 10 scale. You should be working and breathing hard but at a maintainable effort. This is where serious conditioning happens! If you are not yet at a 7, turn that walk into a jog."

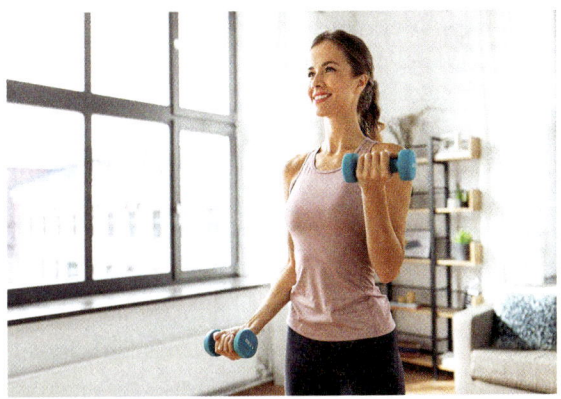

LOAD OR RESISTANCE

An exercise can also be progressed by adding or increasing load or resistance. This can be achieved with dumbbells, resistance bands,

© Ground Picture/Shutterstock

 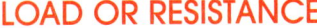

weighted bars, medicine balls, or kettlebells to name a few. It is important to remember that form can be adversely affected when weight is introduced or increased, so you should repeat form cues and monitor participants' movements.

Progressions are often most effective when performed in small increments (Miller, n.d.). An instructor can implement resistance progressions in small increments as participants build strength. For example, have participants perform 10 overhead shoulder presses with 10-pound dumbbells and then perform the final 5 repetitions increasing to 12-pound dumbbells. Or, program 30 seconds of side-to-side shuffles and then add a resistance band for the final 15 seconds of the interval. Encourage participants to reflect on each incremental progression. For example:

> "As you added weight to your overhead press, did you feel any tension in your neck? The goal is to keep the emphasis on the shoulders. So, if you felt your neck take over, let's keep it at 10 pounds next time to optimize our shoulder activation."

This type of input can lead to more beneficial future outputs.

COMPOUND MOVEMENTS

A compound movement is an exercise in which multiple muscle groups and joints are engaged at one time. The more muscle groups engaged, the more complex and challenging the exercise becomes (e.g., barbell row, chest press, or squat). Compound movements require more neuromuscular coordination, stability, and movement efficiency when compared to single-joint movements (e.g., biceps curl, triceps extension, or calf raise). Compound exercises also increase heart rate and calorie expenditure due to the increased energy requirement.

You can progress a single-joint exercise to a compound movement by adding additional movement patterns or joint motions. For example, a biceps curl can become a compound exercise with the addition of a forward-stepping lunge or an overhead press. Similarly, a supine triceps extension can become a compound exercise with the addition of a static bridge hold. You can also create compound movements by adding plyometric activities (e.g., jumping down from a box), the upper body reaches (e.g., lunge with an overhead reach), or different footwork patterns (e.g., fast feet).

BASE OF SUPPORT

Stability is another important consideration for progressing exercise demand, and it is greatly affected by the base of support. The **BASE OF SUPPORT (BOS)** is determined by the area created by the points of contact between an exerciser and a stable surface. A greater BOS is created by more, or more effective, points of contact. For example, standing on two feet provides a greater BOS and, therefore, is more stable than standing on one foot. A position is also more stable when the points of contact are wider. For example, a two-foot basic stance is more stable than a two-foot staggered stance, as seen in a lunge. The point of support is not solely determined by foot placement, though. Points of contact can be your gluteals, knees, hands, elbows, or back. For example, a seated position provides a greater BOS than standing; therefore, it is more stable. A quadruped position with feet, knees, and hands on the ground is more stable than the same position but with one arm and one leg extended. Performing a quadriceps stretch with one hand on the wall is more stable than freestanding. Laying supine with knees bent and feet on the floor provides a greater BOS than prone with legs extended out with feet hovering above the floor. A larger BOS provides more stability; however, when the BOS is decreased, demands for balance, coordination, and muscular engagement are increased, which, in turn, increases the intensity of an exercise. **Table 14.6** provides examples of how to progress an exercise by decreasing the BOS.

TABLE 14.6 Progression Examples Through Base of Support

Foundational Exercise	BOS Progression
Squat	Squat to knee hugger
Overhead triceps extension	Overhead triceps extension in lunge stance
Plank	Plank with single-leg lift
Dumbbell front raise	Front raise with single-leg balance
Seated stability ball biceps curl	Seated stability ball with single-leg lifted Biceps curl
Supine hip bridge	Supine hip bridge with single-leg extension at the top

When progressing BOS, you can encourage participants to create a positive feedback loop by altering support in small increments. For example, when moving from a hip-width, two-foot stance to something less stable, provide incremental options and allow participants to use their body's own feedback to adjust. For example, an instructor could say:

> "Okay, team! We're going to make our squats on this round a little more challenging for our balance. Start by moving one foot back a few inches and allowing that back heel to come up as you drop. If that feels good, try lifting that back foot off entirely and just hover it off the ground a couple of inches. Choose the option that you can stick with for the next 30 seconds. Let's go!"

Base of support can also be altered by introducing **PROPRIOCEPTIVE CHALLENGES** in the form of unstable surfaces, such as a sport beam, foam pad, or BOSU. Note that using an unstable surface can be a safety hazard, and an adequate BOS challenge can be achieved using upper or lower body position modifications instead. Using an unstable surface of any kind may also violate the policies of your facility. It is wise to check with the appropriate staff before introducing unstable surfaces in a group setting. **Table 14.7** outlines the relative challenges of modifications to the base of support.

> **PROPRIO-CEPTIVE CHALLENGES**
>
> Demands placed on the body's ability to sense its position and maintain its stability.

TABLE 14.7 Base of Support Progression

Proprioceptive Challenge	Surface Stability	Lower Body	Upper Body	Full Body
Foundational	Floor	Two-leg	Two arms at the same time	More points of contact with the ground
	Sport beam	Staggered stance	Alternating arms	
	Half foam roll	Single-leg	Single-arm	
	Foam pad	Two-leg (unstable surface)	Single-arm with motion (e.g., trunk rotation)	
	Balance disc	Staggered stance (unstable surface)		
	Wobble board	Single-leg (unstable surface)		Fewer points of contact with the ground
Advanced				

CUEING PROGRESSION

Understanding that safety is the priority means that progressions are not appropriate for all class participants; therefore, it is essential to cue progressions in a way that communicates this message. If an instructor cues progressions as "the better option" or for those who are "more fit" or "more advanced," they can risk alienating class participants or pressuring individuals to progress when it might not be appropriate. In order to minimize this pressure, you will benefit by enacting a positive feedback loop in which participants understand the goal of an exercise, observe the feedback their body is providing, and then utilize that feedback to evaluate if a progression is appropriate. This practice teaches participants to self-monitor and build autonomy.

This concept may seem daunting for a new instructor; however, it can be accomplished through education. Make the most of opportunities to teach class participants the why, not just the what:

- "Why do you utilize the RPE scale to monitor intensity? To ensure the desired workout effect is achieved."
- "Why is pain in the body bad? Because pain can indicate improper form, or a lack of joint stability, reducing safety."
- "Why can't you maintain your balance? Stabilizer muscles are not yet accustomed to working in this way."

With knowledge, participants are empowered to make the right decision for themselves.

To avoid undermining self-empowerment and inclusivity it is best to avoid statements such as the following:

- "If this is too easy …"
- "If you are feeling strong/fit today, you can …"
- "Those of you who are advanced should …"

Instead, state the intensity or goal for the given exercise or interval and then provide modification options to help individuals achieve that result. For example:

- "Twenty more lunges to finish out your leg work for today. At the end of this set, you should have nothing left in those quads. Are you there? If not, hold each lunge at the bottom for a three count before you rise."
- "The goal of the Russian twist is to create tension in your abs and not your back. Try extending your legs straight, as long as you can maintain stress on your abdominals. If your experience back tension, just bring your legs back in."
- "The intensity goal of this interval is an RPE of 8. Are you at an 8? If not, add a jump to that squat."

⚙ PRACTICE THIS

Select a common exercise, such as a supine chest press. Write down proper form for the exercise and how this form relates to the exercise goal. Next, script how you can communicate this goal in clear and concise language. Now, make a list of ways you can progress the selected exercise to increase intensity. Script how you can communicate these progressions focusing on educating and avoiding "better than" language.

Regressions

In contrast to a progression, a regression is a modification that decreases the demand of an exercise or movement combination (Miller, n.d.). Regressions can be described in the same categories as progressions: cardiorespiratory intensity, load or resistance, compound movements, and base of support.

CARDIORESPIRATORY INTENSITY

Monitoring cardiorespiratory intensity through heart rate, RPE, and/or a talk test can prove to be an essential tool in enabling participants of varying fitness levels to all benefit from the same workout. If an RPE of 6 is prescribed, an individual new to exercise can reach the same relative intensity as a seasoned class participant. The instructor can explain that an RPE of 6 feels like a strong working effort that is beginning to feel uncomfortable, and then cue the group to walk, jog, or run to reach, but not exceed, an effort level of 6. In a similar vein, the instructor can inform participants that their effort should not exceed their comfort zone during this portion of the workout; therefore, they should walk if they cannot control their breath. If heart rate monitors are being used, the instructor can recommend specific heart rate zones according to the goal of the effort. For example, cue all participants to select a walk, jog, or run to maintain a Zone 3 effort, and communicate what Zone 3 should feel like. Utilizing a standard of communicating and understanding intensity measurements can provide a method to observe performance and, therefore, provide positive feedback. For example, a participant may think:

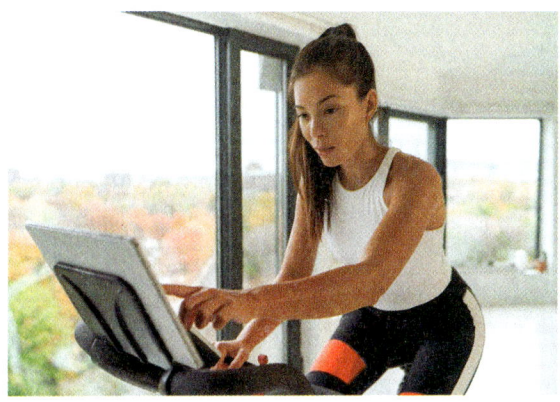
© Maridav/Shutterstock

> "When I run, my RPE exceeds a 6 (output and observation). The instructor said the goal is to maintain a 6. If I walk quickly, I stay at a 6 (output), so in the next class I will walk quickly when the effort demands a 6 (modifying future outputs)."

LOAD OR RESISTANCE

The appropriate load or resistance is mandated by form. If the participant cannot maintain proper form for the number of desired repetitions, the load should be reduced (Mayo Clinic, 2020). Proper form is critical to achieving long-term adherence to exercise, especially among beginners. Beginners may be concerned with and intimidated by the idea of pain or injury. If pain or injury are experienced early in their group fitness journey, they may be less likely to return to class. Therefore, an instructor must be prepared with a variety of regression options.

In the case of load or resistance, regressions take the form of moving to a bodyweight-only version or reducing the weight of the equipment.

COMPOUND MOVEMENTS

An instructor should consider regressing a compound movement when a participant cannot maintain proper form, does not have the strength or muscle coordination to execute all aspects of the movement correctly, or does not understand the complexity of the movement. When this is the case, you can break the complete movement down into its parts. For example, if a group is struggling to master a squat with an overhead press, begin by cueing the group through a proper squat, and then cue them through an overhead press. Once they are able to complete a proper squat and a proper overhead press, then put the two movements together to produce a squat to overhead press. If it is still challenging, a participant may simply hold the dumbbells at shoulder height as they squat. Also, understand that it may take several classes to master each piece of an exercise, and only after ample practice is the group ready for a progression to compound movements.

BASE OF SUPPORT

A lack of proper stability can cause an individual to quickly lose form. Although it is beneficial to challenge balance, if the BOS is such that a participant cannot continue with an exercise as cued, the instructor should suggest a regression. Consider the following examples of BOS regressions:

- Increasing points of contact with the ground (e.g., moving from single-leg to allowing the floating foot to lightly touch down)
- Widening the BOS (within proper form guidelines)
- Moving to a seated position
- Using external support (e.g., wall, barre, chair, or suspension trainer)
- Moving from feet elevated to on the floor (e.g., placing heels on the floor in a V-sit)
- Moving from less stable to more stable surfaces

It may be the case that an individual can regain balance and return to a less stable exercise option after momentarily regressing to regain balance and form.

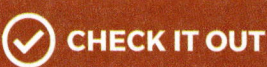

CHECK IT OUT

Simply challenging a participant's balance does not necessarily *improve* their balance. If a participant is struggling as they are trying to balance, the movement is actually reinforcing their failure at balancing. To properly train improved balance and proprioception, instructors must place participants in a position to be successful. That is, balance and stability are improved in *slightly unstable yet still controllable* environments.

CUEING REGRESSIONS

When cueing regressions, an instructor should take extra care to frame their words in a positive manner. At no point should a participant feel less competent, less fit, or less than anyone else in the room. It is essential that participants learn that regressions are just as critical to forming a positive feedback loop as progressions. It is helpful to avoid words such as *easy, simple, beginner,* and *basic.*

Instead, follow the same format as progression cueing: explain the goal or desired outcome, educate the group on how to observe physical feedback, and teach how to modify behavior to alter the outcome. Regressions contribute to successful outcomes for exercisers, not only regarding safety, but also because their efforts are targeting the right intensity and muscle groups. In this way, participants are getting more out of the workout, and performing a movement properly may actually feel *more* challenging. This is why we should avoid saying *regression* with participants and instead use words like *option*, *choice*, or *modification*. For example:

- "In rotational movement, the movement starts from your core. If you are feeling this effort in your lower back instead, set your medicine ball down and focus the effort on your abdominals, or rotate only as far as your core stays engaged."
- "The priority of the jump squat is controlling your landing just before you jump explosively back up. Let's slow down a bit, land softly, hold the bottom for a two-count as you line up your stance, and jump just a few inches off the ground."
- "A deadlift targets the hamstrings and glutes. If the single-leg version feels like your body is more focused on balancing than working those muscles, place both feet down and focus on them."

To keep regressions positive, focus on cueing what to do rather than what not to do. **Table 14.8** provides examples of modification cues that communicate what to do rather than what not to do.

TABLE 14.8 Positive Versus Negative Modifications Cues

Negative Modification Cues	Positive Modification Cues
"Don't use your arms to row."	"As you row, squeeze your shoulder blades together to engage your mid-back."
"Don't lift your hips when you plank."	"Lower your knees to the floor as you draw your belly in and create a straight line from knees to head."
"Don't rush your lunge."	"To get the most out of the lunge, control the whole movement, so slow your lunge to match my count. Ready? Down for two, up for two."
"Try not to lose your balance."	"Try widening your stance a little."
"Don't overdo it."	"Let's match your effort with the work block."

 INSTRUCTOR TIP

Range of motion adjustments can be a quick and easy way to regress a movement without sacrificing intensity or requiring equipment or position changes. For example, if a participant's knees cave inward during the last portion of their squat, simply ask them to squat to the point just before that occurs. Modifications like these quickly keep participants where they are both safe and successful.

Lesson 3: Responding to Unexpected Circumstances and Outdoor Conditions

Unexpected Conditions and Events

An experienced instructor comes to class prepared with the workout fully planned and practiced; however, they should also have the expertise and strategies to accommodate unexpected conditions. These conditions might include new participants, lack of equipment, technical malfunctions, outside distractions, or emergency situations.

> ### ⚠ CRITICAL
>
> When presented with an unexpected condition or event, you should first evaluate the safety of the situation. If there is any safety risk to yourself or others, action should be taken, even if that requires stopping class. Examples include acute injuries, emergency medical situations, emergency weather, or equipment failure. Facilities in which you teach should have outlined and shared all emergency procedures, including emergency response systems, evacuation plans, and accident reporting.

If the situation is not dangerous, such as a malfunctioning audio system or not enough dumbbells to go around, the instructor should try to maintain the flow and structure of the class to the best of their ability. It is beneficial to have backup plans and strategies ready and in place, if possible, to allow for flexibility when needed. This can include using bands or kettlebells if there are not enough dumbbells, decreasing intensity and increasing water breaks if the studio is warmer than usual, shadow boxing if there are not enough heavy bags, or jogging in place if the track is unexpectedly closed. Keep in mind that movement is what matters, which means you might need to be creative if the situation calls for it.

In an unexpected situation, class participants will follow the instructor's lead. If the instructor is negative, complaining about the lack of equipment, perhaps even blaming the facility management, the participants will also react in a negative manner. However, if the instructor avoids blame and focuses on problem-solving, the situation can remain positive. You can even use a challenging situation to create a positive feedback loop. For example, if the original plan was to create a particular intensity by using heavy weights, and there are not enough heavy dumbbells available, the instructor can create a learning opportunity by teaching the group that the same intensity can be created by decreasing the speed of repetitions (i.e., increasing time under tension). So instead of reaching the desired outcome through heavy weights, participants can simply increase the tension created in the muscle groups. This creates a new point of input that can be utilized for future beneficial modifications by participants.

Imagine you are leading a class and the music stops working. Think about the steps you could take to problem-solve and still deliver a great experience. Consider these steps:

- Take the lead and move about the room to reach more participants.
- Acknowledge the situation with a joke.
- Assess participant safety.
- Share your game plan.
- Move forward positively.

Outdoor Environments

Exercising in outdoor environments presents additional considerations. The goal is to ensure a positive participant experience and a safe exercise environment.

Participant Experience

Most indoor group fitness spaces have been designed with the participant experience in mind, specifically considering sound, sight lines, lighting, temperature, and flooring surfaces. Some outdoor fitness spaces are beautifully designed with these elements in mind. Others offer beautiful trees, grass, or sunshine but might not function as well in these areas. Unique environments can offer many benefits, for example, the opportunity to integrate new challenges such as hills, sand, or stairs, along with more space and fresh air. However, adjustments will be needed to make an outdoor class experience effective. Consider the following:

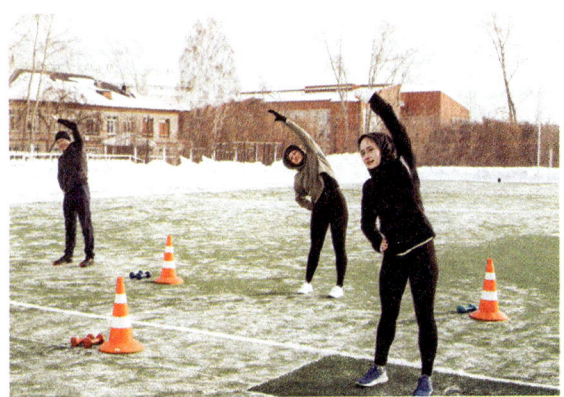

© LenaLavr/Shutterstock

- **Sound.** This includes both the music and the instructor's voice. If the class format is reliant on music to follow the choreography, a proper sound system and speakers will be needed. If music is used as background motivation, perhaps a portable speaker is sufficient. A microphone may be needed to project the instructor's voice, depending on the size of the group. Note that local sound ordinances may limit the use of loud music and microphones during specific times of day. The instructor might also have to contend with outside noises, such as cars or construction. If possible, select your location with this in mind, trying to avoid crowded or loud areas. If this is unavoidable, you may have to repeat cues, speak to the class in smaller groups rather than as a whole, or be prepared to walk around and give personal feedback.
- **Sight lines.** When outdoors, there might not be a fixed front of the class; therefore, you will need to ensure that participants can see you when providing instructions and exercise demonstrations. This can be accomplished by utilizing landmarks in the space such as "eyes on me by the big tree" or "face toward the parking lot for the next set." Take note of visual obstacles that might block you from view. Stand on higher ground, if possible. Repeat instructions from multiple locations. Avoid participants facing busy areas as that can be distracting.

- **Ground surface.** The ground outside might not be as clean, level, or comfortable as an indoor studio floor. Select an area that is as level as possible, then scan the area for any hazards (e.g., rocks, pinecones, or potholes) and remove them, if possible. Remind the group to bring thick mats to outdoor classes and wear supportive shoes.

The goal is to provide a positive exercise experience. Exercising outdoors takes more consideration and time on the part of the instructor. It is recommended that the instructor preview the location prior to class in order to properly plan for the previously mentioned elements. It may be beneficial to share details of the location with participants prior to class and let them know how to come prepared. For example, bring water and a thick mat; wear proper footwear; and have a hat, sunglasses, jacket, or gloves. The instructor should also monitor participants as it applies to the specific environment. Are they warm enough, cool enough, or drinking enough water? Is the ground uneven and causing unsteady footing? Are participants enjoying the setting? Can they hear cues? How can you make the experience better next time?

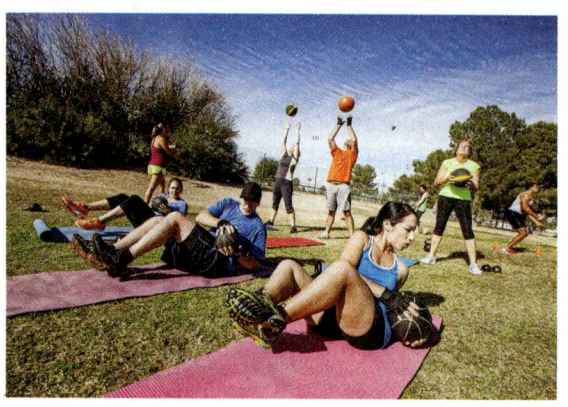

© CREATISTA/Shutterstock

Outdoor Safety and Climate Considerations

When leading a class outdoors, there are some additional safety considerations. The instructor should ensure that they are familiar with the space, including routes to and from the location, available restrooms and water, and any terrain or obstacles they will encounter. Just as when indoors, it is critical to have emergency procedures in place. If the class is not directly outside the facility, the instructor should bring a mobile phone to contact emergency services, if needed.

Outdoor exercise can be performed year-round with some special considerations, including an understanding of how temperature can affect intensity, RPE, and hydration. Research has found that heart rate and RPE are significantly higher in hot weather conditions, and, overall, participants perceive work to be harder and feel worse (Maw et al., 1993). The same study also found that RPE was significantly lower in cold temperatures than in heat. These findings mean that outdoor bouts of exercise in the heat may need to be shortened and include more and longer breaks to accommodate elevated heart rates and perception of effort. However, in the cold, participants may underestimate their effort and overdo intensity without realizing it. In both situations, the instructor should keep a close eye on participant reactions to intensity, continue to ask questions to gain feedback, and make modifications to keep the group safe. Note that the body will naturally acclimatize to varying temperatures over time (de Freitas & Grigorieva, 2015). When exercising outdoors in cold or heat, gradually build workloads in intensity and duration. Colder temperatures may require a longer warm-up period, and warmer climates may call for a longer cool-down to return the body to a more comfortable temperature.

Hydration is also an important consideration when exercising outdoors. Many underestimate the impact of dehydration in cooler temperatures, forgetting that participants lose water through sweating and breathing even in cold environments. Winter winds can also have a drying effect on participants' hydration status (Weiss, 2022). When exercising in heat, hydration is critical because the body cools itself by sweating (Ansorge, 2023). However, if the body becomes dehydrated, it loses its mechanism for cooling, which can lead to heat exhaustion or heat stroke. On hot days, humidity levels should also be considered because high humidity can slow the evaporation of sweat from the skin, reducing the effectiveness of sweating to cool the body (Dougherty, 2011).

Weather conditions such as rain or snow can make outdoor exercise unsafe. Air quality can also adversely affect participants and, therefore, should be monitored. High winds, allergies, and bugs can also make for a negative experience. An instructor must balance out the benefits and challenges of an outdoor workout and decide if it is the best environment for the group.

Equipment

Some facilities have constructed great outdoor class spaces with space for equipment storage. Other outdoor environments require that equipment be transported to and from the location. Whichever situation you are teaching in, plan accordingly to ensure that you have the proper equipment for the format and participants' comfort. Depending on the format, some common outdoor equipment includes cones, agility ladders, resistance bands, jump ropes, suspension trainers, sandbags, and mats. Equipment can be damaged when used outside; therefore, the instructor should regularly check the condition of all equipment to minimize unsafe situations. For example, regularly check resistance bands to spot any weak points or holes that can lead to breakage. Check sandbags for leakage and suspension trainers for points of wear. When selecting outdoor equipment, also consider ease of transportation. Medicine balls and kettlebells may be hard to carry 10 blocks to a local park, for example, making resistance bands a better choice. Also evaluate what is already in place, such as park benches for step-ups or playground equipment for pull-ups.

SUMMARY

Leading a large group of participants with varying needs and abilities can be a challenge. Education can be an effective answer to this challenge. Part of the instructor's role is to teach participants how to monitor the messages their bodies are giving them. They must guide participants in how to use that feedback to make positive improvements and encourage them to take ownership of creating positive feedback loops. An instructor should do their best to create stable environments for the participants to learn but be flexible when unexpected circumstances present themselves. And, most important, if you focus on safety first, your expertise will shine through.

REFERENCES

Ansorge, R. (2023). *Heat exhaustion.* WebMD. https://www.webmd.com/fitness-exercise/heat-exhaustion

Centers for Disease Control and Prevention. (2022). *Perceived exertion (Borg rating of perceived exertion scale).* https://www.cdc.gov/physicalactivity/basics/measuring/exertion.htm

de Freitas, C. R., & Grigorieva, E. A. (2015). Role of acclimatization in weather-related human mortality during the transition seasons of autumn and spring in a thermally extreme mid-latitude continental climate. *International Journal of Environmental Research and Public Health, 12*(12), 14974–14987. https://doi.org/10.3390/ijerph121214962

Dougherty, E. (2011). *Why do we sweat more in high humidity?* MIT School of Engineering. https://engineering.mit.edu/engage/ask-an-engineer/why-do-we-sweat-more-in-high-humidity/

Foster, C., Porcari, J. P., Anderson, J., Paulson, M., Smaczny, D., Webber, H., Doberstein S. T., & Udermann, B. (2008). The talk test as a marker of exercise training intensity. *Journal of Cardiopulmonary Rehabilitation and Prevention, 28*(1), 24–30. https://doi.org/10.1097/01.HCR.0000311504.41775.78

Hattie, J., & Timperley, H. (2007). The power of feedback. *Review of Educational Research, 77*(1), 81–112. https://doi.org/10.3102/003465430298487

Heick, T. (2022). *What's a feedback loop in learning? A definition for teachers.* Teachthought. https://www.teachthought.com/learning/what-is-a-feedback-loop-for-learning/

Goman, C. K. (2022). *Body language of listeners.* Global Listening Centre. https://www.globallisteningcentre.org/body-language-of-listeners/

Jeans, E., Foster, C., Porcari, J. P., Gibson, M., & Doberstein, S. (2011). Translation of exercise testing to exercise prescription using the talk test. *Journal of Strength & Conditioning Research, 25*(3), 590–596. https://doi.org/10.1519/JSC.0b013e318207ed53

Kolata, G. (2001, April 24). 'Maximum' heart rate theory is challenged. *The New York Times.* https://www.nytimes.com/2001/04/24/health/maximum-heart-rate-theory-is-challenged.html

Maw, G. J., Boutcher, S. H., & Taylor, N. A. (1993). Ratings of perceived exertion and affect in hot and cool environments. *European Journal of Applied Physiology and Occupational Physiology, 67*(2), 174–179. http://doi.org/10.1007/BF00376663

Mayo Clinic. (2020). *Weight training: Do's and don'ts of proper technique.* https://www.mayoclinic.org/healthy-lifestyle/fitness/in-depth/weight-training/art-20045842

Miller, K. (n.d.). Exercise progressions and regressions: How to's of scaling movement. *NASM* [Blog]. https://blog.nasm.org/fitness/exercise-progressions-and-regressions-how-tos-of-scaling-movement

Morse, G. (2004). Feedback backlash. *Harvard Business Review.* https://hbr.org/2004/10/feedback-backlash

Moss, C. M., & Brookhart, S. M. (2019). *Advancing formative assessment in every classroom: A guide for instructional leaders* (2nd ed.). ASCD.

Persinger, R., Foster, C., Gibson, M., Fater, D. C. W., & Porcari, J. P. (2004). Consistency of the talk test for exercise prescription. *Medicine & Science in Sports & Exercise, 36*(9), 1632–1636.

Quinn, T. J., & Coons, B. A. (2011). The talk test and its relationship with the ventilatory and lactate thresholds. *Journal of Sports Sciences, 29*(11), 1175–1182. https://doi.org/10.1080/02640414.2011.585165

Recalde, P., Foster, C., & Skemp, K. M. (2002). The talk test as a simple marker of ventilatory threshold. *South African Journal of Medical Sciences. 9,* 5–8.

Reed, J. L., & Pipe, A. L. (2016). Practical approaches to prescribing physical activity and monitoring exercise intensity. *Canadian Journal of Cardiology, 32*(4), 514–522. https://doi.org/10.1016/j.cjca.2015.12.024

Roy, S., & McCrory, J. (2015). Validation of maximal heart rate prediction equations based on sex and physical activity status. *International Journal of Exercise Science, 8*(4), 318–330.

Scherr, J., Wolfarth, B., Christle, J. W., Pressler, A., Wagenpfeil, S., & Halle, M. (2013). Associations between Borg's rating of perceived exertion and physiological measures of exercise intensity. *European Journal of Applied Physiology, 113*(1), 147–155. https://doi.org/10.1007/s00421-012-2421-x

Swain, D. P., & Franklin, B. A. (2002). Is there a threshold intensity for aerobic training in cardiac patients? *Medicine & Science in Sports & Exercise, 34*(7), 1071–1075. https://doi.org/10.1097/00005768-200207000-00003

Weiss, C. (2022). *How to exercise safely during the winter.* Mayo Clinic. https://mcpress.mayoclinic.org/women-health/mayo-clinic-q-and-a-how-to-exercise-safely-during-the-winter/

Wiliam, D. (2017). *Embedded formative assessment* (2nd ed.). Solution Tree.

CHAPTER 15

INSTRUCTING VIRTUALLY

LEARNING OBJECTIVES

The intent of this chapter is to explore instructing virtually, the relevance of virtual instruction to instructors and participants, and how to create an engaging virtual workout. This chapter will also review legal, ethical, and safety considerations when designing and offering virtual workouts.

After reading this content, students should be able to demonstrate the following objectives:

- **Compare** the characteristics and requirements of virtual and in-person instruction.

- **Identify** methods for creating an engaging, motivating virtual group fitness experience.

- **Discuss** legal and ethical considerations for instructing group fitness virtually.

Lesson 1: Virtual Versus In-Person Instruction

Introduction

Virtual group fitness instruction provides fitness professionals with the ability to reach more participants, avoid geographical limitations, and increase their income potential. In the past, having a physical space—and typically an organization with management and marketing—was a prerequisite to teaching group fitness classes. Today, with the evolution and availability of technology, those barriers to entry have largely been eliminated. Theoretically, any instructor with an open room, a smartphone, and a reliable Internet connection can teach virtual group fitness classes. However, teaching group fitness in a virtual setting is much more complex than that. As the popularity of virtual fitness expands and becomes a viable option for many instructors and coaches, it is critical to understand both the opportunities and challenges it presents.

For instructors looking to diversify, sustain, and expand the number of participants they reach in a rapidly growing (and increasingly competitive) market, offering virtual classes can help broaden these efforts. The shift to work-from-home settings combined with the continuous rise of chronic health conditions, such as obesity, diabetes, heart disease, and other lifestyle-influenced conditions, have highlighted the value of adaptable online fitness services for both participants and instructors.

With the ability to teach classes anywhere at any time, virtual instructors can have a substantial influence on the health and wellness of participants at any fitness level. On any given day, a virtual instructor in California can teach class in the morning joined by a lunchtime exerciser in Florida and an evening exerciser in the UK. There has never been a better or more exciting time for credentialed fitness professionals to step into the virtual arena.

However, as exciting as these possibilities may be, aspiring virtual instructors must be aware of the significant distinctions that exist between in-person and virtual instruction. Adapting to new methods of class planning, delivery style, participant engagement, and safety protocols is essential for effective virtual instruction. Additionally, if an instructor is teaching independently, proficiency in technology, business management, and marketing strategies must also be considered.

Whether or not you choose to explore the opportunities presented by virtual instruction, it is important to understand what it is, how it differs from in-person instruction, and how it fits within the greater fitness landscape.

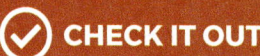

CHECK IT OUT

Not long ago, the fitness industry was centered around locations that included a built-in participant base for fitness professionals: the gym facility. According to the 2019 IHRSA Health Club Consumer Report, more than 71 million people in the United States reported being a member of a fitness center, gym, or studio in 2018 (Rodriguez, 2019). To accommodate such growth, the number of gyms, fitness centers, studios, and fitness professionals who run and staff these establishments has exploded. The U.S. Bureau of Labor Statistics (2020) projects 15% growth in employment for fitness trainers and instructors from 2019 to 2029 (**Figure 15.1**), creating a level of competition that forces fitness professionals to become creative with strategies for setting their business apart. Adding virtual classes to their live teaching schedules can help instructors expand their reach to include a whole new group of participants.

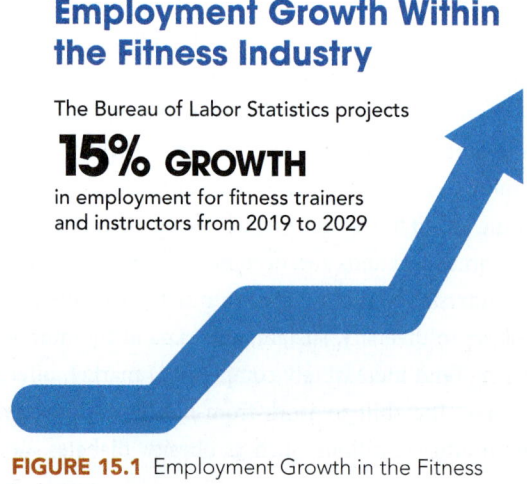

Employment Growth Within the Fitness Industry

The Bureau of Labor Statistics projects

15% GROWTH

in employment for fitness trainers and instructors from 2019 to 2029

FIGURE 15.1 Employment Growth in the Fitness Industry

Offering virtual fitness classes may seem incredibly overwhelming at first. However, do not let the fear of the unknown stop you from taking a positive step toward the innovative world of virtual instruction. To avoid feeling overwhelmed about the requirements needed to transition to virtual instruction, begin by focusing on immediate steps to facilitate this process. For example, start by participating in virtual classes yourself and notice what the instructors do differently. What works? Which elements might be improved? Consider the entire participant experience, from the ease of finding and registering for the class to the way the instructor cues, the quality of the audio, and so on.

Virtual Versus In-Person Instruction

VIRTUAL INSTRUCTORS provide fitness classes and workouts through virtual (online) means, primarily via **LIVESTREAM CLASSES** and **ON-DEMAND CLASSES**. Unlike in-person experiences, where instructors can meet participants face to face, assess their needs, and adapt to them in real time, virtual classes must be planned for and may be delivered to an anonymous, invisible audience. Depending on the platform, it is possible that a virtual instructor will not have any idea how many participants have joined them nor have any information about their experience, skill, or fitness level. Even when participants are known, due to the nature of the digital space, they will often be less visible to the instructor.

To effectively adapt to this reality, virtual instructors must adjust certain elements of their planning and presentation to provide safe, effective, and entertaining classes. These include, but are not limited to, providing very specific class descriptions, prioritizing detailed physical demonstrations, delivering more generalized cues, and employing different engagement strategies. Additionally, without a physical space, established member base, or regularly scheduled classes to attract participants, virtual instructors must find new ways to build a following, develop and maintain relationships, and monitor compliance to avoid injuries and ensure positive outcomes.

Relevance of Virtual Group Fitness Instruction

For instructors and participants alike, digital experiences provide many benefits. Virtual group fitness classes provide flexibility for participants who cannot make it to an in-person class due to closures, proximity, or personal preference. For instructors, various methods of streaming now accommodate unlimited participants in one class, providing them the ability to encourage greater interaction, build larger communities, and increase their income potential by diversifying their offerings. Although there are certainly some disadvantages—notably the absence of in-person connection, individualized coaching, and in

VIRTUAL INSTRUCTORS

Group Fitness Instructors who lead classes in a virtual (online) setting.

LIVESTREAM CLASSES

Virtual (online) group fitness classes that are taught in real time. Participants log in to class at a scheduled time, similar to showing up at a facility.

ON-DEMAND CLASSES

Virtual (online) group fitness classes that are pre-recorded and can be viewed by the user at a time of their choosing.

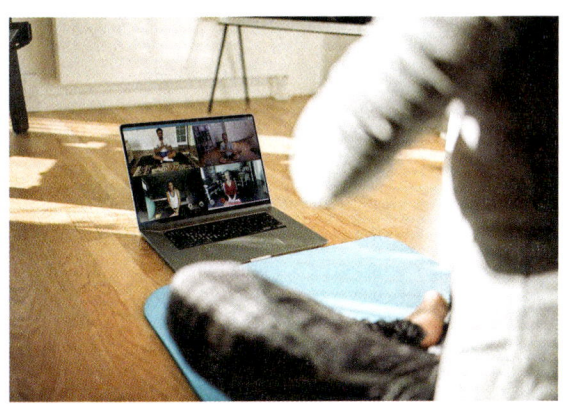
© Jacob Lund/Shutterstock

some cases specialized equipment—the option of offering and participating in digital workouts is game-changing.

Benefits of Virtual Group Fitness

Virtual group fitness offerings can benefit both fitness professionals and participants in several ways. Some of the most enticing include the following:

- Reaching a broader audience as a fitness professional
- More flexibility in scheduling
- More autonomy in programming (if done as an independent instructor)
- Potentially more affordable than in-person classes, especially for participants without a facility membership
- More format availability and shorter class durations (such as 15-, 20-, or 30-minute options) to enable participants to customize their workouts based on personal preferences
- Providing an environment where individuals with anxiety about exercise can participate in a group anonymously without real or perceived pressure to keep up
- Giving participants the ability to work out with a preferred instructor regardless of location
- Encouraging compliance through increased opportunities to participate in both live and virtual classes interchangeably
- Enabling participants with immune system concerns to participate in the environment of their choice

Participants

Virtual classes can benefit existing and prospective participants alike but will appeal to some more than others. Group Fitness Instructors looking to offer virtual classes to new or existing participants will need to understand whether a participant will have their health and wellness objectives met with a virtual experience. Participants who prefer the more individualized instruction, personal accountability, and social connections of a live setting may not be good candidates for virtual classes. However, for a significant cohort of individuals, virtual classes may be their preferred modality and the one in which they find the most success (**Table 15.1**).

TABLE 15.1 Participant Preferences

Participant Group	Motivation Behind Preference
Participants who prefer to stay home	Long commute, packed schedule, lack of childcare, or lack of self-confidence
Participants who have moved	Want to continue relationship with fitness professional or has experienced positive results
Participants who travel frequently	Want to achieve goals while traveling, maintain connection with instructor, or want to stick with their routine
Participants with demanding work schedules	Need to accommodate night or long shifts or focus on health because of alternative schedules
Participants who have health concerns	Immunocompromised, experiencing chronic or terminal illness, or populations with reduced mobility

When participants travel, they should also pack a set of resistance bands. Using bands, bodyweight exercises, and a little creativity, a great workout can be completed even in the most cramped hotel room.

The potential participant types and opportunities identified are merely examples of those who may benefit most from virtual fitness offerings. By appropriately identifying and integrating various technologies with specific needs, virtual fitness can benefit just about any participant, solidifying the service as one of the most versatile and innovative ways to make an impact on the fitness industry as a professional.

Streaming Versus On-Demand Classes

In the domain of digital fitness classes, both on-demand (pre-recorded) and livestreamed offerings are extremely popular with virtual participants (Becvar Weddle, 2020). Although they are similar in many ways, there are also notable differences that affect how they are accessed, delivered, and experienced (Table 15.2).

On-demand workouts are accessible at any time the user wants to exercise. Participants only need to log in, select the pre-recorded workout that suits their needs, and begin. Conversely, livestreamed workouts are delivered live, in real time, just like a regularly scheduled group fitness class in a gym. However, instead of going to a facility, participants can log in to the class wherever they are, regardless of physical location or time zone. In some instances, the instructor is alone, teaching to a camera that is livestreaming and/or recording the workout. In others, the instructor may be teaching simultaneously to a live group as well as to those logging in from afar. Both types of digital experiences provide benefits and challenges.

For participants, both livestream and on-demand classes offer the convenience of exercising wherever they are—whether it is their living room, an unoccupied studio in a facility, or a hotel gym. However, one of the primary differences between the two is variety and accessibility.

TABLE 15.2 Livestream Versus On-Demand Classes

Type	Advantages	Potential Disadvantages
On-demand	▪ Convenience ▪ Format preference ▪ Instructor preference ▪ Potential for progression through a series	▪ Less personal ▪ Repetitive (depending on selection) ▪ Music selection may be limited as a result of royalty-free music constraints
Livestream	▪ Schedule accountability ▪ More personal, group dynamic ▪ Potentially fewer constraints on music selection (if teaching from a facility paying requisite licensing fees)	▪ Schedule availability ▪ Format variety ▪ Unable to revisit favorite workouts

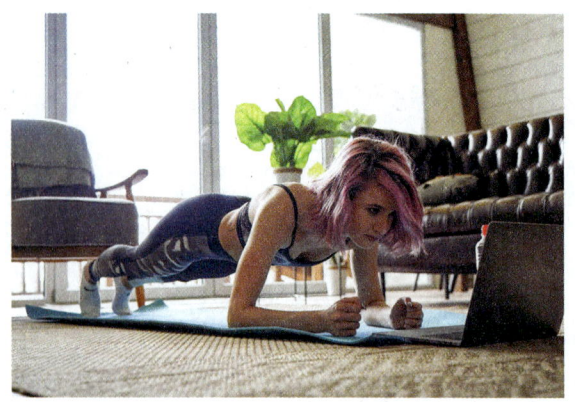

© Ground Picture/Shutterstock

On-demand workouts are pre-recorded and accessible at any time of day, making them especially attractive to those with challenging schedules and specific format or instructor preferences. For example, if an individual only has 30 minutes to work out and they want to do a quick high-intensity interval training (HIIT) session, they can select a class from the on-demand library to meet those specific parameters. If they find that they are especially partial to a certain instructor, they can opt to only do that instructor's classes. If there is a particular workout they really enjoy and want to repeat, they can do it as many times as they like.

In contrast, because livestreamed workouts are unique experiences held at fixed times, participants must be available when the class is offered. Although this may be an obstacle for some, having a dedicated and regular time to attend class may help others maintain a routine and support accountability, much like that of a traditional live class. In addition, participants may appreciate the sense that although they are in different locations, they are still "in it together." Indeed, the absence of traditional social interactions found in live classes, as valuable as they can be for some, may be liberating for others. Participating in group fitness without the group in the same room but still at the same time creates a more private, yet still shared, experience. This option may strongly appeal to individuals with anxiety about going into a gym or studio for any number of reasons (Fable, 2021). And, for those who enjoy the group experience but cannot always be there in person, attending a livestreamed class allows them the opportunity to stay connected to their routine—and potentially to their favorite instructors and community even when they are miles away. An additional option that provides the advantages of both types of offerings is to record a livestreamed class as it is taught and save it for later on-demand use. This allows for an additional revenue stream from a single class and gives participants a chance to revisit the workout, or for those who missed it the first time to attend later.

✓ CHECK IT OUT

Whether offered through a digital-only service, as a digital extension of a commercial facility, or by an individual instructor delivering virtual classes from their home, participation in livestreamed or on-demand workouts often requires a fee. Virtual classes may be included in the membership from a facility, as subscription model, or as an option to purchase class packs (Becvar Weddle, 2020). Depending on the provider and platform, the type, availability, and cost to participate may vary greatly.

Knowledge and Skills Transferrable to Virtual Group Fitness

Regardless of whether participants prefer to use virtual classes exclusively or as another tool in their fitness toolbox, the quality of their experience is largely dependent on the quality of the content and its delivery by the instructor. Fortunately, although there are some significant differences between live and virtual instruction methods, there are also many transferrable skills. With a few shifts in thinking and approach, instructors who desire to make the shift to include virtual classes in their teaching repertoire will find that many of the characteristics that make them great in a live setting will also help them to be successful in a virtual environment.

Character Traits of a Successful Virtual Group Fitness Instructor

A Group Fitness Instructor's passion for motivating and helping participants learn, grow, and achieve goals should be just as evident in virtual experiences as it is in live classes. Great group fitness instructors are energetic, authentic, intentional, and organized (**Figure 15.2**). They are confident communicators and dynamic performers capable of captivating a group and keeping

Energetic

For virtual instructors teaching to a camera in an empty room, one of the most challenging elements can be projecting energy and enthusiasm. No matter the setting, instructors should always use their body language, voice, and facial expressions to keep participants engaged. Movements must be precise, vocal quality should be dynamic, and facial expressions should convey genuine emotion.

Authentic

Participants respond best when they feel that their instructor is genuine and relatable. While it can be challenging to avoid sounding "scripted" when teaching virtually, it is important to maintain an authentic presentation style in order to connect with participants. By looking directly at the camera and teaching to it as if it is a friend or familiar participant (instead of an inanimate object), virtual instructors can create a sense of authentic connection with their virtual audience.

Intentional

Great instructors are intentional in both the movements they select and the way they communicate them. This characteristic is particularly important to effective virtual instruction as it ensures a cohesive flow and promotes compliance when an instructor has no way of knowing if their instructions have been understood. When movements and instructions are logical, deliberate, and clear, it leaves less room for distraction or confusion.

Organized

To be intentional and clear in their delivery, instructors must also be organized and intentional in their planning. In a virtual setting it is much harder to pivot if something does not work or is not well thought out. Planning and preparation for teaching a virtual class should be approached like preparing for a performance. Equipment must be positioned properly, technology must be checked (and re-checked), movement sequences should be rehearsed, and communication of critical cues should be practiced.

FIGURE 15.2 Traits of a Successful Virtual Group Fitness Instructor

them engaged through challenging movements and potential distractions. To be effective in a virtual setting, all these characteristics and skills must not only be present but amplified and augmented in order to connect with and coach participants who are not physically there.

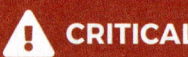

CRITICAL

Having an entrepreneurial spirit is an essential attribute for a virtual instructor looking to attract and retain participants. A proactive mindset keeps you seeking innovative ways to be creative with marketing, social media presence, networking, referral programs, innovative promotion ideas, and gated content to attract new participants. Without this continuous drive for creativity and innovation, it becomes increasingly difficult to stand out in the virtual setting.

Lesson 2: Considerations for Virtual Group Fitness

Changes for Virtual Group Fitness

Although there are many transferrable skills when transitioning from live to virtual instruction, there also some necessary changes in focus. Although having a plan and delivering it in a safe, clear, inclusive manner are vital components of all group fitness instruction, some elements are particularly important and distinct when teaching virtually.

Planning Considerations

One of the most attractive features of virtual classes is that they allow participants to choose from a variety of options that meet their specific needs. When surveyed, virtual participants ranked the type, time, and duration of class along with the equipment and space required as their top reasons for selecting one class over another (Becvar Weddle, 2020). For that reason, just like ordering from a menu in a restaurant, participants will expect the experience to align with the description that convinced them to select it. Instructors must be sensitive to this and deliver their class to meet those expectations.

To do this requires planning regarding the objective of the class, the fitness level for which it is most appropriate, and the required equipment and space that will be required to perform it. When planning a virtual class, instructors should consider the following:

- Do the exercises selected accurately meet the specific goals and objectives stated in the description (e.g., strength, cardio, core, or flexibility)? Although this is important in all group fitness classes, given that many virtual exercisers take an à la carte approach when choosing which workouts to do, it is particularly important that what is delivered aligns with their expectations (Fable, 2021).
- Does the design of the class allow for those objectives to be met within the time allotted? This is especially important if the class is shorter in duration.

- Is the space required to do the workout realistic for a variety of environments? Consider the various spaces participants may be utilizing and plan accordingly.
- What type of equipment, if any, is required? Can effective modifications be made for those participants without it?
- Can the exercises selected be performed or modified by most participants, or should the class indicate a suggested level (e.g., beginner, intermediate, advanced, or all levels)?

Communication and Cueing

One of the major differences between in-person and virtual class delivery is the elevated importance of verbal communication and cueing. Unlike a live, in-person experience where the instructor can see, interact with, and individualize feedback for each participant, the visibility of and familiarity with participants in the digital space ranges from limited to nonexistent. For that reason, it is imperative that virtual instructors embrace a more general approach to cueing than they might in a live setting.

In the live environment where all participants are visible, it is neither necessary nor advisable to articulate all potential errors or form cues if they are not needed. For example, if no one in the room is elevating their shoulders or bouncing on their bike seat, an instructor does not need to say, "Keep your shoulders back and down" or "Avoid bouncing in the saddle." Conversely, in virtual classes, without knowing what each individual participant is doing in the privacy of their home, it is best to err on the side of safety regarding common errors and general form cues.

Similarly, without visibility to the participants' movements or specific knowledge of their individual fitness levels, instructors must assume the need for a multitude of modifications, progressions, and regressions and proactively communicate them. By providing thorough descriptions, clear demonstrations, and lots of options for each exercise, instructors can promote safety, success, and satisfaction for a wide variety of individuals.

Fortunately, although this level of verbal communication might be excessive in a live setting, it is well-suited to the virtual environment. Although it can be counterproductive for an instructor in a live class to overcommunicate without allowing for periods of intentional silence, in the digital world prolonged silence can feel awkward and result in participants feeling lost or disengaged. However, this does not mean that virtual instructors should talk endlessly without a specific message to deliver. Instead, they must be aware that thorough verbal communication is a critical engagement technique in virtual classes and strive to keep it clear, concise, relevant, and consistent (Table 15.3).

TABLE 15.3 In-Person Versus Virtual Communication

In-Person Communication	Virtual Communication
Cue specifically to the participants in the room. Use your knowledge and real-time observations to provide individualized feedback.	Keep cues about form, safety, and technique general. For every move or exercise, point out common errors and share tips to ensure effectiveness.
Provide modifications, progressions, and regressions according to the needs of the group.	Assume the need for modifications, progressions, and regressions and proactively communicate them.
Avoid overtalking. Do not be afraid of moments of silence where participants can focus on the music and listen to their bodies.	Recognize that silence in the virtual space can be awkward, leading to participant anxiety and disengagement.

Environmental and Technical Considerations

Naturally, one of the most significant differences between live and virtual instruction is the role of technology. Everything from a distraction-free environment to a stable Internet connection, from device placement to equipment choices, and from optimal lighting to audio quality must be considered.

For instructors teaching virtual programming from a facility or studio, it is likely that these technical requirements will be supported by the business. However, virtual instructors teaching independently from home or another space will need to find their own solutions to these technical requirements.

SETTING UP YOUR SPACE

Although it is theoretically possible to instruct virtual classes from any location with Internet access, a dedicated space at home is the most common and accessible choice. Ideally, virtual classes should be delivered from or recorded in an organized studio space where all necessary equipment and resources are within easy reach.

Before selecting and setting up a dedicated space at home, it is best to ask the questions in **Figure 15.3**. If the answer to any of those questions is no, the space should be reconsidered or adjustments should be made to it.

ENVIRONMENTAL CONSIDERATIONS

Remember, because a participant's time is precious and paid for, it is very important for the virtual session space to be as distraction-free as possible. A noisy environment is a distracting one. Barking dogs, crying babies, beeping oven timers, and phone notifications can all reduce the value and professionalism of a virtual session. Naturally, unless the session is filmed in a

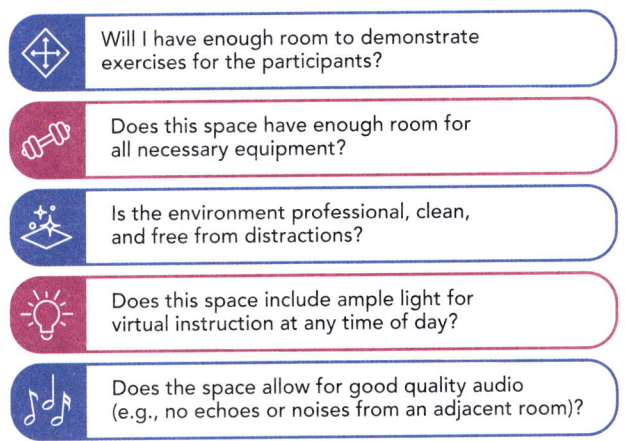

FIGURE 15.3 Setting Up a Workout Space

closed-sound stage, some things are unavoidable and bound to happen; however, it is important to minimize the possibility of distraction wherever possible.

Another trick to minimize distractions in the virtual session room is to set up a visual "do not disturb" signal. Like the "on air" light at a radio station, a sign on the door or closed curtains to shut off the room can go a long way toward letting family know that a virtual class is in progress and to not disturb you if at all possible.

EQUIPMENT CONSIDERATIONS

Your personal equipment needs and the needs of your participants will vary greatly depending on the format you are teaching. Formats that require the least amount of equipment, such as dance-based fitness, cardio kickboxing, bodyweight-based conditioning, HIIT, yoga, and mat Pilates lend themselves well to the virtual environment. However, many participants may also have specialized equipment such as indoor cycling bikes, step benches, stability balls, medicine balls, and dumbbells.

When offering virtual classes, it is vital that clear descriptions have been provided so that participants can assess whether they have what they need to be successful in your virtual session.

CAMERA PLACEMENT

It is essential to have plenty of space between the camera and the demonstration area. At least 6 feet of space between the camera and the instructor is recommended. The room should be big enough to safely perform any necessary demonstrations in full frame, so as to avoid parts of the body being off-camera.

Additionally, make sure all equipment is neatly positioned off to the side. This meets two goals: it sets a professional scene and keeps the equipment within arm's reach when needed. Time is precious for both the participant and the instructor, so none should be wasted by the need to scramble to find equipment.

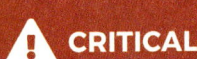 **CRITICAL**

Being fully prepared in advance is essential, and professionalism is key. An instructor would not walk out of the room during an in-person class, nor should this happen during a virtual session.

LIGHTING CONSIDERATIONS

Ample lighting (either natural or artificial) is crucial to instructing in a virtual setting. When taken in dim light, video tends to be lower in resolution and blurry. Although there are some high-end, expensive cameras that can take excellent video in low light, the majority of camera sensors on laptops, tablets, and smartphones do not handle low light well. Although some newer devices now have software-driven night mode for their still cameras, video mode still requires ample lighting for the best-quality outcome. Additional considerations and tips for lighting include the following:

- **Avoid backlighting.** If windows are behind the instructor on camera, the lens will not be able to properly focus on them, resulting in a dark and shadowy appearance.
- **Shoot in front of a solid, neutral-colored wall.** If this option is not available, consider installing blackout curtains, decorative drapes, or blinds to block backlight and create a pleasant background for the video.
- **Front lighting should be projected toward the performer.** Ring lights that integrate with a smartphone or tablet while doubling as a tripod are a great option.

Some free or low-budget solutions to lighting might be as simple as opting to film content in a brighter location on sunny days, an office that has a large amount of natural daylight, or a room with a lamp fixture with a cool white light bulb installed and the lampshade removed. Although these options may be less optimal, they can help the instructor create higher-quality content without investing too much into equipment.

👍 HELPFUL HINT

With budget and portability in mind, instructors may find appropriate lighting solutions in portable ring lights or clip-on smartphone lights that are both compact and effective. Ring lights are typically adjustable (**Figure 15.4**), whereas clip-on lights may not be (**Figure 15.5**).

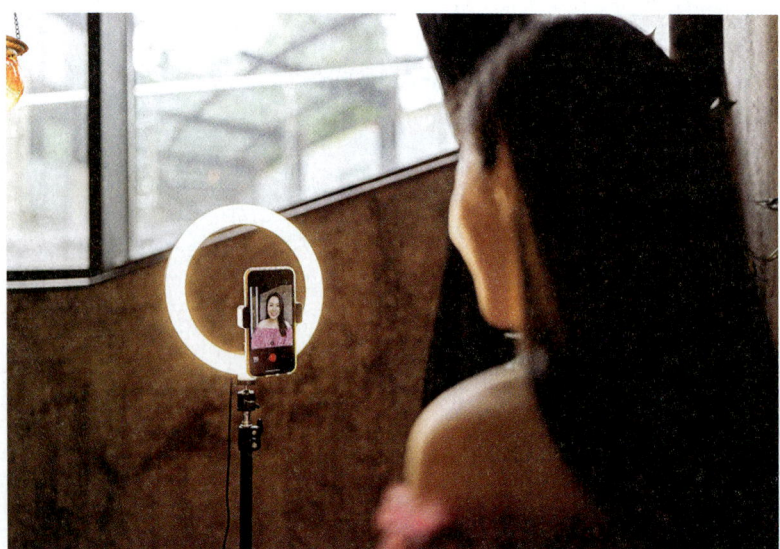

FIGURE 15.4 Ring Light
© Alinabuphoto/Shutterstock

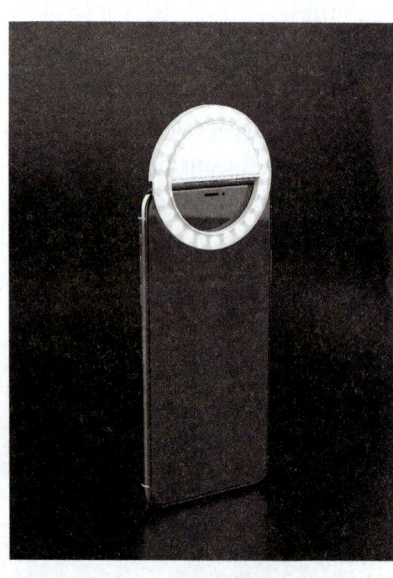

FIGURE 15.5 Clip-On Light
© GO DESIGN/Shutterstock

VIDEO QUALITY CONSIDERATIONS

Given that a large portion of human communication is conveyed through body language (Park & Park, 2018), it is important that participants can see the instructor's movements and facial expressions as clearly as possible. With that in mind, virtual instructors should evaluate the quality of the camera they plan to use.

Considerations when looking for a camera include the following:

- Megapixel (MP) rating
- Resolution
- Budget

Although it is not necessary to have the most expensive, high-end camera to get started, it is worth remembering that in the highly competitive virtual space, more professional-looking video can significantly improve the participant experience.

AUDIO QUALITY CONSIDERATIONS

Whether livestreaming or recording video content, instructors should pay special attention to sound quality. Considering the importance of verbal communication in the virtual setting, having a quality microphone that is connected to the device is critical. Poor audio quality or videos with excessive background noise may result in participants retaining less of the information (Klatte et al., 2013). For that reason, it is not advisable to utilize the microphone on a phone or laptop, but instead to invest in a wireless microphone that connects directly to the recording device (**Figure 15.6**).

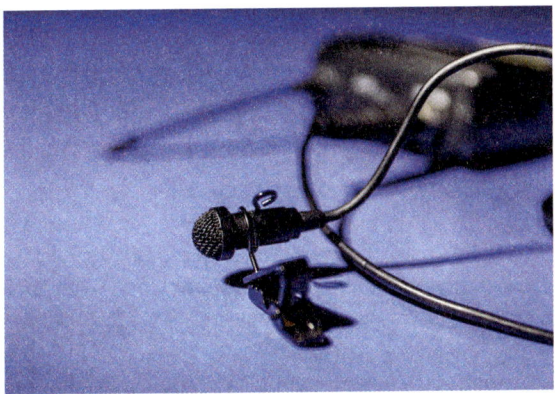

FIGURE 15.6 Wireless Microphones
© Thanes satsutthi/Shutterstock

PRACTICE THIS

A perpetual challenge in any group fitness environment is striking a good balance between music and microphone volume. To ensure the quality of the audio, instructors should always do a dry run and a sound check with the help of a friend or colleague online in another location.

Additionally, it is advisable to do a full rehearsal class with trusted participants. This will not only confirm that equipment works (speakers, lighting, video, etc.), but it is also an opportunity to solicit feedback and learn how to quickly overcome obstacles.

Additional Technology Considerations

Virtual instruction relies heavily on technology, which, when utilized properly, can produce highly effective outcomes. From filming high-quality videos to choosing the appropriate videoconferencing software for livestreams, this section will explore some of the necessary and ancillary technologies needed for virtual instruction. Note that this is only applicable if an instructor wishes to teach independently (i.e., from their home). For instructors teaching virtually as part of a larger organization or facility, these technological considerations will typically be addressed by the business.

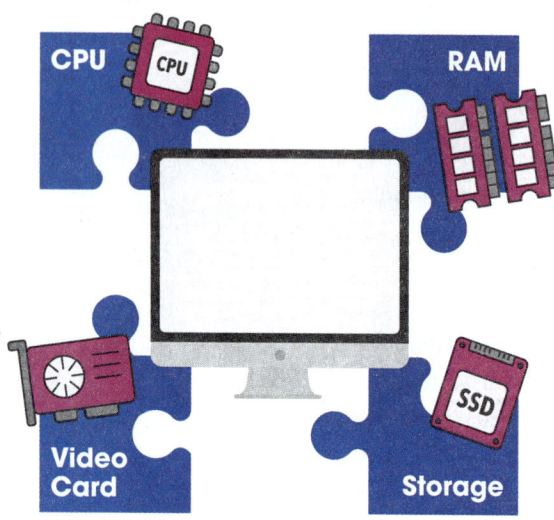

HARDWARE REQUIREMENTS

Hardware includes the physical components that are required for a computer system to function. These physical components include a mouse or trackpad, keyboard, screen or monitor, and speakers, as well as the processing hardware. These parts can be thought of like puzzle pieces (**Table 15.4**).

SOFTWARE REQUIREMENTS

Software components are the actual programs running on a computer system to make it function and operate. For example,

TABLE 15.4 Hardware Requirements

Component/ Consideration	Description
Computer processor	When choosing a computer, it is important to ensure that its processing capability aligns with the intended use of the machine. A personal home computer used for basic computing, some streaming, and Internet access will have significantly different processing needs than a computer intended for small business use. In order to make the best purchase for building a virtual-instructing business, the fitness professional should understand what components and requirements are needed to operate effectively, efficiently, and productively.
RAM	RAM stands for random access memory. It is another piece of the puzzle that makes up a computer system. RAM temporarily stores the information that the computer needs to access immediately or in the near future. Instead of the computer going into a hard drive storage device to pull the data it requires, RAM knows what the computer will need next and keeps that information at hand, ready to be used.
Storage	With virtual instructing, the fitness professional may be responsible for not only handling and organizing participant information, but also managing and storing files such as a business plan, workout demonstration or marketing videos, and social media content. Storage can be local (on your computer or an external hard drive) or cloud based on external servers in other geographic locations.
Graphics	The final piece, a video card or graphics card, is hardware that takes all the data from across a computer system and produces a visible image on the computer monitor or laptop screen. For filming high-quality exercise videos, editing social media content, or creating PowerPoint presentations, the built-in video card that comes with any mid-range desktop or laptop will meet the needs of a virtual coaching business.

software is found in the form of operating systems themselves, such as Windows from Microsoft or iOS from Apple, to programs such as Microsoft Word, Microsoft Excel, video games, and even just music players. **Table 15.5** lists some software considerations for virtual group instruction.

TABLE 15.5 Software Requirements

Consideration	Description
Operating software	The following are the main determining factors when choosing an operating system to fit the needs of a virtual instructing business: ■ Budget ■ Intended use, such as added video editing ■ Ease of use, with peripherals like tablets or wearable fitness trackers ■ Preference, user experience, and interface ■ Hardware
Videoconferencing software	When choosing videoconferencing software, the user should consider factors such as price, participant and meeting time thresholds, mobile app accompaniment, and other features, such as meeting recording. Although many videoconferencing applications are available for free, it is common for them to have restrictions on the number of attendees and meeting runtimes. Several software vendors (Zoom, Webex, Google Meet, Microsoft Teams, and even Facebook) offer the user the ability to upgrade to a paid version, which removes the aforementioned restrictions.
Document processing software (word processing, spreadsheets, etc.)	Word processing software is another common communication tool used by virtual fitness professionals. It can be used for record keeping and business administration activities such as scheduling and invoicing. Spreadsheet software can allow the fitness professional to create workouts, invoice participants, or build participant metric monitoring sheets, among many other uses.
Internet service requirements	The nature of virtual instruction relies on the ability to access the Internet with a reliable connection. Slow or inconsistent connections lead to frustrations for both the participant and the fitness professional and can impact quality of service. You will want to consider the following: ■ Bandwidth ■ Type of Internet (fiber optic, satellite, or broadband)

The Technology Considerations Checklist (Appendix) can be used by aspiring virtual instructors to track technology considerations, notate inventory they may already own, and suggest future technology purchases.

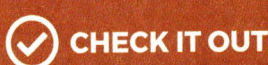 **CHECK IT OUT**

Go online and search for "Internet Speed Test," and then test your current Internet speed. If it is running at less than 25 Mbps, it may be time for you to upgrade your Internet package or service provider.

Using these checklists, fitness professionals should be able to determine what hardware and software requirements are met, how much bandwidth is needed to run a business, and what operating systems are preferred when purchasing a computer. However, although these are components that contribute to producing and delivering higher-quality content, it may also be feasible to start small and then upgrade as budget allows.

Lesson 3: Obstacles, Challenges, and Engagement Strategies

Virtual Instruction Challenges

Although virtual instruction offers many benefits for both fitness professionals and participants, fitness professionals should understand and acknowledge the constraints that come with providing virtual services. Fitness professionals looking to augment their services by offering virtual options will need to address additional obstacles and challenges faced in the virtual environment. Aside from the technical requirements when teaching virtual classes, instructors need to identify and acknowledge that there are differences between interacting in person versus virtually with the participant.

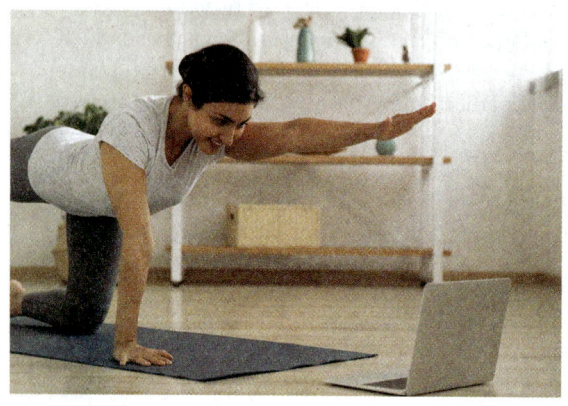

© Fizkes/Shutterstock

Participant Engagement

A virtual environment makes it easier for participants to disengage, making participant retention markedly more difficult. Therefore, fitness professionals looking to offer virtual services will face new challenges with participant engagement. Unlike in-person activities, the virtual instructor will need to seek creative solutions to ensure that participant engagement is upheld. Allowing your authenticity as a warm, dynamic professional to shine will go a long way to keeping participants on board.

Participant Safety

As with in-person classes, the participant's safety should remain a top priority. When offering virtual classes, it is imperative that instructors deliver programming that prioritizes participant safety while being conducive to the virtual environment.

When teaching a virtual group fitness class, instructors should keep the following in mind to help minimize risk of injury:

- Instructors cannot see the participants (or if they can, they cannot see every angle).
- Instructors cannot assist with hands-on adjustments or corrections and should not provide programming that requires them.
- Instructors should be diligent about providing form cues and methods for participants to gauge their intensity on their own.

- Instructors should be extra careful to demonstrate exercises correctly and thoroughly, pointing out safety concerns such as abnormal discomfort.
- Virtual instructors should never assume their participants' abilities.

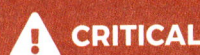

⚠ CRITICAL

Virtual instruction presents an especially significant challenge when it comes to participant safety. It is critical that instructors check in frequently with participants to remind them of the importance of self-monitoring and provide them with tips on how to do it effectively. First aid and CPR cannot be delivered in a virtual setting. Ensure that the local emergency medical response system can be activated and reach any participant if necessary.

Workout Design

Whatever the format or modality, instructors designing programming for virtual classes must consider how to keep it achievable and adaptable to a wide range of participants. Unless it is a select group or specialized program where the instructor has knowledge of each participant's abilities, limitations, and access to equipment, instructors should adhere to the following best practices for virtual workout design:

- Avoid complex movements that are difficult to cue verbally.
- Avoid high-risk movements that increase potential for injury.
- Keep equipment needs simple and limited.
- Choose exercises and movements that can be easily modified, progressed, or regressed.

Creating an Engaging Virtual Experience

The exponential growth in the digital fitness space has created countless opportunities for prospective participants to engage in all types of virtual classes. Consumers can choose from a wide array of virtual workouts that range from the highly produced, professional experiences offered by well-funded subscription services to the countless (and often questionable) free workout videos posted on the Internet. Depending on their taste, format preferences, and budget, virtual participants can typically find and engage in exactly the type of experience they desire. Although this is great news for participants, carving out a niche in the highly competitive virtual space can be daunting for instructors. Not only has it highlighted vast differences between the high-quality experiences provided by the big digital platforms and those that are decidedly less professional, but it has also flooded the market with content and increased the level of competition among virtual fitness instructors. To stand out in today's digital space, virtual instructors must create experiences that are specific, consistent, well-organized, and entertaining (Fable, 2021). To deliver engaging virtual classes, instructors must adapt their presentation style for a virtual audience, learn to motivate and connect with participants they cannot see, and build community among participants who cannot see each other.

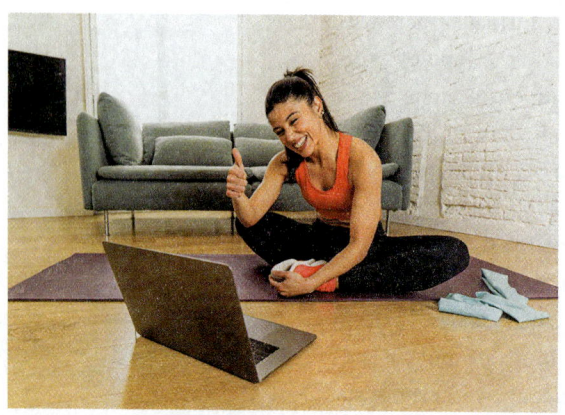
Record yourself teaching a practice virtual class with your phone or on a virtual meeting platform and then evaluate yourself. Notice your body language, focus, word choice, clarity of cues, and other presentation elements. Use what you learn by observing yourself to hone your virtual teaching skills (and share it with a friend or mentor for additional feedback).

Presentation Style and Engagement Methods

When teaching virtual classes, instructors cannot feed off the energy of the group or adapt to real-time feedback from the participants. They do not know if anyone laughs at their jokes or has responded to their questions with an enthusiastic "Whoo!" Instead, they must rely on other tactics to ensure that their presentation is engaging and fun. Fortunately, while engaging with an invisible crowd may be new to many group fitness instructors, it is a reality that performers in the entertainment industry confront regularly. By applying methods used by entertainers in mediums such as television or film, virtual group fitness instructors can effectively engage with participants in the digital exercise environment. Although many of these tactics should also be applied in live classes, they must be taken to a new level when teaching virtual classes.

PREPARATION

Preparing for a digital class might be likened to preparing for a film shoot. Before an actor can portray a character, they must learn their lines. Before a dancer can perform with precision and grace, they must learn the choreography. In the same way, a virtual instructor must plan—and often rehearse—every detail of the workout to ensure they can deliver it flawlessly. When an instructor does not need to think about what is coming next (or refer to notes), they can be fully present in their performance. Although it may seem excessive, this level of preparation will instill the instructor with a captivating confidence that transcends the digital divide, promoting participant trust and engagement.

PRESENCE

Trained performers understand the importance of exuding larger-than-life energy when they are onstage or onscreen. Virtual instructors must learn to do the same. Energy (or a lack thereof) in movement, vocal tone, and facial expressions will be exaggerated when all eyes are fixed on the performer. To keep participants engaged and energized, virtual instructors should hold themselves with confidence, execute precise movements, speak using dynamic tones, and use their facial expressions to convey genuine emotion.

FOCUS

Unlike the live setting where an instructor will scan the room and make comfortable eye contact with each participant during class, in a virtual setting, this may not be possible. When an instructor is teaching alone to a camera, they must look and speak directly into it. If the instructor's gaze is above the camera or bouncing around, it will appear as though they are disengaged or distracted. Conversely, when they look and speak directly into it, participants on the other side will perceive that they are speaking to them. This is an important distinction that instructors must embrace and execute when teaching virtually.

RELATABILITY

Another important but challenging aspect of creating engaging virtual experiences is retaining a sense of authenticity. Just as participants in live classes gravitate toward instructors who are genuine, vulnerable, and uniquely themselves, the same holds true in the virtual world. Even when presenting to individuals they cannot see, instructors must do their best to avoid sounding artificial or impersonal. It may be challenging at first, so practice is essential. This can be accomplished by recording and evaluating the areas for improvement.

WORD CHOICE

As noted earlier, excellent verbal communication skills are important in a virtual setting. To keep participants engaged and to avoid the awkwardness of silence, virtual instructors should talk almost continuously during class. For that reason, they must ensure that what they are saying is worth listening to.

Communication of goals, exercises, and drills must be clear, concise, and consistent and include relatable sensational cues that allow participants to evaluate themselves during each exercise (**Table 15.6**). When providing options, regressions, or progressions, instructors should be descriptive and thorough, providing participants with enough information to allow them to make the best decision for themselves.

TABLE 15.6 Sensational Cueing Examples

Instead of this …	Try this …
"This is hard!"	"You should feel breathless during this effort" or "This effort should feel unsustainable. You can do it for 20 more seconds, but if you feel like you could go longer, you have more to give."
"These should burn!"	"You should feel a noticeable burning sensation in the top of your thighs and glutes, but if you only feel it in your knee, check your alignment or back off."
"You got it!"	"You know you're doing it right if you feel it in back of your upper arms without pain in your shoulder or elbow."
"Keep it steady."	"You should feel like you could do this for a while. You might not want to have a long conversation, but if you can't speak more than a couple words before taking a breath, you are working too hard."

Finally, a discussion of intentional word choice would not be complete without mentioning the avoidance of repetitive filler words or pet phrases such as "Good job!" "You got it!" or "Awesome!" (which can be particularly annoying considering that the instructor has no way of knowing if they have actually got it, and it is preserved for posterity if the class is recorded). Although all instructors are susceptible to falling into the pet phrases trap, in the digital setting it can be especially obvious (Fable, 2021). To ensure that participants remain engaged with the workout and the instructor, word choice should be deliberate, positive, and, most of all, make participants feel that the instructor is speaking directly to them.

Using "if, then" statements can be an effective strategy to help participants make appropriate movement or intensity choices. For example, "If you feel pain in your knee instead of your quads working, check your alignment or reduce your range of motion" or "If you are still breathless from the last interval, tap this one out and join us when your breath is under control."

MUSIC SELECTION

Although effective music selection and utilization is imperative in all group fitness classes, it is especially important in virtual classes. Without the social connections inherent to the live setting, music can be one of the most critical factors for participant enjoyment. Instructors should approach their music selection like a director approaches the soundtrack for a movie. It should align with the energy, intensity, and mood of each class segment, providing an intentional emotional backdrop for the workout.

Additionally, participants have been shown to be more satisfied with an instructor who is visibly connected to the music selected (Wininger & Pargman, 2003). By showcasing their own connection to the music and inviting participants to do the same, instructors can create a sense of shared appreciation and improve engagement even without face-to-face interaction.

Use of music in virtual group fitness can present confusing legal gray areas, particularly the use of popular music by original artists. To avoid legal action and copyright violation, instructors should only use music from reputable organizations that specialize in this category and produce music for this purpose.

Motivating and Connecting

Although motivating and connecting with participants in the virtual environment presents challenges, it can still be accomplished by employing strategies that work particularly well in online classes. These include, but are certainly not limited to, effective goal setting, gamification or challenges, and fostering authentic connections:

- **Goal setting.** Accomplishing goals is a powerful motivator. Although everyone will have different personal goals based on their unique experience, personality, and circumstances, by communicating specific yet achievable goals in the moment as well as over time, instructors can help participants to stay motivated. Example in-the-moment goals might include something like "Try to do one more push-up in this round than the last one" or "Make it your goal to smile throughout this entire set of squats. I will do the same!" In-the-moment goals need not be complicated or excessively challenging to be an effective motivator, but they should be specific. Long-range goals might include inviting participants to commit to a certain number of workouts per week, to perform an exercise progression (e.g., 10 push-ups on their toes) by a certain date, or even to complete a full series of progressive workouts.

- **Gamification and challenges.** Related to goal setting, research has shown that gamification and challenges (i.e., achieving a set number of steps each day) can positively influence motivation to engage in physical activity (Cho et al., 2021). By applying related concepts, such as setting up and tracking participant attendance over a defined period or creating a leaderboard for a specific challenge, instructors can help participants stay motivated to remain consistent. Rewards might include a free class or other incentives such as a badge on their community profile. The use of technology and social media in the online environment can make these types of challenges easy to implement and foster engagement between participants through friendly competition.
- **Authentic connections.** In addition to motivating virtual participants, fostering authentic, personalized connections will keep them engaged and feeling as though they are valuable to you (Fable, 2021). By letting participants know who you really are, they will begin to see you as a real human being with feelings, challenges, and unique interests just like theirs. Sharing class-appropriate, personal stories relevant to a motivational message, playing favorite songs, or even referring to movies, television shows, or books you love can open a window into your world that will help them feel connected. Then, you might choose to connect your in-class message to a social media post and invite them to share their own related stories or accomplishments. In this way, even though separated by physical distance, participants may begin to feel more connected not only to you, but to the others in the class as well.

Building Community Virtually

Social media is one of the most effective ways to build community in the virtual environment. By utilizing regular social media posts that include educational tidbits, playlists, motivating messages, teasers for upcoming workouts, and calls for participants to share milestones, instructors can build a robust online community that enhances the virtual class experience and entices participants to engage with each other. Effective tactics might include, but are certainly not limited to, the following:

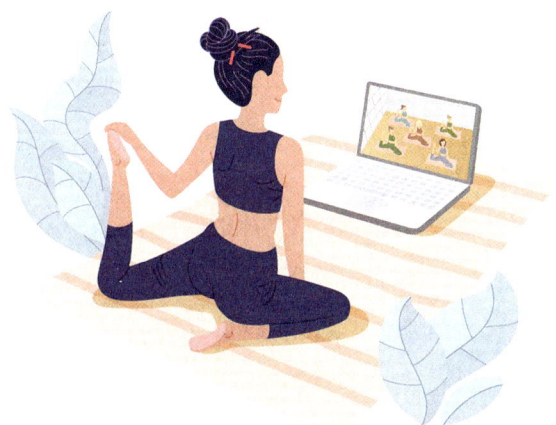

© Indie Design/Shutterstock

- Sharing the goal or theme of upcoming classes
- Polling the group to discover favorite music or exercises
- Teasing upcoming playlists
- Providing suggested workout options for days without classes
- Shouting out participants who post their results after class
- Creating opportunities for participants to identify a virtual workout buddy from class
- Setting up a virtual happy hour for class participants to meet you and each other

Given the role that social media plays in the lives of so many individuals today, it is safe to say that, in many ways, online communities can be every bit as connected as those in real life. And, considering that users of digital exercise platforms are most likely tech savvy in other areas of their lives, creating a virtual community connected to a virtual exercise class is a natural next step.

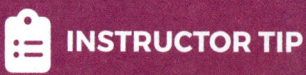
Ongoing Role of Social Media in Virtual Instruction

Although effective use of social media is a valuable tool for all instructors to build and connect with their community, for virtual instructors, the use of social media is an especially critical component. Without a physical space to share information and interact with participants, social media is often the primary method of marketing, communication, and community building.

Given its importance, virtual instructors should carefully consider how to best market and build their online fitness brand using various social media platforms. Popular strategies include the following:

- Daily or weekly scheduled posts and updates
- Short teaser videos
- Invite-only pages for participants to share and connect
- Live announcements or Q & A sessions

However, although virtual communication and social media offer many benefits, fitness professionals who offer, or plan to offer, virtual programming must also understand both the advantages and disadvantages of virtual communication (**Table 15.7**) which also includes email, messaging, and videoconferencing. The fitness professional should take stock of the range

TABLE 15.7 Communication Platforms

Platform	Description
Email	Using email for participant communication comes with many benefits, including accessibility. Email provides a clear one-on-one platform for talking between participants and fitness professionals and builds a foundation for confidentiality and trust in the relationship.
Online communities and apps	Online communities or apps can include private company memberships or social media platforms like Facebook. With private company membership, a fitness professional can have their own membership site or app where individuals can access their information and update and share results with their instructor and/or a larger community. Individuals can receive support, links, and updates just as with the private community; however, there are few ways to track data or performance.
Text messaging	Fitness professionals can use texting to provide or receive immediate answers to questions or for reminding participants of daily goals. Reminder messages are particularly useful as some studies show that they may help increase attention toward health goals (Schwebel & Larimer, 2018).
Video calls and conferencing	Various smartphone applications and online conferencing services enable fitness professionals to interact with and watch their participants perform workouts and relay comments or advice based on body language and nonverbal cues. Moreover, fitness professionals can visually demonstrate correct movement technique like they would in person.

of potential issues they might face using a virtual instructing platform and evaluate which method(s) of communication will work best for their needs.

Lesson 4: Other Virtual Considerations

Legal and Ethical Considerations for Virtual Group Fitness

All fitness professionals, including those providing virtual services, are expected to adhere to their scope of practice, which includes the services professionals are allowed to provide in accordance with their qualifications or licensure. Whatever service a Group Fitness Instructor provides, they must do so within the scope of practice aligned to their credentials. The limitations and boundaries of that scope can be found within their credentials already obtained. Although operating in a virtual environment does not change the scope of practice, it can provide some additional challenges.

Even though participants will be working with a fitness professional remotely, obtaining the correct forms and signatures remains an activity of utmost importance.

Required Legal Forms

Group Fitness Instructors providing virtual classes are responsible for the following legal forms and documents:

- **Liability release and safety waiver.** Exercise of any kind includes the risk of injury. Each participant must attest that they will perform at-home exercise in the safest possible way, acknowledge the inherent risk of physical activity, and release the fitness professional of any liability. Agreements of this nature are industry standards for gyms and health clubs when participants enroll in membership.
- **Contractual agreement.** This document covers items that include billing practices and cancellation policies that keep participants accountable.
- **Physical Activity Readiness Questionnaire (PAR-Q) with a health history questionnaire.** The PAR-Q is a simple self-screening tool that can and should be used by anyone who plans to start an exercise program. Fitness professionals or coaches typically use it to determine the safety or possible risk of exercising for an individual based on past health history, current symptoms, and other risk factors (Appendix). These forms can be emailed to a participant or provided for download on a business website. Once completed, the forms can be scanned and sent back, or hard copies mailed directly. Even when retaining paper copies, it is good practice to add scanned copies to each participant's personal digital folder as well. All forms need to be completed and signed before the first class is held.

Safety Considerations and Emergency Response

It is the instructor's responsibility to make the workout as safe as possible to prevent accidents and participant injury. However, even with appropriate precautions and planning, the possibility exists that something could go wrong. Unlike the live environment, where the instructor is there in person to respond to emergencies according to the protocols of the facility, virtual instructors must instead react quickly to notify the participant's local authorities and/or an emergency contact. For this reason, each participant should provide the instructor with a street address, emergency contact, and local police department phone number. If the participant is attending class from a different location, they should also inform the instructor of the location change.

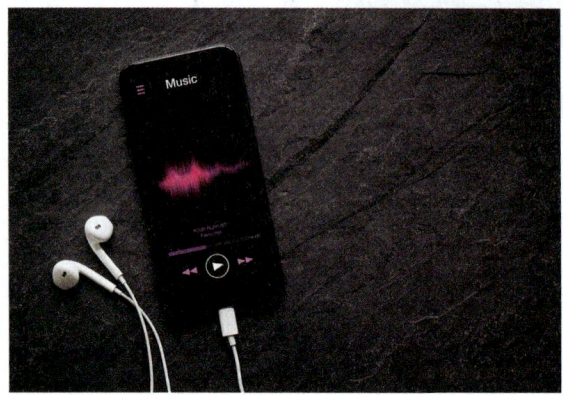

© Kaspars Grinvalds/Shutterstock

Music Use in the Virtual Environment

Using music legally is an important consideration in all group fitness environments but is especially complex in the virtual space. The legal requirements differ for workouts that are pre-recorded (on-demand) versus those that are livestreamed. The legal requirements also differ for independent instructors and those teaching as part of a commercial program or facility. Given the value that music has in classes, it is important that instructors understand which music they can legally utilize for their virtual offerings.

Critically, instructors must understand that paying a streaming service for private utilization (e.g., listening to music at home or while you work out alone) is different from paying the considerable licensing fees required for public performance (e.g., teaching group fitness to it, live or virtually). Instructors who teach live classes in facilities where they are allowed to use licensed music (e.g., music by original artists) may only do so if the facility has paid the requisite fees to the appropriate associations. This becomes even more complicated in the virtual space. For example, even if a large company has paid the fees for in-person classes, if those classes are recorded and made available on demand, it is a violation of that agreement. If an independent instructor opts to record and post a virtual class using music for which they have not paid the licensing fees, they are subject to serious legal consequences. Furthermore, if they attempt to livestream a class on a social media platform using music for which they have not paid the licensing fees, they are subject to the class being interrupted without warning.

To be protected and in compliance with the law, instructors should adhere to the following guidelines:

- For virtual classes taught as an employee of a larger entity, carefully consult the facility's management to determine which music you can legally utilize depending on the virtual medium (livestream or on-demand). If in doubt, only use music that is designated royalty-free.
- For independent instruction, unless you have personally paid the (very costly) appropriate fees and acquired the requisite licensing, only utilize royalty-free music for all types of virtual offerings.

Licensed Workouts, Programs, or Formats

Just as in the live environment, utilizing licensed workouts, programs, or formats in virtual classes without the appropriate licensing, affiliation, and /or express permission from the creator is not only unethical but also illegal. Instructors who teach licensed programming in a live setting should not assume that the same programming can be taught virtually without the knowledge and permission of the owner, even if they are paying the in-person licensing fees.

Any instructor teaching a licensed program (whether currently or formerly) should not attempt to utilize that content outside of the defined parameters. Doing so, particularly online, may result in swift and costly legal consequences. It is important to consult with the content creator to verify virtual instruction is covered under the licensing agreement.

Independent Versus Facility-Based Instruction

With the immense growth in the virtual space, it is no surprise that many instructors have entered the arena. However, for instructors who desire to teach virtually on their own while also teaching in a facility (or teaching virtually as part of an organization), this can present a conflict of interest. If an instructor who teaches in a facility is also providing virtual classes independently, they must not market their virtual offerings to the paying members of the facility. Although it can be tempting to invite regular participants from live classes in a facility to independent virtual classes, this behavior is unethical and may result in termination of employment and/or legal action.

SUMMARY

Virtual instruction allows fitness professionals to serve participants who may have otherwise been out of reach due to their preference, proximity, or availability. On the surface, it seems like the logical next step for every fitness professional, but virtual instructing will not work for everyone. Just as different classes and format styles appeal to different participants, virtual instruction will appeal to some instructors more than others.

Although it may seem that virtual instruction lacks the human connection and interaction afforded by in-person classes, one can also argue that it also enables a new level of connection with participants who were previously excluded for one reason or another. When executed effectively, the virtual experience provides participants and instructors with a new and more accessible way to work together to achieve goals and build community. Whether providing pre-recorded on-demand workouts or leading livestream classes, group fitness instructors can use virtual instruction as a means to reach a larger population.

REFERENCES

Becvar Weddle, A. (2020). *Virtual workout trends during shelter-at-home*. MindBody Business. https://www.mindbodyonline.com/business/education/blog/virtual-workout-trends-during-shelter-home

Cho, I., Kaplanidou, K., & Sato, S. (2021). Gamified wearable fitness tracker for physical activity: A comprehensive literature review. *Sustainability, 13*(13), 7017. https://doi.org/10.3390/su13137017

Fable, S. (2021, October). Digital fitness lessons with impact. *IDEA Fitness Journal.* https://www.ideafit.com/business/digital-fitness-lessons-with-impact/

Klatte, M., Bergström, K., & Lachmann, T. (2013). Does noise affect learning? A short review on noise effects on cognitive performance in children. *Frontiers in Psychology, 4,* 578. https://doi.org/10.3389/fpsyg.2013.00578

Park, S. G., & Park, K. H. (2018). Correlation between nonverbal communication and objective structured clinical examination score in medical students. *Korean Journal of Medical Education, 30*(3), 199–208. https://doi.org/10.3946/kjme.2018.94

Rodriguez, M. (2019, Sept.) Report: Health club, gym, & studio usage reach all-time high [Press release]. IHRSA. https://www.ihrsa.org/about/media-center/press-releases/report-health-club-gym-studio-usage-reach-all-time-high/

Schwebel, F. J., & Larimer, M. E. (2018). Using text message reminders in health care services: A narrative literature review. *Internet Interventions, 13*, 82–104. https://doi.org/10.1016/j.invent.2018.06.002

U.S. Bureau of Labor Statistics. (2020). *Occupational outlook handbook: fitness trainers and instructors.* https://www.bls.gov/ooh/personal-care-and-service/fitness-trainers-and-instructors.htm

Wininger, S. R., & Pargman, D. (2003). Assessment of factors associated with exercise enjoyment. *Journal of Music Therapy, 40*(1), 57–73. https://doi.org/10.1093/jmt/40.1.57

CHAPTER 16

YOUR JOURNEY AS A GROUP FITNESS INSTRUCTOR

LEARNING OBJECTIVES

The intent of this chapter is to go over next steps as you prepare for your final exam and explore employment opportunities as a Group Fitness Instructor.

After reading this content, students should be able to demonstrate the following objectives:

- **Identify** next steps for a Group Fitness Instructor.
- **Discuss** continued self-care and career maintenance and development strategies.

Lesson 1: The Exam

Introduction

As you near the end of this portion of your professional education, with all the knowledge you have gained, you might be starting to question what comes next. In this chapter, next steps will be covered as you journey into your teaching career. This includes preparing for your exam, securing a job as an instructor, and creating longevity in your career. Deciding to start with the AFAA Group Fitness Instructor credential will launch a successful career in group fitness. In this course, you have learned the following:

- About the group fitness industry and aspects of a career in group fitness
- The fundamentals of exercise science and how to apply it in a class setting

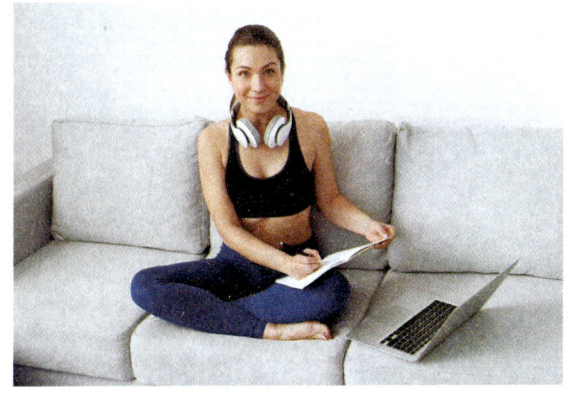

© Viktoriia Hnatiuk/Shutterstock

- How to design and plan classes that are effective and fun
- How to lead classes and create engaging experiences for all participants

Now it is time to apply what you have learned!

Preparing for Your Exam

Even when you are fully prepared, exams can still be stressful. Taking the steps to review the skills, content, and knowledge gained in this text will prepare you for success on the exam. Additionally, understanding the logistics and process of taking your exam can increase confidence and reduce stress.

Study Tips

When studying to become a Group Fitness Instructor, there is a lot of information to absorb, but making sure you understand the learning objectives from each chapter will ensure that you understand the essential concepts of the course. Reviewing the key terms presented throughout the course will help you understand the format and content to be assessed on the exam, including the various sections. Knowing how to apply the knowledge you have gained will help on the exam and beyond. You should also leverage other resources from the AFAA Group Fitness Instructor material such as the study guide, quizzes, and practice exams. This will build confidence as well as highlight any areas that may need additional review. Some additional study tips include the following:

- Practice the concepts and methods provided in the text.
- Plan to study over a period of time to avoid cramming at the last minute.
- As you review the text, rewrite the information in your own words.
- Remove distractions such as smartphones and televisions.
- Teach someone else the information you have learned, paying special attention to complex or challenging topics.
- Do your best to be relaxed while studying to improve focus.

Exam Preparation

Being prepared for your exam will reduce stress and help the day run smoothly. Some tips for being prepared for your exam include the following:

- Take the exam soon after you finish this course while the information is fresh in your mind.
- Make sure to have a good night's sleep before the day of your exam.
- Leave enough time to travel to the test location or set up online to avoid the stress of rushing.
- Eat a nutritious meal before the exam.

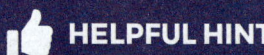 **HELPFUL HINT**

Applying the study and preparation tips will provide you with the opportunity to perform your best and achieve the best outcome on the exam.

Seeking Employment as a Group Fitness Instructor

Once you have passed your exam, received your credential, and feel comfortable designing group fitness classes, you are ready to start looking for employment, if that is the route you choose. Earlier you learned about different types of facilities and employment opportunities available to Group Fitness Instructors. Choosing an opportunity to pursue is the next step. Depending on your experience level, looking for a job at a facility that has an established group fitness program will provide opportunities to learn from peers and possibly receive additional training. Some of the additional training that you might want to look for when considering a job is the opportunity to shadow classes and/or team teach. **SHADOWING** provides an opportunity to get used to being in front of participants or on a stage without the pressure of actually teaching but still practicing demonstrating movement. Team teaching is an opportunity to teach a few minutes, a block, or a few songs without the pressure of teaching a full class. Many larger facilities have these opportunities available for new instructors. Additionally, if you already attend classes regularly at a facility, that may also be a great place to look for a job.

Applying for a job as an instructor can often be done online or in person. Many fitness facilities have online portals that allow individuals to apply directly to their location. Most facilities will require a CPR/AED certification in addition to a format-specific or Group Fitness Instructor credential. Contacting a group fitness director or manager directly and having a conversation regarding your experience can be beneficial, especially at the start of your group fitness career.

SHADOWING

Participating on stage with the class instructor without teaching.

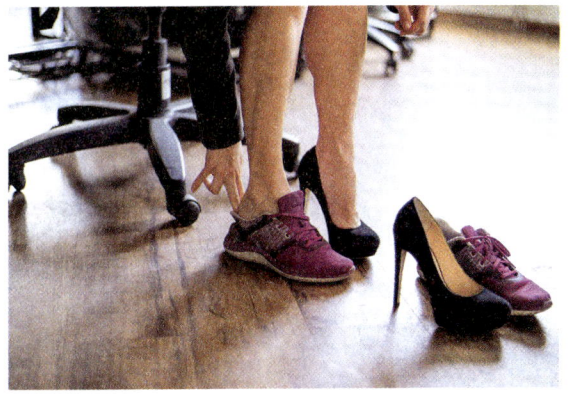
© Reshetnikov_art/Shutterstock

Auditioning and Interviewing

After you have identified and applied for a job, you may be asked to participate in an interview. When interviewing for a Group Fitness Instructor position, it is important to be prepared and professional. It is acceptable to wear professional looking activewear, but avoid wearing workout clothes. It is also very likely that you will audition as part of the hiring process, and the group

 HELPFUL HINT

When putting together audition material, it is important to present a section or class that you are confident in, with elements that showcase your ability as an instructor. It is not essential to pick the hardest section of a class. Using material that shows your ability to coach, demonstrate, and connect with participants will highlight your skills as an instructor.

fitness director or manager will schedule a time to do so. Having a prepared section and the proper attire with you at an interview will prepare you for any situation. You may be asked to audition by teaching to the group fitness manager; in this case, they may participate, or they may just observe. You could also be asked to teach a small section of material in a group audition, teaching to other instructors. Another possibility is teaching a section of a live class with another employed instructor or teaching a full class to participants. Being prepared for any of these options will ensure that you perform your best.

Designing Group Fitness Classes

Once the components of group fitness classes and workouts are understood, you can create your own library of workouts. You don't need to wait until you pass the exam or gain employment to start designing classes, but you should decide what you would like to teach. Some of the questions to ask yourself include the following:

- Do I want to teach pre-choreographed, pre-formatted, or freestyle classes?
- What type of format do I want to teach?
- What is the objective of my class?
- Do I understand what is needed in each of the five components of my class?
- Do I know what type of music I need for my class?
- Do I know the exercises or movements for the format I want to teach, or can I find them?

If you can answer these questions, you can start to design a class workout.

The first thing to do is to decide what type of class or classes you would like to teach. By outlining your workout strategy for each class type, you will be able to see the similarities and differences between them (**Figure 16.1**). Even though the steps for putting classes together differ for each type, once the music and exercises are selected, scripting and practicing your workout will be very similar.

Selecting a format is the next decision to make when building a workout. A few things to consider when choosing a class format are the demographics of your area; the availability of additional training, if needed; and available job opportunities. However, choosing a format based on what is the best fit for you, your personality, and your skill set is going to create a class, regardless of format, that is authentic and enjoyable to teach. When selecting a format, it is

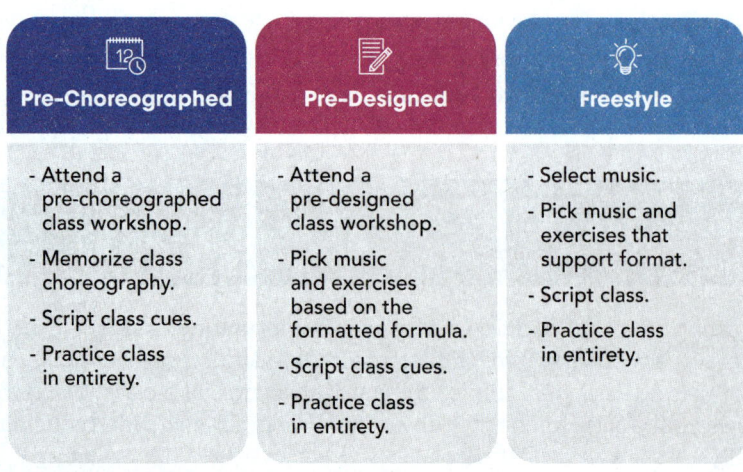

FIGURE 16.1 Steps for Class Planning by Class Type

important that you have experienced that format for yourself and that you enjoy the workout. If *you* do not enjoy the class format, it can be challenging, especially in the beginning, to deliver a class that will also be enjoyable to your participants.

Once you have selected your format, determining a class objective will create a road map for your class outcomes. This will guide everything from exercise and music selection to relevant cues that lead your participants as they achieve those objectives. For example, a class objective for a strength-based class could include the following:

- A total-body workout using assorted weights on a barbell
- A lower body workout with additional emphasis on core muscles using kettlebells
- A workout to build upper body strength using various modalities

Additionally, your class objective can be broken down into an outline of the class applied to sections based on blocks of time or with each song. Using the upper body example, the following outline could be created:

- Movement prep
- Body of the workout
  - Bodyweight exercises
  - Resistance band exercises
  - Dumbbell exercises
- Transition

Another example of the same outline might be the following:

- Movement prep
- Body of the workout
  - Chest exercises
  - Back exercises
  - Triceps exercises
  - Biceps exercises
  - Shoulder exercises
- Transition

⚙ PRACTICE THIS

Creating a class objective can vary depending on the format. For example, a cardio kickboxing class may have a different objective than a Zumba class or a yoga class. However, some class objectives can be applied across many formats. Using the following class formats, practice creating class objectives that are specific to a particular format and objectives that can be used for most or all of them:

- Step
- Kettlebell
- Cardio dance
- Pilates
- Boot camp
- Indoor cycle

After creating a class objective that aligns with the format, the five components of the workout will be designed: the intro, movement prep, body of the workout, transition, and outro. At this point, start to build the body of the workout for the class, followed by the movement prep and transition, and finally the intro and outro. It is important that the components are cohesive, work together to achieve the class objective, and are true to the class format. Understanding how each component feeds into the next will create a class that flows seamlessly and will build confidence in your participants.

Planning an entire class can feel overwhelming, but breaking down the body of the workout into smaller pieces based on time, exercise focus, or song, can make the planning smoother and build class flow. Different methods for class planning include the following:

BLOCKING METHOD

BLOCKING METHOD

Creating blocks of work based on time intervals or repetitions. These blocks can stand alone or can be repeated in a number of sets.

- You can use the blocking method to create blocks of work based on time or repetitions.
- In the blocking method, exercise can be performed to the beat of the music or the music can be used as background motivation. This method is often used in high-intensity interval training (HIIT) or boot camp formats.
- Set blocks can be built with a number of exercises, each with a specific number of repetitions. These sets are repeated a number of times, generally three to four times. Set blocks are commonly used in resistance-based formats.

SONG METHOD

SONG METHOD

Creating blocks or sections of work that last the duration of a song. This can be done by utilizing 32-count phrasing or applying exercises to song mapping.

- You can use the song method to create sections of class using a song as the duration for that block of work.
- Single-song planning can apply a section of work or exercise focus to a single song and a new section of work to the next song, and so on. Single-song planning is used in Zumba, step, and other heavily choreographed classes.
- Song building is a method that teaches a movement or series of movements and continues to build on that for the entire class. Song building is commonly used in dance cardio formats.

⚙ PRACTICE THIS

Before creating an entire class, pick five exercises and put them together in a single song, time block, and set block. Evaluate which one was the most entertaining, which had the best flow, and any impact on the intensity level of each section.

With both of these class planning methods, music can be used to drive the tempo of movement. When using the music to regulate tempo, it is important to review the recommended tempo ranges for class formats and select music that allows time for full, effective range of motion. When using the song method to plan exercise, understanding music mapping and 32-count phrasing can create class flow by aligning movement changes to music changes or to 32-count blocks of music. These movement changes can be a new exercise or dance move, or they can be a tempo change. Using the changes in the music to change tempo can create excitement and energy, even if you are teaching the same exercise through the entire song.

Selecting exercises can be like putting together a puzzle; the right pieces must fit together to create the class or it can be confusing. Having a format selected works as a guide for you, and

When participating in a class that flows from the beginning to the end without a problem, it can feel as though the experience is organic and unique. However, this can be challenging to achieve. Creating class flow is a skill that an instructor builds over time and is fine-tuned with planning, practice, and experience. It is also created in the details. Consider the following techniques you can use to create flow:

- Choose exercises that work well together.
- Create highs and lows in the workout with exercise and intensity selection.
- Balance and blend music with intense, emotional, and energetic tonalities.
- Use different voices (conversational, building, intense, and silent) to create energy or grab attention.

the five components of the workout show where to put the pieces. As you grow as an instructor, your library of workouts will continue to build robust, fun, effective, and safe classes. And after selecting exercises, progressions and regressions can be added so the class will reach a wide range of fitness levels. When starting out, however, it is important to identify resources for safe and effective exercises. When searching for creative content, remember to use credible sources only. When referencing social media and the endless supply of information on the Internet, it is easy to come across bad information. Credible sources that should be used include respected organizations or individuals that create evidence-based and researched content.

Once you have designed your group fitness class, consider doing a practice run with real participants. If you are not currently employed, ask friends and family to practice the class. This will provide insight and perspective that you may not see based on practicing alone. Ideally, practice your class with participants who have a range of fitness levels, abilities, and interests.

Instructor Self-Care

A career in group fitness is rewarding and fun, but it can take a physical and mental toll. Applying the knowledge gained in this text will help you navigate and avoid some of the strain that occurs over your career. Instructors are susceptible to and have a higher rate of overuse injuries (Bratland-Sanda et al., 2015) and perceived burnout (Prochnow et al., 2020). This underscores why self-care is an essential practice for a career in group fitness. Taking care of your body with proper nutrition, technique, alignment in and out of class, as well as body work such as massage (Best & Crawford, 2017) or stretching to reduce discomfort, can keep you healthy and teaching longer. Equally as important is protecting your voice and hearing. Being conscientious of this in the beginning will extend the longevity of your career.

Engaging in self-care and staying healthy can prevent professional burnout. Consider the following tips for professional self-care:

- Take time to rest and recover when needed.
- Set boundaries, such as a maximum number of classes per week or set days/times you are unavailable.

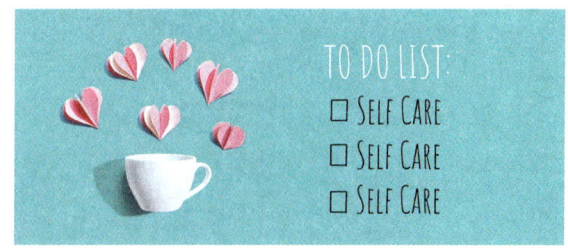

© TierneyMJ/Shutterstock

- Teach programs that you love to teach and find intrinsically enjoyable.
- Work in environments where you feel valued and safe.

Professional burnout is common and can be challenging to work through. It is important to listen to your body and, should you feel like you are heading toward burnout or are already there, discuss with your supervisor about taking some time for yourself to rest and recover, allowing you to come back refreshed and feeling your best.

👍 HELPFUL HINT

In order to avoid burnout, consider learning new formats or participating in fitness opportunities outside the group fitness studio, such as attending conferences, mentoring new instructors, or writing educational group fitness content. This is a great way to continue your work with fitness and renew your joy of teaching without being physically taxing on your body.

Lesson 3: Continuing Education

Continuing Education and Development

Continuing education is an essential part of group fitness to stay current in the industry and expand professional skill sets. It is also a great way to stay professionally motivated and invigorated. New methods of training and new formats are constantly being created, and, to stay relevant, it is necessary to advance your knowledge and skill set just as you would with any career. Continuously building your knowledge base through continuing education is a requirement to maintain your credential, but it also reveals more opportunities as an instructor and creates a fulfilling career path. Developing your skills can lead to positions such as:

- **Master trainers**: Educate new instructors and teach specializations.
- **Presenters**: Present group fitness classes to audiences all over the world.
- **Group fitness managers and directors**: Run a group fitness program at a facility, regional, or national level.
- **Group fitness content creator or program creator**: Write materials for industry education or create or choreograph programs.

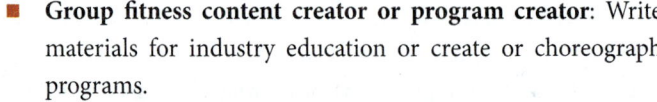
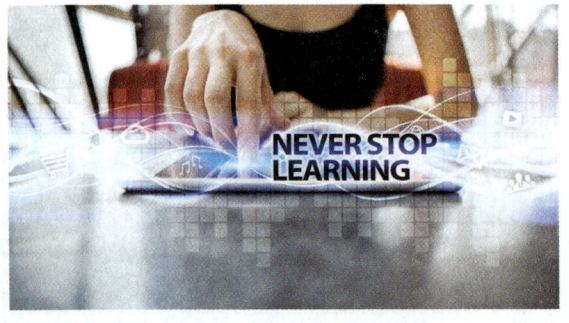

© Wright Studio/Shutterstock

Opportunities to continue learning and developing as an instructor can include both informal and formal education sessions. Some informal methods of development include attending other instructors' classes for inspiration, team teaching and exchanging feedback, and recording and reviewing yourself teaching. Formal methods of continuing education include professional workshops and conferences as well as trainings on general group fitness methods and/or specializations.

When attending formal education, keep in mind that continuing education units (CEUs) are required to maintain your AFAA Group Fitness Instructor credential. Often, an education session will provide the information needed to submit their course CEU value toward your recertification or renewal. Most educational events will advertise the CEUs that are included. If a CEU value is not provided, it is possible to submit the course information and educational material to AFAA for review and approval of CEU credit.

Specializations

An additional opportunity for career advancement and growth is to earn specializations. Specializations can start with a broad overview of a format or topic and become focused as you continue to learn. If you plan on teaching a specific format, you will be required to teach the format to meet any outlined expectations. Many fitness organizations offer trainings that specialize in formats, advanced instructor techniques, and branded equipment. Specialization within group fitness will increase your skills as an instructor and make you a more desirable candidate to potential employers.

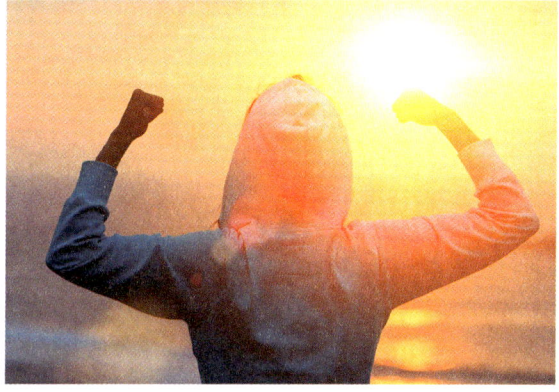
© Dirima/Shutterstock

SUMMARY

Completing this content is a significant and exciting step in your group fitness career. With the information presented, you now possess an understanding of what is required of an effective and engaging Group Fitness Instructor. Using the content provided, you can start to build classes and, most important, build the kind of fitness career you have always wanted. Your next step is to prepare for your exam to become an AFAA Group Fitness Instructor. Once you have passed the exam and have gained employment, it is time to put all your hard-earned skills and knowledge to work! Congratulations!

REFERENCES

Best, T. M., & Crawford, S. K. (2017). Massage and postexercise recovery: The science is emerging. *British Journal of Sports Medicine, 51*(19), 1386–1387. https://doi.org/10.1136/bjsports-2016-096528

Bratland-Sanda, S., Sundgot-Borgen, J., & Myklebust, G. (2015). Injuries and musculoskeletal pain among Norwegian group fitness instructors. *European Journal of Sport Science, 15*(8), 784–792. https://doi.org/10.1080/17461391.2015.1062564

Prochnow, T., Oglesby, L., Patterson, M. S., & Umstattd Meyer, M. R. (2020). Perceived burnout and coping strategies among fitness instructors: A mixed methods approach. *Managing Sport and Leisure, 27*(5), 484–498. https://doi.org/10.1080/23750472.2020.1825986

APPENDICES

AFAA's Code of Professional Conduct

AFAA has established a code of ethics and guidelines in order to protect the public and the profession. Candidates are expected and AFAA-credentialed professionals are required to agree to and follow the AFAA Code of Professional Conduct, stated below.

Professionalism. Each AFAA Professional must provide optimal professional service and demonstrate excellent participant care in their practice. Each professional must:

1. Abide fully by this AFAA Code of Professional Conduct and continue to abide by the applicable provisions of the Testing Rules of Conduct;
2. Conduct themselves in a manner that merits the respect of the public and other colleagues;
3. Treat each colleague and participant with the utmost respect and dignity;
4. Not make false or derogatory assumptions concerning the practices of colleagues and participants;
5. Use appropriate professional communication in all verbal, non-verbal, and written transactions;
6. Provide and maintain an environment that ensures participant safety that, at a minimum, requires that the AFAA Professional must:
   a. Not diagnose or treat illness or injury unless for basic first aid or if the professional is legally licensed to do so and is working in that capacity at that time;
   b. Hold a current cardiopulmonary resuscitation (CPR) and automated external defibrillator (AED) certification at all times.
7. Refer the participant to the appropriate medical practitioner when, at a minimum, the AFAA Professional:
   a. Becomes aware of any change in the participant's health status or medication;
   b. Becomes aware of an undiagnosed illness, injury, or risk factor; or
   c. Becomes aware of any unusual participant pain and/or discomfort during the course of the class that warrants professional care, in which case the professional will immediately discontinue the class for that participant.
8. Refer the participant to other healthcare professionals when nutritional and supplemental advice is requested unless the AFAA Professional has been specifically trained to do so or holds a credential to do so and is acting in that capacity at the time;
9. Maintain a level of personal hygiene appropriate for a health and fitness setting;
10. Wear clothing that is clean, professional, and appropriate to the work environment;
11. Remaining in good standing and maintain current credential status by acquiring all necessary continuing education requirements.

Confidentiality. Each AFAA Professional must respect the confidentiality of all participant information. In their professional role, the professional must:

1. Protect the participant's confidentiality in conversations, advertisement and any other arena unless otherwise agreed upon by the participant in writing or, when necessary due to a medical occurrence or when legally required; and
2. Protect the interest of participants who are minors by law or unable to give voluntary consent by securing the legal permission of the appropriate third party or guardian.

Legal and Ethical. Each AFAA Professional must comply with all legal requirements within the applicable jurisdiction. In their professional role, the professional must:

1. Obey all local, state, federal, and provincial laws, regulations and professional rules;
2. Accept complete responsibility for their actions; and
3. Respect and uphold all existing copyright, trademark and intellectual property right laws.

AFAA may revoke or otherwise take action with regard to the credential of an individual who is or has been convicted of, plead guilty to, or plead nolo contendere (no contest) to a felony or misdemeanor or has been found through legal process to have been negligent or responsible for injury or harm in performing in their professional capacity or have misrepresented their qualifications to provide services, including opinions or advice, to the public.

Business Practice. Each AFAA Professional must practice with honesty, integrity, and lawfulness. In their professional role, the professional must:

1. Maintain adequate liability insurance;
2. Accurately and truthfully inform the public of services rendered and their qualification to render such services;
3. Honestly and truthfully represent all professional qualifications and affiliations;
4. Advertise in a manner that is honest, dignified and representation of services that can be delivered without the use of provocative and/or sexual language and/or pictures;
5. Maintain accurate financial, contract, appointment, and tax records including original receipts for a minimum of four years; and
6. Comply with all local, state, federal, and regional laws and employer rules regarding harassment and discrimination, including sexual harassment.

Class Planning Sheet

Class Name:	Instructor:

Vision	
Format	
Time	
Music	
Equipment needs	
Pre-class set up	
Movement prep	
Body of workout	
Transition	
Outro	

Class Intro Template

Hey everyone! Welcome to _class name_. I'm _your name_, and I'll be guiding you through this _length_-minute class. Today we're going to be using _equipment_. Please let me know if you'd like my help as you _pick out/set up_ your _equipment/station_. Today we're going to focus on [vision] and prioritize movements that _objectives_.

> _One sentence that helps participants understand how the class will feel (muscles burning, calming, breathlessness, etc.)._

If we ever get to an exercise that's not appropriate for your body, _tell them how to get your attention_ and I'll come give you a modification.

> _One sentence or energetic phrase to set the tone for the experience before beginning class._

Class Outro Template

Great work, everyone! Today we *tell them what they accomplished*, which is great for *tell them the benefits of it*. Way to *tell them something the group did well*! I know that *identify something that really challenged them* got really tough, but take pride in *identify how they succeeded at it*. Before you leave, please *direct them how to clean their space and equipment*. I hope you join me for *share what other classes and times you teach at that facility*. If you have any questions for me, please *tell them where to find you after class*. I'm *your name*, and I'm so glad you joined me for class today. Have a great one!

Technology Considerations Checklist

Hardware Checklist

Identify current hardware. If the equipment does not meet recommended ratings, consider upgrading it. It will ensure that a quality service is being provided to the participant.

Component	Recommended Minimum Requirement	Current Equipment Ratings	Pass? Yes/No
CPU speed (GHz)	2.4 GHz or faster		
RAM/memory (GB)	8–16 GB		
Internet speed test	25 Mbps		
Smartphone video resolution	1080p high definition or greater		
Smartphone camera megapixel rating	10 megapixels or higher		

Software Inventory Checklist

Organize what software to use.

Software Program	Suggestions	Chosen Program
Spreadsheets	Google Sheets, Numbers by Apple, or Microsoft Excel	
Word processing	Google Docs, Microsoft Word, or Pages by Apple	
Videoconferencing	Google Meet, Zoom, WebEx, Skype, or Microsoft Teams	
Component	**Yes/No**	**Notes**
Digital camera or smartphone		
Tripod		
Microphone		
Lighting fixture		

PAR-Q+

2023 PAR-Q+

The Physical Activity Readiness Questionnaire for Everyone

The health benefits of regular physical activity are clear; more people should engage in physical activity every day of the week. Participating in physical activity is very safe for MOST people. This questionnaire will tell you whether it is necessary for you to seek further advice from your doctor OR a qualified exercise professional before becoming more physically active.

GENERAL HEALTH QUESTIONS

Please read the 7 questions below carefully and answer each one honestly: check YES or NO.	YES	NO
1) Has your doctor ever said that you have a heart condition ☐ OR high blood pressure ☐?	☐	☐
2) Do you feel pain in your chest at rest, during your daily activities of living, OR when you do physical activity?	☐	☐
3) Do you lose balance because of dizziness OR have you lost consciousness in the last 12 months? Please answer NO if your dizziness was associated with over-breathing (including during vigorous exercise).	☐	☐
4) Have you ever been diagnosed with another chronic medical condition (other than heart disease or high blood pressure)? PLEASE LIST CONDITION(S) HERE: _____	☐	☐
5) Are you currently taking prescribed medications for a chronic medical condition? PLEASE LIST CONDITION(S) AND MEDICATIONS HERE: _____	☐	☐
6) Do you currently have (or have had within the past 12 months) a bone, joint, or soft tissue (muscle, ligament, or tendon) problem that could be made worse by becoming more physically active? Please answer NO if you had a problem in the past, but it does not limit your current ability to be physically active. PLEASE LIST CONDITION(S) HERE: _____	☐	☐
7) Has your doctor ever said that you should only do medically supervised physical activity?	☐	☐

✓ **If you answered NO to all of the questions above, you are cleared for physical activity.**
Please sign the PARTICIPANT DECLARATION. You do not need to complete Pages 2 and 3.

- ▶ Start becoming much more physically active – start slowly and build up gradually.
- ▶ Follow Global Physical Activity Guidelines for your age (https://www.who.int/publications/i/item/9789240015128).
- ▶ You may take part in a health and fitness appraisal.
- ▶ If you are over the age of 45 yr and NOT accustomed to regular vigorous to maximal effort exercise, consult a qualified exercise professional before engaging in this intensity of exercise.
- ▶ If you have any further questions, contact a qualified exercise professional.

PARTICIPANT DECLARATION
If you are less than the legal age required for consent or require the assent of a care provider, your parent, guardian or care provider must also sign this form.

I, the undersigned, have read, understood to my full satisfaction and completed this questionnaire. I acknowledge that this physical activity clearance is valid for a maximum of 12 months from the date it is completed and becomes invalid if my condition changes. I also acknowledge that the community/fitness center may retain a copy of this form for its records. In these instances, it will maintain the confidentiality of the same, complying with applicable law.

NAME _____ DATE _____

SIGNATURE _____ WITNESS _____

SIGNATURE OF PARENT/GUARDIAN/CARE PROVIDER _____

⬤ **If you answered YES to one or more of the questions above, COMPLETE PAGES 2 AND 3.**

⚠ **Delay becoming more active if:**

- ✓ You have a temporary illness such as a cold or fever; it is best to wait until you feel better.
- ✓ You are pregnant - talk to your health care practitioner, your physician, a qualified exercise professional, and/or complete the ePARmed-X+ at www.eparmedx.com before becoming more physically active.
- ✓ Your health changes - answer the questions on Pages 2 and 3 of this document and/or talk to your doctor or a qualified exercise professional before continuing with any physical activity program.

2023 PAR-Q+

FOLLOW-UP QUESTIONS ABOUT YOUR MEDICAL CONDITION(S)

1.	**Do you have Arthritis, Osteoporosis, or Back Problems?**	
	If the above condition(s) is/are present, answer questions 1a-1c If **NO** ☐ go to question 2	
1a.	Do you have difficulty controlling your condition with medications or other physician-prescribed therapies? (Answer **NO** if you are not currently taking medications or other treatments)	YES ☐ NO ☐
1b.	Do you have joint problems causing pain, a recent fracture or fracture caused by osteoporosis or cancer, displaced vertebra (e.g., spondylolisthesis), and/or spondylolysis/pars defect (a crack in the bony ring on the back of the spinal column)?	YES ☐ NO ☐
1c.	Have you had steroid injections or taken steroid tablets regularly for more than 3 months?	YES ☐ NO ☐

2.	**Do you currently have Cancer of any kind?**	
	If the above condition(s) is/are present, answer questions 2a-2b If **NO** ☐ go to question 3	
2a.	Does your cancer diagnosis include any of the following types: lung/bronchogenic, multiple myeloma (cancer of plasma cells), head, and/or neck?	YES ☐ NO ☐
2b.	Are you currently receiving cancer therapy (such as chemotheraphy or radiotherapy)?	YES ☐ NO ☐

3.	**Do you have a Heart or Cardiovascular Condition? This includes Coronary Artery Disease, Heart Failure, Diagnosed Abnormality of Heart Rhythm**	
	If the above condition(s) is/are present, answer questions 3a-3d If **NO** ☐ go to question 4	
3a.	Do you have difficulty controlling your condition with medications or other physician-prescribed therapies? (Answer **NO** if you are not currently taking medications or other treatments)	YES ☐ NO ☐
3b.	Do you have an irregular heart beat that requires medical management? (e.g., atrial fibrillation, premature ventricular contraction)	YES ☐ NO ☐
3c.	Do you have chronic heart failure?	YES ☐ NO ☐
3d.	Do you have diagnosed coronary artery (cardiovascular) disease and have not participated in regular physical activity in the last 2 months?	YES ☐ NO ☐

4.	**Do you currently have High Blood Pressure?**	
	If the above condition(s) is/are present, answer questions 4a-4b If **NO** ☐ go to question 5	
4a.	Do you have difficulty controlling your condition with medications or other physician-prescribed therapies? (Answer **NO** if you are not currently taking medications or other treatments)	YES ☐ NO ☐
4b.	Do you have a resting blood pressure equal to or greater than 160/90 mmHg with or without medication? (Answer **YES** if you do not know your resting blood pressure)	YES ☐ NO ☐

5.	**Do you have any Metabolic Conditions? This includes Type 1 Diabetes, Type 2 Diabetes, Pre-Diabetes**	
	If the above condition(s) is/are present, answer questions 5a-5e If **NO** ☐ go to question 6	
5a.	Do you often have difficulty controlling your blood sugar levels with foods, medications, or other physician-prescribed therapies?	YES ☐ NO ☐
5b.	Do you often suffer from signs and symptoms of low blood sugar (hypoglycemia) following exercise and/or during activities of daily living? Signs of hypoglycemia may include shakiness, nervousness, unusual irritability, abnormal sweating, dizziness or light-headedness, mental confusion, difficulty speaking, weakness, or sleepiness.	YES ☐ NO ☐
5c.	Do you have any signs or symptoms of diabetes complications such as heart or vascular disease and/or complications affecting your eyes, kidneys, **OR** the sensation in your toes and feet?	YES ☐ NO ☐
5d.	Do you have other metabolic conditions (such as current pregnancy-related diabetes, chronic kidney disease, or liver problems)?	YES ☐ NO ☐
5e.	Are you planning to engage in what for you is unusually high (or vigorous) intensity exercise in the near future?	YES ☐ NO ☐

2023 PAR-Q+

6. **Do you have any Mental Health Problems or Learning Difficulties?** This includes Alzheimer's, Dementia, Depression, Anxiety Disorder, Eating Disorder, Psychotic Disorder, Intellectual Disability, Down Syndrome

If the above condition(s) is/are present, answer questions 6a-6b   If **NO** ☐ go to question 7

6a.	Do you have difficulty controlling your condition with medications or other physician-prescribed therapies? (Answer **NO** if you are not currently taking medications or other treatments)	YES ☐ NO ☐
6b.	Do you have Down Syndrome **AND** back problems affecting nerves or muscles?	YES ☐ NO ☐

7. **Do you have a Respiratory Disease?** This includes Chronic Obstructive Pulmonary Disease, Asthma, Pulmonary High Blood Pressure

If the above condition(s) is/are present, answer questions 7a-7d   If **NO** ☐ go to question 8

7a.	Do you have difficulty controlling your condition with medications or other physician-prescribed therapies? (Answer **NO** if you are not currently taking medications or other treatments)	YES ☐ NO ☐
7b.	Has your doctor ever said your blood oxygen level is low at rest or during exercise and/or that you require supplemental oxygen therapy?	YES ☐ NO ☐
7c.	If asthmatic, do you currently have symptoms of chest tightness, wheezing, laboured breathing, consistent cough (more than 2 days/week), or have you used your rescue medication more than twice in the last week?	YES ☐ NO ☐
7d.	Has your doctor ever said you have high blood pressure in the blood vessels of your lungs?	YES ☐ NO ☐

8. **Do you have a Spinal Cord Injury?** This includes Tetraplegia and Paraplegia

If the above condition(s) is/are present, answer questions 8a-8c   If **NO** ☐ go to question 9

8a.	Do you have difficulty controlling your condition with medications or other physician-prescribed therapies? (Answer **NO** if you are not currently taking medications or other treatments)	YES ☐ NO ☐
8b.	Do you commonly exhibit low resting blood pressure significant enough to cause dizziness, light-headedness, and/or fainting?	YES ☐ NO ☐
8c.	Has your physician indicated that you exhibit sudden bouts of high blood pressure (known as Autonomic Dysreflexia)?	YES ☐ NO ☐

9. **Have you had a Stroke?** This includes Transient Ischemic Attack (TIA) or Cerebrovascular Event

If the above condition(s) is/are present, answer questions 9a-9c   If **NO** ☐ go to question 10

9a.	Do you have difficulty controlling your condition with medications or other physician-prescribed therapies? (Answer **NO** if you are not currently taking medications or other treatments)	YES ☐ NO ☐
9b.	Do you have any impairment in walking or mobility?	YES ☐ NO ☐
9c.	Have you experienced a stroke or impairment in nerves or muscles in the past 6 months?	YES ☐ NO ☐

10. **Do you have any other medical condition not listed above or do you have two or more medical conditions?**

If you have other medical conditions, answer questions 10a-10c   If **NO** ☐ read the Page 4 recommendations

10a.	Have you experienced a blackout, fainted, or lost consciousness as a result of a head injury within the last 12 months **OR** have you had a diagnosed concussion within the last 12 months?	YES ☐ NO ☐
10b.	Do you have a medical condition that is not listed (such as epilepsy, neurological conditions, kidney problems)?	YES ☐ NO ☐
10c.	Do you currently live with two or more medical conditions?	YES ☐ NO ☐

PLEASE LIST YOUR MEDICAL CONDITION(S) AND ANY RELATED MEDICATIONS HERE: _____

> ## GO to Page 4 for recommendations about your current medical condition(s) and sign the PARTICIPANT DECLARATION.

APPENDIX F

2023 PAR-Q+

✅ **If you answered NO to all of the FOLLOW-UP questions (pgs. 2-3) about your medical condition, you are ready to become more physically active - sign the PARTICIPANT DECLARATION below:**

▶ It is advised that you consult a qualified exercise professional to help you develop a safe and effective physical activity plan to meet your health needs.

▶ You are encouraged to start slowly and build up gradually - 20 to 60 minutes of low to moderate intensity exercise, 3-5 days per week including aerobic and muscle strengthening exercises.

▶ As you progress, you should aim to accumulate 150 minutes or more of moderate intensity physical activity per week.

▶ If you are over the age of 45 yr and **NOT** accustomed to regular vigorous to maximal effort exercise, consult a qualified exercise professional before engaging in this intensity of exercise.

🛑 **If you answered YES to one or more of the follow-up questions** about your medical condition:
You should seek further information before becoming more physically active or engaging in a fitness appraisal. You should complete the specially designed online screening and exercise recommendations program - the **ePARmed-X+ at www.eparmedx.com** and/or visit a qualified exercise professional to work through the ePARmed-X+ and for further information.

⚠ **Delay becoming more active if:**

✓ You have a temporary illness such as a cold or fever; it is best to wait until you feel better.

✓ You are pregnant - talk to your health care practitioner, your physician, a qualified exercise professional, and/or complete the ePARmed-X+ **at www.eparmedx.com** before becoming more physically active.

✓ Your health changes - talk to your doctor or qualified exercise professional before continuing with any physical activity program.

- You are encouraged to photocopy the PAR-Q+. You must use the entire questionnaire and NO changes are permitted.
- The authors, the PAR-Q+ Collaboration, partner organizations, and their agents assume no liability for persons who undertake physical activity and/or make use of the PAR-Q+ or ePARmed-X+. If in doubt after completing the questionnaire, consult your doctor prior to physical activity.

PARTICIPANT DECLARATION

- All persons who have completed the PAR-Q+ please read and sign the declaration below.

- If you are less than the legal age required for consent or require the assent of a care provider, your parent, guardian or care provider must also sign this form.

I, the undersigned, have read, understood to my full satisfaction and completed this questionnaire. I acknowledge that this physical activity clearance is valid for a maximum of 12 months from the date it is completed and becomes invalid if my condition changes. I also acknowledge that the community/fitness center may retain a copy of this form for records. In these instances, it will maintain the confidentiality of the same, complying with applicable law.

NAME _____ DATE _____

SIGNATURE _____ WITNESS _____

SIGNATURE OF PARENT/GUARDIAN/CARE PROVIDER _____

— For more information, please contact —
www.eparmedx.com
Email: eparmedx@gmail.com

Citation for PAR-Q+
Warburton DER, Jamnik VK, Bredin SSD, and Gledhill N on behalf of the PAR-Q+ Collaboration. The Physical Activity Readiness Questionnaire for Everyone (PAR-Q+) and Electronic Physical Activity Readiness Medical Examination (ePARmed-X+). Health & Fitness Journal of Canada 4(2):3-23, 2011.

Key References
1. Jamnik VK, Warburton DER, Makarski J, McKenzie DC, Shephard RJ, Stone J, and Gledhill N. Enhancing the effectiveness of clearance for physical activity participation; background and overall process. APNM 36(S1):S3-S13, 2011.
2. Warburton DER, Gledhill N, Jamnik VK, Bredin SSD, McKenzie DC, Stone J, Charlesworth S, and Shephard RJ. Evidence-based risk assessment and recommendations for physical activity clearance; Consensus Document. APNM 36(S1):S266-s298, 2011.
3. Chisholm DM, Collis ML, Kulak LL, Davenport W, and Gruber N. Physical activity readiness. British Columbia Medical Journal. 1975;17:375-378.
4. Thomas S, Reading J, and Shephard RJ. Revision of the Physical Activity Readiness Questionnaire (PAR-Q). Canadian Journal of Sport Science 1992;17:4 338-345.

The PAR-Q+ was created using the evidence-based AGREE process (1) by the PAR-Q+ Collaboration chaired by Dr. Darren E. R. Warburton with Dr. Norman Gledhill, Dr. Veronica Jamnik, and Dr. Donald C. McKenzie (2). Production of this document has been made possible through financial contributions from the Public Health Agency of Canada and the BC Ministry of Health Services. The views expressed herein do not necessarily represent the views of the Public Health Agency of Canada or the BC Ministry of Health Services.

Copyright © 2023 PAR-Q+ Collaboration 4/ 4
01-11-2022

Reprinted with permission from the PAR-Q+ Collaboration (www.eparmedx.com) and the authors of the PAR-Q+ (Dr. Darren Warburton, Dr. Norman Gledhill, Dr. Veronica Jamnik, Dr. Roy Shephard, and Dr. Shannon Bredin).

Citations:

Warburton D, Jamnik V, Bredin S, Shephard R, Gledhill N. The 2022 Physical Activity Readiness Questionnaire for Everyone (PAR-Q+) and electronic Physical Activity Readiness Medical Examination (ePARmed-X+). Health & Fitness Journal of Canada 2022;15(1):54-57. https://hfjc.library.ubc.ca/index.php/HFJC/article/view/815

Warburton DER, Gledhill N, Jamnik VK, Bredin SSD, McKenzie DC, Stone J, Charlesworth S, Shephard RJ, on behalf of the PAR-Q+ Collaboration. The Physical Activity Readiness Questionnaire for Everyone (PAR-Q+) and electronic Physical Activity Readiness Medical Examination (ePARmed-X+): Summary of consensus panel recommendations. Health & Fitness Journal of Canada 2011;4:26-37.

32-count phrasing A common musical structure used in group fitness where musical sections are arranged in 32-count blocks to create choreography that can easily be broken down into exercise sequences.

5 components of a workout The five essential elements that provide a scientifically sound and holistic group exercise experience: intro, movement prep, body of the workout, transition, and outro.

A

Acetyl coenzyme A A byproduct formed from metabolism of glucose, fatty acids, and amino acids that is used for the production of adenosine triphosphate (ATP).

Activities of daily living (ADL) The fundamental tasks needed to manage basic self-care activities, such as bathing, dressing, grooming, meal preparation and feeding, and homemaking.

Acute program variables Aspects of a training program that dictate the stimulus provided.

Adenosine triphosphate (ATP) The unit of energy created, stored, and used by the body to support all functions of living, including exercise and physical activity.

Aerobic Literally means "with oxygen"; refers to the metabolic pathway for creating energy in the presence of oxygen.

Aerobic (oxidative) system One of the body's three energy systems. This energy system is fueled by fats, carbohydrates, and proteins and requires oxygen. It can produce a seemingly limitless supply of energy but it does so at a slower rate than the other two systems.

AFAA 5 questions A series of considerations to aid in evaluating the safety, efficacy, and appropriateness of exercise selection.

Agility Ability to maintain center of gravity over a changing base of support while changing direction at various speeds.

Agonist Muscle that works as the prime mover of a joint exercise.

Anaerobic Literally means "without oxygen"; refers to the metabolic pathway for creating energy without the presence of oxygen.

Anaerobic threshold The exercise intensity at which glycogen via the anaerobic glycolysis energy system becomes an exerciser's dominant fuel source.

Antagonists Muscles that oppose the prime mover.

Association The act of focusing intently on internal feedback while performing a task, such as breath rate or muscle activity.

Associative cues Cues that turn the focus inward to concentrate on the feedback cues from the body.

Asynchronous An application of music where there is no conscious synchronization between the tempo or meter of the music and an individual's movement.

Ataxia Impaired coordination due to damaged nerves.

ATP-PC system One of the body's three energy systems. This anaerobic system produces energy very rapidly but in extremely limited amounts. It is fueled by adenosine triphosphate (ATP) and phosphocreatine. Also known as the ATP-CP and phosphagen systems.

Auditory cueing The use of verbal communication to share information.

Auditory learning Deriving information by listening.

Autonomy The understanding and ability to directly affect an outcome.

B

Balance Ability to maintain the body's center of gravity within its base of support.

Base of support (BOS) The area encompassed by the points of contact between an exerciser and a stable surface.

GLOSSARY

Beat The audible, metrical division that occurs within the foundational layer of music.

Beat drop The dramatic release of progressive tension within a song. Typically occurs two to three times within a song.

Beats per minute (BPM) A musical term that refers to measurement of the tempo (speed) of music.

Bioenergetics The study of the three energy systems, also referred to as metabolic pathways, that produce adenosine triphosphate (ATP).

Blocking method Creating blocks of work based on time intervals or repetitions. These blocks can stand alone or can be repeated in a number of sets.

Body composition The relative proportion of fat mass and fat-free mass in the body.

Body mass index (BMI) Formula for screening weight categories in which an individual's weight (in kg) is divided by the square of their height (in meters).

Body of the workout Majority of the fitness class; exercises with a singular or integrated focus on cardiorespiratory fitness, muscular endurance, flexibility, mindfulness, or fun.

Brand-specific format A specialized group fitness training to prepare instructors to teach formats that require knowledge and skill beyond the scope of a primary certification, such as indoor cycling.

Broad objectives Class objectives that are open-ended and vague, usually referenced in the written description.

C

Cardiac output ($\dot{Q}$) Heart rate multiplied by stroke volume; a measure of the overall performance of the heart and the amount of blood the heart pumps over a period of time.

Central nervous system (CNS) Division of the nervous system comprising the brain and the spinal cord. Its primary function is to coordinate activity of all parts of the body.

Chin tuck A neutral position of the head and neck (cervical spine) where the chin is level and head is pulled straight back so the ears are aligned over the shoulders.

Class objective A specific, clearly defined milestone that acts as a stepping stone along the journey toward achieving the desired outcome.

Class template The outline of a group fitness class format that divides the class into blocks of work and provides guidance for the instructor as they choose which movements and exercises to fill in as they write the workout.

Class vision A broad intention that guides the specific decisions the instructor makes as they plan the class.

Communication touch points Moments of interaction that build rapport, trust, and connection through positive communication.

Compound movement An exercise in which multiple joint segments and muscle groups are engaged during the exercise.

Concentric A muscle action that occurs when a muscle develops tension to overcome a resistive force, resulting in the shortening of the muscle.

Conditioned A state in which the body has proportionately adapted to imposed demands through practice and repeated exposure.

Constructive feedback Feedback that provides information regarding an individual's actions that can be used to improve performance and build successful behaviors.

Continuing education unit (CEU) A unit of education required by AFAA to maintain certification. To remain current, AFAA instructors must earn 15 CEUs every 2 years.

Crossfade A setting in a music playback device or application that blends the end of one song into the beginning of the next, making the transition sound seamless.

D

Dissociation The act of mentally separating or disconnecting from a physical task and focusing on other external elements, such as sounds or visual input.

Dissociative cue Cues that turn the focus outward to offer distraction from internal cues or discomfort.

Distress The body's physiological response to a stressor resulting in negative experiences, feelings, and mental states.

Dynamic balance Ability to maintain equilibrium through the intended path of motion when external forces are present.

Dynamic stretching The active extension of a muscle, using a muscle's force production and the body's momentum, to take a joint through the full available range of motion.

Dyspnea Difficulty or trouble breathing.

E

Eccentric A muscle action that occurs when a muscle develops tension while lengthening.

Endorphins Chemicals produced by the nervous system to cope with stress.

Endurance The ability to sustain a given effort for an extended period of time or to resist fatigue.

Energy systems Three distinct but interrelated metabolic processes the body uses to create energy based on physiological demand: ATP-PC system, the glycolytic (anaerobic) system, and the aerobic system.

Eustress The body's physiological response to a stressor resulting in improvement, positive adaptation, or positive experience.

Exercise Physical activity that is usually planned, structured, generally repetitive in nature, and intended to induce some

level of overload on the body's physiological systems.

Exercise selection Process of choosing exercises that allow for achievement of the desired adaptation.

F

Fitness Any activity or exercise that elicits general improvements in at least one of the health-related parameters of fitness.

Flexibility The present state or ability of a joint to move through a range of motion.

Flow The ability to create a seamless experience for participants where they connect to the music, moves, and the class as a whole.

Freestyle Method of choreography based on the instructor's personal preference, skill set, and knowledge.

Frontal plane Plane of motion that divides the body into anterior and posterior halves.

Function Integrated, multiplanar movement that involves acceleration, stabilization, and deceleration of the forces our bodies encounter each day.

G

General adaptation syndrome How the body responds to imposed demands to accommodate future application of similar stressors. Characterized by the three stages of alarm, resistance, and exhaustion.

Glucose A simple sugar that is the main fuel for the body's

cells. It is produced by the breakdown of complex carbohydrates.

Glycogen A complex carbohydrate stored in the muscles and liver that is used in energy production.

Glycolytic (anaerobic) system One of the body's three energy systems. This anaerobic system produces energy rapidly through anaerobic glycolysis, which uses carbohydrate as fuel to produce energy.

Golgi tendon organs (GTOs) Receptors sensitive to the change in tension of the muscle and the rate of that change.

Group fitness as a service Offering group fitness classes with no extra fees—considered as a benefit of membership.

H

Health Any movement, activity, or exercise where physiological adaptations include some quantitative or qualitative measure of health (e.g., blood pressure or blood sugar).

Heart palpitations Heart flutters or rapid heartbeat.

Heart rate (HR) Rate at which the heart pumps, usually measured in beats per minute (bpm).

Heart rate reserve (HRR) Also called the Karvonen method; a formula used to calculate exercise target heart rates that takes into account maximal heart rate and resting heart rate: $[(HR_{max} - HR_{rest}) \times$ Desired intensity percentage] + HR_{rest} = Target heart rate.

Heart rate training zones Often calculated as a percentage of maximal heart rate. Heart rate values are divided into functional ranges used to gauge intensity and develop particular forms of cardiorespiratory fitness.

Heat cramps Muscle spasms that are painful. It could be a warning signal or sign of a heat-related emergency.

Heat exhaustion More severe than heat cramps and usually occurs after a long period of strenuous exercise or work in the heat and/or humidity.

Heat stroke The most severe heat emergency; usually occurs after the signals of heat exhaustion are ignored. Dangerously elevated internal temperatures cause vital body systems to fail.

Hypertension Chronically high blood pressure as defined by a systolic pressure above 130 mm Hg and/or a diastolic blood pressure above 80 mm Hg.

Hypertrophy Skeletal muscle fiber enlargement.

Hypothermia Condition that occurs when the body can no longer generate enough heat to maintain normal body temperature.

I

Initial training Education taken to qualify to teach a specific group exercise format designed by a particular brand or organization.

Integrated fitness Comprehensive approach combining all exercise components to help a participant achieve higher levels of function.

Interpersonal communication Communication that takes place between two individuals, characterized by a back-and-forth exchange of information while alternating the roles of sender and receiver.

Interval training Training that alternates lighter exertion or recovery periods with higher intensity exertion periods.

Intrapersonal communication Communication with oneself, including self-talk, visualization, memory, and the use of imagery.

Intrinsic motivation The driving force behind actions taken for inherent enjoyment, interest, and the pleasure of doing them and the satisfaction one receives from them.

Intro Instructor engagement with participants and an explanation of the workout and class expectations.

Isometric When a muscle is exerting force equal to the force being placed on it, leading to no visible change in the muscle length.

K

Kinesiology The study of human body movement.

Kinesthetic cueing The use of physical movement and feedback to communicate information.

Kinesthetic feedback Information about body position and movement as provided by internal feedback mechanisms such as stretch receptors.

Kinesthetic learning Obtaining information through physical action.

Kinetic chain A concept that comes from engineering that compares the segments of the human body to the links in a chain, with each joint affecting those above and below it.

L

Lactate A byproduct of anaerobic energy production. Also known as lactic acid.

Lactate threshold The point during high-intensity activity when the body can no longer meet its demand for oxygen and anaerobic metabolism predominates.

Livestream classes Virtual (online) group fitness classes that are taught in real time. Participants log in to class at a scheduled time, similar to showing up at a facility.

M

Macronutrients Nutrients required in large amounts in the diet; include carbohydrate, fat, and protein.

Maximal heart rate (HR_{max}) The fastest rate an individual's heart can beat in 1 minute.

Mechanoreceptors Sensory receptors responsible for

sensing change of position in body tissues.

Metabolic pathway A series of chemical reactions that either break down or build up compounds in the body.

Metabolic response A reaction by the body to a stimulus or influence.

Metabolism All of the chemical reactions that occur in the body that are required for life. It is the process by which nutrients are acquired, transported, used, and disposed of by the body.

Mind–body connection The relationship between the brain and the physical body whereby a person's thoughts, emotions, beliefs, and attitudes can affect their physical functioning and performance.

Modality Form or mode of exercise that presents a specific stress to the body.

Modification An alteration to an exercise or movement, including progressions, regressions, and alternative movement options.

Mood The emotional state of an individual.

Movement prep Exercises to increase body temperature and blood flow and prime the body for the workout demands.

Muscle contraction Series of steps that result in the muscle producing force.

Muscle spindle A receptor that senses the amount and rate of stretch in muscle tissue.

Musical phrase A single unit of music that creates a regular pattern and that typically

makes sense when heard alone.

Music mapping The process of identifying the basic elements of a song such as the intro, verse, chorus, and other notable features so that they may be applied in class design.

N

Neural drive The signals from the nervous system that activate muscle fibers.

Neuromuscular efficiency The ability of the neuromuscular system to enable all muscles to work in a coordinated manner in all planes of motion.

Neutral spine Ideal alignment of the spine's curves to allow for safety, structural support, proper distribution of forces, and optimal muscular activation.

Niche A specific area of expertise that is focused for a specific audience.

Non-stop mix A format of fitness music that is seamlessly mixed together without gaps between songs. It is often mixed together at a consistent BPM throughout with one song flowing to the next. Also referred to as a continuous mix.

Nonverbal communication Conveying information without the use of words.

O

Obesity A complex, chronic noncommunicable disease involving an excessive amount of body fat; classified by a

body mass index (BMI) of 30 or greater.

On-demand classes Virtual (online) group fitness classes that are pre-recorded and can be viewed by the user at a time of their choosing.

Osteoporosis A skeletal condition of decreased bone mass and increased risk of fracture.

Outro Final class segment to conclude the class, praise participants' effort, and invite participants back to the next class.

Overtraining Condition in which the individual trains too much, which results in a decrease in function and performance.

P

Parasympathetic nervous system The portion of the autonomic nervous system that helps the body to return to a resting state.

Participant-centered Creating, modifying, and teaching workouts for the needs and goals of your participants.

Pedaling cadence Often used interchangeably with revolutions per minute (RPM) in reference to pedaling speed.

Periodization Division of a training program into smaller progressive steps, with built-in recovery phases.

Peripheral nervous system (PNS) All of the nerve fibers that branch off from the spinal cord and extend to the rest of the body.

GLOSSARY

Personal branding Efforts made through interpersonal interaction and online presentation that communicate your vision, values, talents, expertise, and beliefs.

Personalized cueing Providing cues that focus on personalized feedback or instruction based on an individual's situation.

Perturbation A disturbance of equilibrium; shaking.

Physical activity Any movement involving larger or multiple muscle groups that results in increased expenditure of calories.

Plyometric training Uses quick, powerful movements involving an eccentric contraction followed immediately by an explosive concentric contraction.

Positive feedback Feedback that communicates approval of a behavior and motivates an individual to continue the current behavior.

Positive feedback loop A system in which output is used as an input to improve on and create beneficial effects on future behavior.

Posterior chain Group of coordinating muscles along the back of the body (i.e., the hamstrings, glutes, and back).

Post-natal The period just after delivery of a baby.

Power The amount of force produced in a given amount of time.

Pre-choreographed All components of a class are created by a single person, business, or organization with a connected theme, brand, or experience.

Pre-designed A template that provides an overall class direction, theme, or experience that allows instructors to control other variables.

Primary certification/ credential A foundational group fitness certification that addresses the essential knowledge, skills, and abilities that every group fitness instructor should possess to operate within their scope of practice.

Principle of adaptation The long-term changes to the human movement system in response to the demands imposed by exercise or physical activity.

Principle of overload To create physiological changes, an exercise stimulus must be applied at an intensity greater than the body is accustomed to receiving.

Principle of progression An option that allows the fitness class participant to increase complexity, impact, or intensity of a movement or movement patterns.

Principle of specificity The type of exercise stimulus placed on the body will determine the expected physiological outcome.

Progression A modification that increases the difficulty of an exercise or movement combination.

Progressive overload Gradually increasing the demand of an exercise or workout over time in order to make small, consistent improvements in a person's overall fitness.

Proprioception The body's ability to naturally sense its general orientation and relative position of its parts.

Proprioceptive challenges Demands placed on the body's ability to sense its position and maintain its stability.

Prosocial behavior A social behavior intended to benefit others (like helping, sharing, or cooperating) or society as a whole, including conformity to acceptable social behaviors or rules.

Public communication One individual addresses a large group.

Pyruvate A byproduct formed during glycolysis, the metabolic process that breaks down glucose and produces adenosine triphosphate (ATP).

Q

Quickness Ability to react to a stimulus with an appropriate muscular response without hesitation.

R

Radio edit A version of a song edited for radio airplay. It may be shorter than the original version and often will have explicit lyrics removed or muted.

Range of motion (ROM) The amount of motion available at a specific joint.

Rating of perceived exertion (RPE) A subjective measurement of physical activity intensity that uses a numeric scale to rate exercise intensity.

Recertification/renewal Continuing group fitness education to remain in good standing as an AFAA instructor.

Regression A modification that decreases the difficulty or demand of an exercise or movement combination.

Remix A version of a song that has been re-worked, often for the purpose of being played in dance clubs. Frequently, the BPM is changed (typically sped up), and the song may also be extended. Remixes can be very useful in group fitness for this reason.

Repetition One complete movement of a single exercise.

Resting heart rate (HR$_{rest}$) The number of heart beats per minute while at complete rest.

Retention tool A service that is offered to connect members to a location and keep them coming back.

Revolutions per minute (RPM) A measure of pedaling speed, or cadence.

Rhythm A pattern of repeated movement or sound.

Rhythm response A concept that references the natural tendency to move in sync with music.

Royalty-free A category of music licensing where the user typically pays a fee only once to play the music unlimited times.

S

Sagittal plane Plane of motion that divides the body into right and left halves.

Sarcomere Individual contractile unit of muscle made up of actin (thin) and myosin (thick) filaments.

Sarcopenia Age-related loss of muscle mass and strength.

Scope of practice Knowledge, skills, abilities, processes, and limitations for which an instructor should be held accountable.

Self-myofascial rolling (SMR) A self-induced rolling technique to inhibit overactive muscles and improve flexibility.

Set A group of consecutive repetitions.

Shadowing Participating on stage with the class instructor without teaching.

Small group communication An interaction of more than two people but a number small enough to allow all participants to interact.

Somatic nervous system The portion of the nervous system that is under voluntary control.

Song method Creating blocks or sections of work that last the duration of a song. This can be done by utilizing 32-count phrasing or applying exercises to song mapping.

Specialty certification Formats created and managed by businesses, education providers, corporate club chains, private studios, and even individual instructors in specific fitness disciplines or with specific equipment.

Specific objectives Class objectives that are clear, explicit, and often change for each individual class.

Speed The straight-ahead velocity of an individual.

Static balance Ability to maintain equilibrium in place with no external forces.

Static stretching The process of passively taking a muscle to the point of tension and holding the stretch for a minimum of 30 seconds.

Strength The ability of the neuromuscular system to produce force; the maximal amount of force that can be produced.

Stress The body's physiological response to a stressor, which can be an event or condition.

Stretch tolerance A person's ability to experience the physical sensations associated with stretching and increase their comfort at end-range.

Stretching An active process to elongate muscles and connective tissues in order to increase the present state of flexibility.

Stroke volume (SV) Amount of blood pumped out of the heart with each contraction.

Sympathetic nervous system The portion of the autonomic nervous system that helps the body to respond to stress. Also known as the fight-or-flight response.

Synchronous When movement is purposely done in time with music.

Syncopated An unexpected rhythmic feel that occurs when the rhythmic emphasis is placed off the main beat; commonly used in genres such as salsa, swing, reggae, and dubstep.

T

Talk test A self-evaluation of intensity associated with the ability to talk while exercising.

Tanaka formula A formula used to estimate an individual's maximal heart rate: $HR_{max} = 208 - (0.7 \times Age)$. Percentages of HR_{max} are used to create training zone estimates.

Target heart rate A predetermined exercising heart rate.

Tempo The speed of music, or how fast it is played; typically measured in beats per minute (BPM).

Thermoregulation The ability to maintain body temperature within a healthy range despite the surrounding environment.

Three-dimensional cueing Cueing that integrates the three learning styles: visual, auditory, and kinesthetic.

Time signature A convention in written music that denotes how many beats are contained in a measure.

Training frequency Number of days per week that an exercise is performed.

Training intensity An individual's level of effort compared with their maximal effort; usually expressed as a percentage.

Transition A series of movements and exercises meant to guide the body back to a resting state, often while gently moving and stretching the muscles and joints that were heavily used during the body of the workout.

Transverse plane Plane of motion that divides the body into superior and inferior halves.

V

Valsalva maneuver Exhaling against a closed glottis.

Verbal communication Interaction through the use of words, orally or written.

Verbal cueing progression A progressive cueing approach that categorizes types of verbal cues and lays them out in the order in which they should be delivered: movement cues, mastery cues, and then motivational cues.

Virtual instructors Group Fitness Instructors who lead classes in a virtual (online) setting.

Visual cueing The use of physical movement to communicate information.

Visual learning Utilizing sight to take in information.

INDEX

INDEX

INDEX